The Dynamics of Connection

The Dynamics of Connection

How Evolution and Biology Create Caregiving and Attachment

David C. Bell

LEXINGTON BOOKS
A division of
ROWMAN & LITTLEFIELD PUBLISHERS, INC.
Lanham • Boulder • New York • Toronto • Plymouth, UK

Published by Lexington Books
A division of Rowman & Littlefield Publishers, Inc.
A wholly owned subsidiary of The Rowman & Littlefield Publishing Group, Inc.
4501 Forbes Boulevard, Suite 200, Lanham, Maryland 20706
http://www.lexingtonbooks.com

Estover Road, Plymouth PL6 7PY, United Kingdom

British Library Cataloguing in Publication Information Available

Library of Congress Cataloging-in-Publication Data
Bell, David C., 1944–
The dynamics of connection : how evolution and biology create caregiving and attachment / David C. Bell.
p. cm.
Includes bibliographical references and index.
ISBN 978-0-7391-4352-0 (cloth : alk. paper)
1. Caregivers. 2. Nurturing behavior. I. Title.
RA645.3.B456 2010
362'.0425—dc22 2009054093

The paper used in this publication meets the minimum requirements of American National Standard for Information Sciences—Permanence of Paper for Printed Library Materials, ANSI/NISO Z39.48-1992.

Printed in the United States of America

Dedication

To Linda, who married me when I didn't know about emotions.

To Michael, Eric, and Claire, who opened my eyes.

Table of Contents

Preface

When my first child was born and I looked into his eyes . . . something happened. I felt a pull and a determination toward my child, but I didn't know what had happened or what it meant. So I began to read the parenting literature. I was looking for an explanation of why parents nurture children to account for my feelings and my determination. There were descriptions of how parents parent (Baumrind, 1968; Belsky, 1984), including descriptions of "good enough" parenting (Winnicott, 1965a). But there were no investigations of why parents would go to the trouble, the fear, the frustration of parenting. When I was in graduate school, I studied the exchange and power (including social norm) theories that were the dominant social explanations of family life at the time. But they didn't feel right. I didn't feel like I was being paid to hold, feed, and change my children. Nor did I feel coerced like I was following someone else's rules. Another common claim was that parenting was "natural," because it evolved and women did it without thinking about it. But I wasn't a woman, and still I wanted to take care of Michael, then Eric, and then Claire.

So what was going on? Why did a relatively level-headed person go to the effort and expense of raising three children? I sure wondered.

When Michael was eleven and Eric four, my wife and I decided to take the family to Japan for a year, which became two. We studied Japanese families in the ways we had previously studied American families. My experiences in Japan introduced me to the concept of *amae* (Doi, 1981; Lebra, 1976). I observed what might be called "total immersion parenting." Mothers slept with their infants and young children in the same bed; the children were kept with the mother just about twenty-four hours a day, except on weekends, when the kids might spend most of the day with the father. Parents were observant (mothers would notice when the child was beginning to get hungry or needing a change of diaper and thus would provide what the child needed before the child ever got to the crying stage) and tolerant (children were "spoiled," as Americans say; they were never as far as I could tell punished). This Japanese parenting, like my own, was never "natural" in the sense of easy; it was very hard work, very motivated work.

I began to understand this paradox because of a problem that occurred in the research my wife Linda and I conducted with our Japanese colleagues. We had interviewed Japanese families using procedures we had developed in the United States and we had developed a coding scheme for describing taped family interactions. One of our instruments was a thermometer-like scale for measuring each family member's power on a range of one to fifteen. The Japanese coders initially were confused by this scale. They asked us what we meant by "power." We used what is the most common meaning of "power" in American social science: "Power is the extent to which one gets what one wants." The coders were satisfied with this definition and proceeded to code family interactions. But we came to a family where the husband, feeling apparently confused by the task, withdrew from the family discussion until he could see how it went, at which time he reentered the conversation. Linda and I coded him low in power because he did not influence the discussion much, but the Japanese coders surprised us by giving him a high score for "power." We were very confused by this development, and we questioned the coders on how they could rate him high in power. "Because," they said, "at first he did not want to participate and was allowed to withdraw; then when he wanted to participate, he was welcomed." When we objected that this is not power, they pointed out that he got what he wanted. From this lesson, I learned that people don't have to be controlling to get what they want. They can get it by being what an American might think of as being weak.

It was in these discussions that I began to see the centrality of the concept of *amae* in Japanese culture. I also could see in this concept a resolution of some problems I had been having with understanding power in American families as well. *Amae* focuses on getting what you want, not by trading and not by controlling, but by depending. This view of depending emphasizes the importance of other people, and our relationships with people, to our ability to achieve our satisfactions. It suggests that instead of viewing relations with people as instruments for getting what we want, it is equally valid to see relationships as places where we want to give.

Another significant influence on my thought was John Bowlby (1969/1982). Bowlby noted that a psychological system in a child to elicit child care (what he called "attachment") and a corresponding system in the parent to give care ("caregiving") have definite survival advantages. Brain research on a wide variety of vertebrates (synthesized by Panksepp, 1998) showed that neural circuits for both attachment and caregiving can be found in all mammals studied.

The discovery of these motivational brain circuits has shown that the feeling I had holding my son and looking into his eyes was an internally generated and genuine feeling of love. Most of us in families care for our children and for one another because of this love. The general expectations that we will nurture one another come from the general preponderance of such nurturance in families, but in most cases these expectations probably do not cause this nurturance. At the same time that our love leads us to support and nurture family members, it can also lead us to overcontrol and overprotect when our own prejudices, fears and anger keep us from accurately perceiving their needs.

The challenge to family theory and family research is to investigate and eventually understand the actions and the intersections of the multiple motivations that produce families. Although social norms are certainly of importance in the regulation of social life, it turns out that at a fundamental brain level, humans *want* to nurture and help others, at least those to whom they have a special caring relationship. The implications of this natural phenomenon are only beginning to be explored by researchers studying dating and relationship formation, marriage, and parental nurturance.

Unlike American and European authors who described the dependency of the child as powerlessness (i.e., children don't get what they want), the Japanese viewed the dependency of the child as the reason why children were the ones in the family that got the highest proportion of their needs met. The Japanese concept of *amae* made more sense than power for understanding families. Americans seem to believe that people get what they want by trading for it (exchange) or coercing someone to get it (power). Children in Japan, and adults as well, get what they want by asking. This concept of active dependency, so alien to my American mind, made a lot of sense to me as a fundamental part of families. It took me a while to realize that active *amae* dependency and Bowlby's concept of attachment had a lot in common, although attachment theory seemed to me at the time to be more concerned with pathology and loss of relationships than with their formation or positive operation. Furthermore, attachment theory tended almost completely to ignore the caregiving side of the parent-child and adult-adult relationship. Again, there was no consideration in this literature for why anyone should nurture another.

When my wife Linda and I began to write about the family, our competencies were clearly differentiated. I remember that she wrote the first draft of a paper on family individuation. My reaction was that her paper was terribly vague and fuzzy. So I rewrote the paper, clarifying her concepts and explanations. In a display of both restraint and indignation that has allowed our marriage to be exciting and yet endure, Linda informed me that my concepts were clear and my explanations were elegant. If only, she commented, they weren't so wrong.

They were, she conceded, correct as far as they went, but they were so precise and restricted that they accounted for a vanishingly small proportion of what goes on in the family individuation process.

Hah, I retorted, your explanation is so vague and, well, fuzzy that it doesn't make any point.

Over the two years that it took us to write this paper (which never did get published), the stability of our marriage was tested at many points (which is also related to why we never revised the paper). But as attribution theory tells us, people who put that much effort into a relationship are bound to conclude that the relationship must be worth it.

I am a sociologist who found theory construction exciting in graduate school. Linda got her PhD in social psychology, but underwent additional training in family therapy. When she looks at the family, she sees individual histories and motives and defenses organized in a systemic family pattern. When I look at data on the family, I see regularities and principles in the form of concepts and propositions. The trick is to express principles and explain regularities in a way that corresponds as closely as possible to the way that people experience the processes we explain. And for family processes, I am convinced that the experience is generally emotional. The confusion, ambivalence, and uncertainty that characterizes the lived experiences of parents are ways that people work out the emotions that arise in families.

Two skills are of crucial importance in explaining human behavior. The first is the ability to be clear, to define concepts and describe processes in a way that illuminates rather than obfuscates. The second crucial skill is a "feel" for interactions and relationships. The left brain/right brain complementarity of these two skills suggests how rare this combination is. I have been fortunate because my modest strengths in the first area are amplified and corrected by Linda's strengths in the second area. This has taught me that "good theory" must not only be clear and elegant, it must also be real. It must conform to the reality experienced by the people we study. It is not enough to develop elegant theories that conform to the data. It is in addition necessary to include in our explanations an awareness of the experience of the processes we study.

I am fundamentally indebted to Takeo Doi, who first described the central importance of *amae* in Japanese culture and took the chance to communicate the experience of *amae* to a Western audience. Over several years struggling with his account in the context of experiencing *amae* in Japan, his explanations were finally able to penetrate my individualistic mind. Koji Suzuki, Dr. Doi and Takeshi Takatomi provided me with the opportunity to work at the (Japanese) National Institute of Mental Health for two years where these ideas began to come together. Koji T. Munakata, my colleague and co-worker at NIH, with his Osaka personality and wit, challenged me to see Japanese life in its multifaceted variety rather than as the stereotypes that inevitably emerge from summary descriptions. Hisako Dendo and Kaoru Kawanami were among the Japanese coders of family interactions who, when they had difficulty understanding what we meant by "power" in family interactions, induced us to add "*amae*" to the important processes of family interaction. And I must thank many other people with whom I have shared conversations that improved my understanding of *amae*. These include Fumiye Miho, Yoji Nakata, Shinichi Nakamura, Noriko Nakamura, and Izumi Sasama Shimpo.

Janet Chafetz and Helen Ebaugh offered me encouragement, and offered extensive comments on several chapters. I did not always take their advice. Alan Richard pushed me to discover the depth of my debt to Bowlby, and then worked with me to develop and extend the theoretical system I present here. Isaac Montoya provided a comfortable and supportive environment where I could pursue these ideas. Mary Cox offered meticulous editorial corrections.

There is no way this work could have been written without Linda G. Bell, my wife and collaborator. Thanks to Linda for staying with me through a seemingly interminable series of drafts. I took most of her advice. Not only did she initiate the research project on family interaction that we ultimately replicated in Japan, but it was her instigation that actually got us to pick up the children and go to Japan. My family isn't like the families of some other authors. My family did not absolve me from family responsibilities during the writing of this book. I did a lot of work in fifteen minute stretches punctuated by chauffeuring, listening, cooking, washing, holding, tutoring, story-reading, and those various other incidents that weave the fabric of family life.

Chapter 1. The Riddle of Nurturance

The nurturance that occurs in and out of families has been a puzzle for the social sciences. A number of relatively unconvincing theoretical orientations have attempted to apply standard self interest explanations to the family: exchange, adaptation, power, social bond. What is needed is a theoretical orientation that gives the emotional nature of relationships a central place.

The most basic of all nurturance experiences is the child's experience. It is the happiest experience that many people ever have. American social science, however, has a bizarre and pessimistic view of childhood. Most of the traditional accounts have stressed the frustration and helplessness of the infant and child and the child's associated struggle for mastery and control. Many accounts have also described the parental experience as essentially helpless and/or reactive: parents have been seen to follow cultural prescriptions and scripts, pursue culturally defined rewards, or enact unconscious biological imperatives. I want to take a different look at parental behavior, through a lens more congruent with parental experience.

Healthy families, unlike most other groups in our lives, are emotional places. Family members love one another, shout at one another, hug one another, fight one another, and comfort one another. The family is a place where feelings rather than calculations can predominate. The family is home. It is not just the place where, as Sandburg says, "when you have to go there, they have to take you in." It is not just a haven in a lonely world (Lasch, 1977). It is where people love. And yet the healthy family does not just involve positive feelings and emotions. Family members feel hurt, they feel ignored and betrayed. What makes a family healthy is not the absence of these feelings, but the ability of the family to acknowledge these feelings, to experience them, and to recover, to love again.

The infant and child I want first to understand, the one who grows up in a healthy family, is happy. He has many needs and wants, and for most of his day these needs and wants are met. When he is hungry, he is fed; when he is soiled, he is cleaned; when he is tired, he sleeps; when he wants contact, he is held. If he wants something, all he has to do is ask; whatever his level of communication competence, he is generally understood and nurtured. This child feels loved. He feels safe and secure. What he needs, he gets. Of course, not all children feel loved and secure. Later, we will examine these experiences as well. But for now, we will look at positive experiences.

As the child grows in a healthy family, she becomes empowered. As she develops skills, she is permitted and encouraged to exercise them. Her development is her choice. She wants to grow—but sometimes even an eleven year old needs to be tucked into bed. She grows without pressure and without stifling. She learns to master herself and to achieve. And above all, she learns to cherish others, at first her parent(s), siblings, and grandparents, later others. She learns, spontaneously, to see others and to love them and worry about them. As her skills and maturity increase, she comes more and more to love and nurture others.

On the parent's side, parenthood is a burden. It can sometimes be a joyous burden, but it is a burden nevertheless. The burden does not come mostly from outside, from laws or rules or others' expectations. It comes mostly from inside, from the parent's awareness of his limitations, conjoined with his feelings of responsibility. Parenthood starts with the parent's feelings of warmth and contact with this very special child, feelings of concern and awareness of this child's needs. As the parent sees the child's needs, he feels his responsibility for meeting them, and he provides for these needs as best he can. One of the inevitable feelings of the healthy parent is the feeling of guilt and inadequacy as he discovers that he can never quite get it completely right, never quite meet all the child's needs.

And yet for all the feelings of inadequacy and guilt that are bound into the experience of parenting, there is also joy and fulfillment. For all the parent's mistakes and misjudgments, her child grows and thrives. Her love and concern for her child produce a child she can be proud of. Experiencing her child's gratitude and love, she feels the warmth of emotional contact and the glow of achievement. As her child grows and becomes more competent, she comes more and more to trust and depend on her child. The child now tells her what he needs and not only cares for himself but cares for her as well in the increasingly elaborate ways of which he is capable. The parent not only cherishes; she feels cherished.

In most accounts of parental caregiving, the caregiver has traditionally been assumed to be a mother, based on cultural patterns in Britain and the United States. Most theory in the social sciences over the past hundred years has taken mothers and mothering for granted (Bell & Richard, 2000a; Epstein, 1988; Harding, 1991; Millman & Kanter, 1987). Gendered accounts of parenting have presented women's nurturing behavior as an unproblematic female characteristic, a characteristic that can be assumed without explanation (Epstein, 1988; Harding, 1991; Millman & Kanter, 1987). Parents, it has been said, have a "need" to nurture (Solomon & George, 1996), and nurturance is functionally required for species survival (Bowlby, 1969/1982), so there was little interest in coherent social explanations of women's behavior. Mother's love was sacred (Hinde, 1982), so like all sacred subjects, Bowlby's "normative sensitive mother" (1988, p. 9) and Winnicott's "good enough mother" (1965a, 1965b) did not need to be explained. Women's nurturing behavior was merely assumed to be "natural."

I do not want to give the impression that there have been no attempts to explain parenting, because there have been many. Most of these accounts are quite superficial. Because parenting is taken as so natural, theorists usually "explain" parenting in a few sentences as biological, as a matter of exchange, as coercion, or as enforced or internalized norms. Many of these accounts, by taking parenting as innate or unproblematic, have tended to trivialize the difficult conflicts and choices that parents experience. A great deal of empirical work has been performed to describe the quality of caregiving among parents whose children are secure or insecure (Bretherton, 1980; Moncher, 1996; Rothbard & Shaver, 1994). These and other authors have described what empirically makes a "quality" caregiver (one whose children are secure)—these parents are sensitive and responsive to their children. However, almost no detailed theoretical work has been done to explain *why* "quality" caregivers choose to act as they do.

A Short Detour into Explanation

Why do parents endure the disruptions and frustrations of parenthood and give nurturance to their children? The explanation of a phenomenon is based on understanding the logic by which the phenomenon operates. Social scientists understand people through theory. A theory consists of both (1) a causal explanation and (2) an application of the explanation to the real world. What makes constructing and understanding theory particularly difficult is that the development and refinement of causal logic is accomplished in a theory alongside of the application of the causal logic to some empirical situation. Causal logic and empirical relevance are both requirements of theory.

We can enhance the exposition and development of causal logic by distinguishing the theoretical orientation from the theory proper (Bell, 2008). Theoretical orientations are strictly logical in content (in spite of being inspired by our experience); theories apply the causal logic to a specific class of empirical situations. In this book, we will focus both on theoretical orientations and on theories.

Theoretical Orientations and Theories

The fundamental content of explanation is causal process (Bell, 2008; Hage, 1972). The advantage of identifying the theoretical orientation as an entity conceptually separate from a theory is that it clarifies the importance of process. An orientation is generally based on a single mechanism or process: a process of interpersonal exchange, a mechanism of conditioning, a process of power exertion, a mechanism of perception, a process of norm conformity, a process of class conflict, and so on. Theoretical orientations make up that part of the theoretical system that focuses solely on causal logic. They are constructed so as to be universal, logically consistent definitions and assertions that may, in principle, be applied anywhere. As a result, the vocabulary of the theoretical orientation is restricted to abstract, non-empirical terms. An orientation refers to "actors" rather than "people," "parents," or "Americans." It refers to "systems" instead of "democracies" or "families." In this way, orientations try to avoid smuggling in unexamined assumptions that lie behind our empirical categories.

Assertions are statements that describe the causal relations between theoretical concepts. A formal assertion usually takes the form

The greater the *X* the greater (or less) the *Y*, because . . .

where *X* and *Y* are (theoretical, unobservable) variable concepts and the "because. . . " clause describes the causal process that produces the stated relationship between the concepts. The because clause provides a "theoretical linkage" (Hage, 1972), a "process" (Merton, 1967), a "cause" (Babbie, 1989; Burr, Hill, Nye, & Reiss, 1979; Chafetz, 1978; Stinchcombe, 1968) and an "explanation" (Kerlinger, 1973). Without the "because" clause, an assertion is a claim without substantiation. It is the because clause that carries the causal logic of the theoretical assertion. A wide range of assertions will be described later in this chapter.

In this book, I will focus on the connection theoretical system that combines the caregiving theoretical orientation and the attachment theoretical orientation, an extension of Bowlby's original formulation of the logic of attachment.

Theory. An orientation, for all its logical elegance, is not very useful unless it has some relevance to the real world. It is in a *theory* that the abstract causal logic of a theoretical orientation is applied to the real world. A theory is a *theory of* some empirical phenomenon (Merton, 1967). Using this terminology, there is no such thing as "attachment theory" per se. What is often called "attachment theory" is by this terminology an "attachment theoretical orientation." A theory that applies the causal logic of attachment to the class of children is an attachment theory of childhood. By their very nature, theoretical orientations describe universal, logically true processes that can be applied to any empirical situation. And since there are many orientations, there can be many processes potentially in operation in any particular empirical situation. It is probable that in most situations there will be multiple processes operating. Thus in most settings we have the opportunity to employ multiple theoretical orientations to understand the complexity of human behavior. The application of any particular orientation to explain a given behavior is voluntary. That is, the investigator is free to base an explanation of any given behavior on any orientation that appeals. This choice is, of course, conditioned by cultural and personal experience. Nevertheless, the investigator has—in principle—wide latitude in selecting what she believes to be a useful theoretical orientation. We have the option to explain the movements of the planets by divine intervention (Ptolemy), by magnetic attraction and repulsion (Keller), by the attraction of gravity (Newton), or by the curvature of space (Einstein).

There is no reason, of course, why a particular theory necessarily has to take its causal process from a single theoretical orientation. There are very few "pure" situations that can be fully understood as involving the operation of only one process. Even what seems to be a simple situation may involve multiple processes. For example, a theory of childhood is strengthened by including social learning processes in addition to attachment processes. However, to create such a theory requires that both the causal logic of attachment and the causal logic of social learning be well understood and that the application of both logics be carefully traced in child development. However, sometimes, two logics are clearly complementary and can be combined in a single analysis. In this book, I will highlight the complementary contributions of caregiving and attachment logics within a given theory. Thus I will create a *connection theory of parental nurturance of children* (a caregiving theory to explain parental actions and a complementary attachment theory to explain child actions) and a *connection theory of adult relationships* (consisting of caregiving and attachment theories of both partners). That is, I will create a theory of parental nurturance that abstracts the causal logics of caregiving and attachment from all of the other causal processes that happen in the real world in order to see what part of multiplex reality that can be accounted for by this complementary pair of logics. And then I will use the causal logics of connection to create a theory to explain an important aspect of adult relationships.

Process. A description of process is of crucial importance in understanding behavior. That is why the assertions and theoretical propositions in this book will contain a "because" clause to describe the process. It is not responsible to ignore process, and is certainly not appropriate to *assume*, without investigation, that a particular process operates. Just because an abstract theoretical orientation *can* be applied to any concrete situation does not mean that it *should* be so applied. Furthermore, the processes that theorists propose should be consistent with the experience of those whose behavior the theories are trying to explain. We will be well rewarded if we look diligently into each situation and use the experience of the participants to create explanations that are meaningful to them. There will be settings in which the participants are not aware of the process, and situations in which there is one way of understanding an experience that is meaningful to the participants but another way of understanding that is meaningful to a scientific observer. But such situations are probably the exception rather than the rule, and certainly must be justified explicitly.

EXPLAINING PARENTAL NURTURANCE

My goal in this book is to understand nurturance. I want to understand the child's experience of nurturance and the effects of this experience on the child. And I want to understand the parent's nurturance. I want to know not only *how* parents nurture children but also *why* they nurture. What is the dynamic logic that moves parents to act for their children? Fundamental to this work is its grounding in a connection theoretical system. Coming out of the matched caregiving and attachment theoretical orientations, I develop theories to explain parental nurturance, caregiving, and attachment.

I take nurturance to be behavior for the purpose of benefiting another. More specific content will be given to the concept of nurturance in Chapter 6. But for now this will be sufficient. Nurturance does not refer to all action that benefits the other, but only to action that is purposively directed toward the other's benefit. Nurturance may or may not involve sacrifice; the status of the nurturer's own benefit is not part of the definition of nurturance.

Parenting is a tough job. Parents are responsible for turning children into civilized adults. This is accomplished by parenting, a complex mix of love, frustration, nurturance, discipline, listening, restraint, and sacrifice. Without the constant and conscientious nurturance of children by parents, humans would have died out long before they learned to use tools. Parental nurturance is one of only a few fundamental functional requirements for human species survival.

And yet this most crucial of functions has aroused very little curiosity among social scientists. Family scientists have mostly taken parental nurturance for granted. This is not to say that family scientists have ignored nurturance. Quite a bit has been written about parental nurturance of children. Much has been written about how parents nurture, and about how parents ought to nurture. However, little has been written about *why* parents nurture. And what has been written has generally been quite superficial. Processes originally used to explain other quite different phenomena have been applied quite casually to parents. As I noted above, any theoretical orientation *can* be applied to create a theory of parental nurturance; however, it is equally clear that not all theoretical orientations *should* be used for this purpose.

One of the problems in understanding the nurturance of children by parents is that our experiences are self-contradictory. We remember our childhoods as the best of times (we were loved) and the worst of times (we were frustrated and controlled). We experience parenting as joyous (watching a precious child grow into her or his potential) and constricting (we always have to be there and to sacrifice our time and energy for our children) and frustrating (we often make mistakes).

Some theories of parenting

There have been many explicit theories of parental nurturance and a greater number of implicit theories of parental nurturance. Many of the explanations that I will describe in this chapter have a surface plausibility. They use logics that have been found applicable in a wide variety of contexts. These explanations of parenting were plausible to me, too—until my first child was born. I was in graduate school at the time and I found that my son Michael was much more interesting than my dissertation. My wife was in a demanding clinical internship, and I had the opportunity—the often exhausting, frustrating, daunting, exhilarating, terrifying opportunity—to parent. What I found was that the conventional explanations for parenting, however attractive they were at a distance, did not apply to me and Michael.

Exchange. Exchange theoretical orientations and their theories of parental nurturance are based on ideas largely imported into sociology, social psychology, and anthropology from economics. The logic of exchange is represented by the metaphor of the barter. I give you something you want and in return you give me something I want. Exchange is thus a transaction between two relatively equal, calculating, maximizing participants. Within this general idea of exchange, a number of distinct versions of exchange logic have been created. Six such versions are summarized in Table 1.1. Nevertheless, for all their surface plausibility, these exchange explanations were unsatisfying to me. When Michael smiled, I felt "repaid" for the nurturance I gave. Yet the logic of exchange said that I must be nurturing Michael *because* of the smile—and that he was smiling *because* of my nurturance. In my own experience, I was gratified to get that smile, but it was clear to me that I nurtured him because he needed it, not because I was trading my nurturance for his smile. Thus I could not find that our relationship was explained as an exchange relationship.

Note 1.1. Ego and Alter

In discussing the various theoretical orientations that have been applied to parental nurturance, we run into the problem of distinguishing unambiguously the two persons involved in a relationship. Because the fundamental logic of the various theoretical orientations applies to abstract actors, we do not want to use specific observable terms (like "parent" or "child") for the persons because observable terms have multiple cultural and other meanings that obscure the clarity of the explanatory logic. Therefore I use generic terms to describe the two persons involved (and in nonhuman species, the two animals): "ego" for one partner and "alter" for the second partner. An extensive discussion and evaluation of these theoretical orientations is given in Bell (2008).

Table 1.1. Exchange theoretical orientations

Assertion of the theoretical orientation	Application to parenting
Direct social exchange assertion. The greater the value of the social rewards received by ego from alter, the greater the value (to ego) of social benefits ego provides to alter, because in a direct transaction between equal, self-interested actors, the way to receive greater rewards from a self-interested alter is to agree to give greater benefits (Blau, 1986; Coleman, 1990; Hechter, 1987).	A parent nurtures a child because the child "pays" for it (Simons, Whitbeck, Conger, & Melby, 1990; York & Wachtel, 1982).
Implicit social exchange assertion 1 (retrospective). The greater the value (to ego) of the rewards provided to ego by alter in the past, the greater the value (to ego) of the benefits ego provides to alter... **Implicit social exchange assertion 2 (prospective).** The greater the value of the rewards that ego anticipates that alter will provide at a later time, the greater the value of the benefits ego provides to alter... ... **(for both assertions)** because in the presence of a norm of reciprocity even self-interested actors must give benefits to "repay" rewards (Blau, 1986; Burns, 1973; Homans, 1974; Nye, 1979, 1982; Walster, Walster, & Berscheid, 1978).	(1) A parent nurtures a child in order to reciprocate because the child rewarded the parent at some time in the past. (2) A parent nurtures a child because the parent expects that the child will reciprocate and reward the parent at some point in the future (Becker, 1960; Levinger, 1982; Rossi & Rossi, 1990).
Indirect social exchange assertion. The greater the value of the reward to be provided to ego by an agent of alter, the greater the value (to ego) of the benefits ego provides to alter, because when a benefit to alter is a benefit to the agent, the agent will give proportional rewards to ego (Blau, 1986).	A parent nurtures a child because the parent is rewarded by the other parent as an agent of the child (Bahr, 1982; Belsky, 1984; Nye & McLaughlin, 1982; Parsons & Bales, 1955).
Generalized exchange assertion 1 (retrospective). The greater the value of the rewards provided to ego by some member(s) of society in the past, the greater the value (to ego) of the benefits ego provides to alter now, because a norm of generalized reciprocity requires that each actor repay previous rewards to someone. **Generalized exchange assertion 2 (prospective).** The greater the value of the rewards that ego anticipates will be provided to ego at a later time by some member(s) of society, the greater the value of the benefits ego provides to alter now, because in the presence of a generalized norm of reciprocity, a self-interested actor can expect to receive reward at a later time for benefits provided to another in the present (Ekeh, 1974; Lévy-Strauss, 1969; Nye, 1982).	(1) A parent nurtures a child in order to reciprocate for the nurturance the parent received as a child from the parent's own parents. (2) A parent nurtures a child because the parent anticipates being nurtured by someone else in the future (Aldous, 1977).

Adaptation (Reinforcement). Other explanations, popular in sociology and psychology, focus on adaptation. Adaptation theoretical orientations and theories are based on rewards, or "reinforcements." A reinforcement is a net reward attached to a given action. For example, if you put rat food at the end of a maze and put a rat in, the rat will at first randomly search the maze until it finds the food. The rat's reward (the food) is contingent on performing a specific behavior (finding the end of the maze). All other behaviors receive no net reward. Initially the rat does not know the contingencies, but if you repeatedly put the rat at the start of the maze with food at the end, the rat will eventually learn to perform, and to perform efficiently, those actions that get it to the end of the maze and the food reward. In the simple case, there is only one action that receives a net reward. In the general case, there can be many actions that receive different levels of net reward. In the work on animals, a list of actions and their associated net rewards is a "contingency schedule" or a "reinforcement schedule" (Table 1.2). Adaptation logic said that I nurtured *because* I had previously been rewarded by behaviors such as Michael's smile. The problem with that as an explanation was that the logic claimed that I would only increase my nurturance if I had the promise of greater reward. And yet the times I found myself doing the most nurturance were exactly those times when there was the least reward (like the times at two a.m. I would endlessly walk Michael around the room against my shoulder while he was cutting a tooth).

Power and Social Norms. Power theoretical orientations and theories (Table 1.3) are based on inequality and exploitation. When people are equal, each has a free choice in methods of achieving their interests. People can refuse transactions that do not benefit them, so all transactions that occur are beneficial to all parties. But with inequality, choice is more limited. The stronger person can force outcomes that the weaker person would not voluntarily accept. The weaker person still has a preference for free exchanges, but the rationally self-interested stronger person has an incentive to maximize exploitation and has no incentive for restraint (under the assumption of strict self interest). The greater the inequality, the greater the opportunity for exploitation (Scanzoni & Szinovacz, 1980). Exploitation and coercion define power.

The metaphor of power often "feels" right when one is a parent. A parent has the ability to spank or otherwise punish a child to control the child's behavior. And a parent can feel coerced to provide nurturance. It can feel like power when two parents struggle over nurturing the child. When our children were infants, my wife Linda and I divided the childcare day at four: she, a morning person, had responsibility from four

Table 1.2. Exchange theoretical orientations

Assertion of the theoretical orientation	Application to parenting
Reinforcement adaptation assertion. The more net rewards the environment provides to ego for a given action, the more ego will perform the action, because a self-interested actor wishes to maximize rewards (Skinner, 1953; Thibaut & Kelley, 1959).	A parent nurtures a child because there are rewards for nurturing a child.
Social control adaptation assertion. The more net rewards authoritatively allocated to ego by society for a given action, the more ego will perform the action, because a self-interested actor wishes to maximize net rewards assigned by the authoritative environment (Hirschi, 1969).	A parent nurtures a child because society gives rewards for nurturance (LaRossa & Reitzes, 1993; Nye, 1979).
Personal control adaptation assertion. The more net rewards allocated to ego by alter for a given action that conform to alter's values (expressed in the reinforcement schedule alter creates for ego), the more ego will perform the action, because a self-interested actor wishes to maximize rewards (Klein & White, 1996; Mead, 1934; Parsons & Shils, 1951; Vannoy & Philliber, 1992).	A parent nurtures a child because of rewards the other parent gives for nurturing the child.
Social learning adaptation assertion. The more net rewards that ego perceives will be provided to ego for a given action, the more ego will perform the action, because ego, a self-interested actor, wishes to maximize net rewards from the environment. Ego perceives the structure of social rewards from vicariously and symbolically experienced reinforcements received by others (Bandura, 1977; Bandura & Walters, 1963; Kohlberg, 1966).	A parent nurtures a child because the parent (as a child) observed that parents were rewarded for nurturing children (Simons, Beaman, Conger, & Chao, 1993).
Structural role assertion. The more similar actors' role positions, the more similar their actions, because actors in the same role position develop the same motivations and interests, and these similar motivations and interests produce similar actions and thus similar social expectations (norms) (Durkheim, 1933; Toennies, 1961).	A parent nurtures a child because, like other parents, the parent follows the role of parent (Chodorow, 1978; Solomon, 1989).
Institutional control assertion. The more advantages an actor perceives for enforcing a social role norm, the more the actor will enforce the norm, because actors desire to use the rules and resources of the institution of the family to regulate actions that perpetuate their advantages under the institution (Giddens, 1979; Hill & Hansen, 1969).	A father nurtures a child because the mother wants him to share responsibility for the child (Allen & Hawkins, 1999; Maurer & Pleck, 2006).
Symbolic interaction adaptation assertion. The more net rewards allocated to ego by alter for actions that conform to alter's values and expectations, the more ego will perform the action. Ego can negotiate with alter to modify alter's values and expectations (Heiss, 1981; Joas, 1987; Mead, 1934).	A parent nurtures a child because the parent and child have negotiated nurturance (Chafetz, 1990).

a.m., while I, a night person, had responsibility until four a.m. If Michael awoke at eleven p.m. or two a.m., he was my responsibility to feed, change, rock; at four a.m. or six a.m., he was Linda's responsibility. I remember one time Michael awoke crying at 3:45 a.m. I found myself balancing Michael's need, my exhaustion, and Linda's exhaustion. I think we both lay there listening to Michael cry and wanting to sleep. It seemed like hours, but it was probably only a few minutes, and I don't remember which of us got up to rock Michael (but since I don't remember, it was probably Linda who got up).

It is very popular in sociology to assert that parents nurture children because of social norms. But this explanation leaves much to be desired. I remember putting Michael into one of those carriers that held him at my chest to take a walk. He was two or three weeks old the first time, and I was so full of being a parent—and on top of that a male parent. I remember about three times in the park on that day some older women (I was thirty and each of them must have been over sixty) would come up and admire Michael, but would then berate me for risking a child his age out of doors. I remember trying to be respectful to these women—I tried once to discuss the issue but quickly gave up—but I didn't change my behavior. If these occasions weren't what sociologists mean by social sanctions, then I don't know what is. And yet these normative sanctions were ineffective. I remember taking Michael to the park when he was a year old and sitting around with the "other mothers" to watch our children play. I wasn't following social norms then (fathers didn't go to the park on weekdays). If anything, I was helping to create an emerging social norm of father involvement. After Eric was born seven years later, I saw more fathers at the park.

I do remember another time being aware of social norms. I remember Michael was teething, and I walked him around and around his room while he cried. Rocking wouldn't work. Only rhythmic walking and bouncing could still his cries. But it wouldn't end. He wouldn't let me sit down or even slow down. I become aware then of social norms. After a half hour of this it felt I was at the end of my rope. After another fifteen minutes I didn't think I would stay on my feet. After another fifteen minutes I was exhausted, frustrated, and angry. I remember thinking that it would show him if I threw him against the wall. I wanted to throw him, to punish him for my exhaustion and pain. I understood in that moment how abuse can occur, how a caring parent could hurt a child. But I didn't throw him. I was aware that I could be punished for injuring my child. But even more than that, I was aware of how I would feel afterward, of how guilty and ashamed I would feel—and how much I would hurt Mi-

Table 1.3. Exchange theoretical orientations

Assertion of the theoretical orientation	Application to parenting
Direct physical power assertion. The greater alter's threat of the sanction of physical violence to ego, the more benefits ego will provide to alter, because ego wishes to reduce the threat of sanctions (Lenski, 1966; Russell, 1938; Weber, 1946, 1947; Wrong, 1988).	A parent nurtures a child to avoid violence from the child.
Direct negative power assertion. The more (negative) sanctions toward ego controlled by alter, the more benefits ego will provide to alter, because ego wishes to reduce the probability that alter will employ the sanctions against ego (Bachrach & Baratz, 1963; Bierstedt, 1974; Goode, 1971; Lasswell & Kaplan, 1950; Nye, 1980; Osmond, 1978; Safilios-Rothschild, 1976; Secord & Backman, 1964; Smith, 1970).	A parent nurtures a child to avoid punishments from the child (Glasser, 1984; Lerner, 1957; Scanzoni & Szinovacz, 1980).
Direct social power assertion. The greater the stream of (positive) rewards toward ego controlled by alter, the more benefits ego will provide to alter, because ego wishes to reduce the probability that alter will withhold future rewards (Blau, 1986; Emerson, 1962; French & Raven, 1968; Friedrich, 1963; Molm, 1990).	A parent nurtures a child because of the threat that the child might discontinue rewards (Wrong, 1988).
Indirect power assertion. The more sanctions toward ego controlled by an agent for alter, the more benefits ego will provide to alter, because ego wishes to reduce the probability that the agent will employ the sanctions against ego.	A parent nurtures a child to avoid punishments from the other parent (Chafetz, 1990; LaRossa & LaRossa, 1981).
Normative power assertion. Given a norm of a social system, the more sanctions toward ego controlled by the system of which ego is a fixed member, the more ego will follow the norm, because ego wishes to reduce the probability that some member of the system will employ the sanctions against ego (Blake & Davis, 1964; Brickman, 1974; Greenberg, 1980; Homans, 1950; Nye, 1982; Shaffer, 1983).	A parent follows the norm of nurturing a child to avoid sanctions from members of society (Gecas, 1976; Hill, 1971; Lamb, 1978; LaRossa & LaRossa, 1981; Nye, 1980).
Normative socialization power assertion. Given a norm, the more sanctions toward ego controlled by an agent of the system *when ego is receptive*, the more ego will follow the system norm, because ego has internalized the norm and thus ego will give self punishments for failure to follow the norm (Bahr, 1982; Burgess, Locke, & Thomes, 1971; Cahill, 1983; Dager, 1964; Katz, 1979; Nye, 1979).	A parent follows the norm of nurturing a child to avoid self-imposed sanctions for not following the norm (Emde, 1992; Fogel & Mistry, 1986; LaRossa, 1986; Parsons, 1951).
Power as cause assertion. The more resources controlled by alter, the more benefits ego will give to alter (Mishler & Waxler, 1968; Olson & Cromwell, 1975; Straus, 1964).	A parent nurtures a child because of the child's resources (McDonald, 1980).

chael. And in my mind it was my feelings, not my potential punishment, that kept me walking, carrying, rocking until Michael finally fell asleep.

Something else

Although the most popular theories in the social sciences are based on the assumption of fundamental self interest, sociologists and other social scientists have historically been aware that there is more to social life than self interest. From the earliest social scientists (indeed from the first social philosophers), there has been an awareness of multiple (usually dual) views of reality. These views represent a consensus among major social thinkers that social reality is complex and that reality is governed by self interest and, as Brickman (1987) notes, by "something else."

Many sociologists and other social scientists have given descriptions of the "something else" that stands opposite the self interest view. The non-self-interest terms describe premodern nonwestern societies as against modern western ones; they describe women as against men; and they describe the private world of the family as against the public worlds of economics, politics and law. Societies based on cooperation are described by the terms *Gemeinschaft* (Toennies, 1961), mechanical solidarity (Durkheim, 1933), partnership (Eisler, 1987), and community (Nisbet, 1990). Cooperative, nurturant relationships are characterized as justice (Plato, 1952), bestowal (Singer, 1966/1984, 1984-1987, 1987), communion (Bakan, 1966; Clark & Mills, 1979; Weber, 1947), affect (Kantor & Lehr, 1975), status (Kemper, 1978), object relations (Mitchell, 1988), expressiveness (Parsons & Bales, 1955), altruism (Thomas, 1989), *agape* (Nygren, 1953), care (Gilligan, 1982), commitment (Bellah, et al., 1985), connectedness or connection (Hess & Handel, 1959; Jordan, Surrey, & Kaplan, 1991; Miller, 1986), and solidarity (Schwartz & Merten, 1980).

Attempts have been made by these authors and others to go beyond self interest to conceptualize the "something else" that makes families different. Human beings are social animals. They form temporary and permanent relationships. Some of these relationships can be adequately conceptualized as epiphenomena of self interest using exchange, adaptation, or power explanatory logics. But many social scientists believe that there is something more than individual self interest that motivates relationships. They believe that relationships have their own logics that are not derivable from self interest. Some of these other logics are described in Table 1.4. Some of these "social bond" logics were proposed over a hundred years ago by Durkheim, Weber, Marx and Giddings. However,

Table 1.4. Exchange theoretical orientations

Assertion of the theoretical orientation	Application to parenting
Identity bond assertion. The more similarity ego perceives between ego and alter, the more ego will want to meet alter's needs, because similarity creates a feeling of unity and interchangeable interests, and thus for ego to meet alter's needs is similar to meeting ego's needs (Duck, 1994; Giddings, 1896; Pitts, 1964; Schwartz & Merten, 1980; Solomon, 1989).	A parent nurtures a child because the parent feels a sense of unity with the child (Pitts, 1964; Solomon, 1989).
Belonging bond assertion. The greater ego's bond of belonging with alter, the more benefits ego will provide to alter, because ego's bond of belonging with alter makes ego both open and sympathetic with alter and alter's interests and needs (Durkheim, 1933; Etzioni, 1993; Giddens, 1979; Marx, 1968; Parsons & Shils, 1951; Stryker, 1994; Weber, 1946, 1947).	A parent nurtures a child because of the parent's sense of belonging with the child (Parsons & Bales, 1955).
Therapeutic assertion. Given ego's training, the greater ego's knowledge of the needs of alter and skills to meet those needs, the greater ego's nurturance of alter, because knowledge of alter's needs activates ego's motivation to nurture, and meeting alter's needs is the goal of ego's motivation (Allen, 1977; Argyris & Smith, 1985; Batson, 1990; Cancian, 1987; Eisler, 1987; Kottler, 1986; Kuykendall, 1983; Sensat, 1979).	A parent nurtures a child because of the parent's knowledge of parenting (Batson, 1990).
Women's voice assertion. The more an actor has an uninterrupted nurturing experience in childhood (like girls do), the more comfortable the actor will be with giving nurturance, because an uninterrupted nurturing experience makes the actor comfortable with relationships (Chodorow, 1978; Gilligan, 1982; Gilligan, Ward, & Taylor, 1988; Lyons, 1990; Rochlin, 1980).	A mother nurtures a child because of her uninterrupted nurturing experience in childhood (Apter, 1990; Chodorow, 1978; Dinnerstein, 1976).
Moral assertion. The greater an actor's internalization of moral (i.e., altruistic) principles, the more the actor's behavior will meet the needs of others, because behavior follows belief, and the principle of morality is that others' needs be met (Bellah, Madsen, Sullivan, Swidler, & Tipton, 1985; Blustein, 1982; Etzioni, 1988; Kelsey, 1981; Kunz, 1998; Levinas, 1969; Levinas & Kearney, 1986; Thomas, 1989).	A parent nurtures a child because it is the right (moral) thing to do (Doherty, 1997; Hawkins & Dollahite, 1997).

the social bond theoretical orientations have generated very little empirical research into the behavior of parents.

Belonging and the Social Bond. As a parent, I find the therapeutic or praxis logic to be somewhat descriptive of my parenting. The better I understood Michael's needs and the greater my level of skill, the more I could nurture him. A problem with this logic for a parent, however, is that it ignores feelings. As a parent, I knew about the needs of many children other than my own, but I seldom attempted to meet their needs unless it could be done with a kind word at the park. Instead, I was aware of meeting Michael's needs because of the way I felt about him. It was these feelings that also explained why I nurtured my wife and was nurtured by her. "Belonging" or "identity" bonds seem to capture some of the feeling of "bonding" that I felt. However, these concepts were so abstract and bloodless—so sociological—that they seemed to miss the point. There were times when it was painful to be rejected by Michael when I stood firm and refused to give in to one of his passions, for a toy or candy or something else not good for him, so I can't say that the logic of belonging is inapplicable, but its applicability is episodic and often only on the surface. The more important point is that in the face of these rejections and threats of rejection, I still was likely to stick to what I thought Michael needed. The idea of an identity bond is very abstract. It is certainly true that I was aware that Michael was much like me, with red hair and my crooked little toe, but there was no blurring of boundaries: I knew clearly who was who. Nevertheless the metaphor of identity, while not literally accurate, captured some of the sense of being "one."

If there are so many explanations of parental nurturance already proposed, at least implicitly, why is there a need for any new explanations? The main criticism against all of the above theories is that they ignore large parts of parental experience; they ignore feelings. Most explanations claim that parents nurture children based on calculations of personal self interest (exchange, adaptation, power). For those readers who are satisfied with these explanations, there is no reason to read on. For those who think that there has to be more, we will explore explanations that focus on the "something else."

Organization of this book

The vocabulary of theoretical orientations will be important as we turn to the origins of nurturance. By stripping away the distractions of the empirical, we will be able to look with some clarity at some of the logical processes by which sociologists, psychologists, anthropologists and others have tried to explain the origins of nurturance. In what follows in this book, I will work at all three levels of explanation: orientation, theory, empirical description. The primary purpose and goal of this book is to develop and describe a theoretical system that explains the dynamic causal logic of connection out of the theoretical orientations of caregiving and attachment. However, this is not intended as an arid exposition of logic. I will frequently digress and discuss empirical observations in anecdotal and empirical samples to try to convince you of the reasonableness of the causal processes I describe. To do this I will explicitly create theories of connection. Two such theories will be developed in some detail. The first is a theory of childhood socialization scattered throughout Chapters 5, 6, and 7. The second is a theory of relationship formation (from dating to commitment, and perhaps to dissolution) in Chapter 8.

In the next chapter, I turn to an explanation of parenting that has developed a strong following. Attachment theory has generated an extensive empirical literature of childhood experiences and parenting. In Chapter 2, I will show how John Bowlby used both evolutionary and cybernetic thinking to create attachment theory.

Chapter 2. Bowlby's Account of Attachment and Caregiving*

(with Alan J. Richard)

John Bowlby's theory of attachment and caregiving has energized research on the parent-child relationship. His evolution-based psychological model of attachment (how the child depends on the parent for protection) has improved through several versions. However, his complementary vision of caregiving (how the parent nurtures the child) has not been fully developed, lacking a convincing emotional motivation for parental caregiving.

The work of John Bowlby (1969/1982) has generated a great deal of excitement in the fields of parenting and child development by formulating several key concepts for understanding relationships. The concept of attachment is the most widely recognized of these. A large number of monographs and collections have explored this conceptualization (e.g., Ainsworth, Blehar, Waters, & Wall, 1978; Bowlby, 1969/1982, 1973, 1980; Cassidy & Shaver, 1999; Feeney & Noller, 1996; Mikulincer & Shaver, 2007; Parkes & Stevenson-Hinde, 1982; Rholes & Simpson, 2004b; Simpson & Rholes, 1998; Sperling & Berman, 1994). Although Bowlby's work focused on relationships between very young children and their parents, the Bowlbian attachment concept also has informed the development of new theories of adult relationships. In this chapter, we identify the strengths and some weaknesses of Bowlby's attachment theory. Attachment theory has a well developed theory of childhood attachment. We will see that a major strength of Bowlby's system is its explanation of the child's role in parental nurturance. A weakness, however, is the underdeveloped explanation of caregiving.

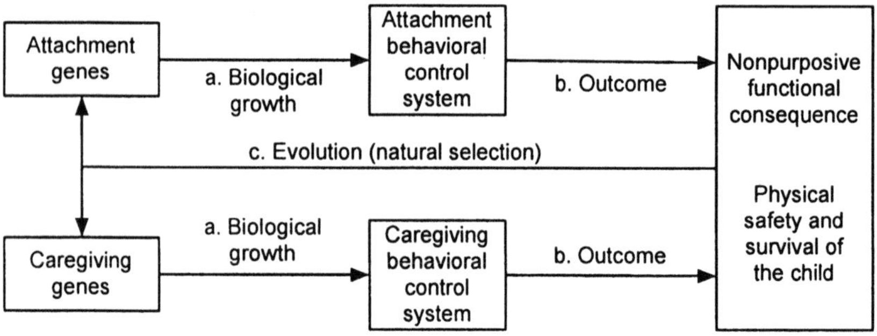

Figure 2.1. Evolution of Behavioral Control Systems in Attachment Theory.

Bowlbian attachment logic treats the species as a system. In his analysis of attachment, Bowlby (1969/1982) situates the human species in its "environment of evolutionary adaptedness" (EEA), that is, during the millions of years of human evolution up to the introduction of agriculture a few thousand years ago. Bowlby focuses in particular on the danger of predators in this environment. Bowlby's partial answer to the question of how the human species survived an environment of predators is that an attachment behavioral control system in the child (asking for proximity to the parent) and a caregiving behavioral control system in the mother (achieving proximity to the child) combined to protect children effectively from predators.[1] Bowlby's EEA places the critical period of caregiving and attachment evolution during the Pliocene and Pleistocene geologic epochs starting about five million years ago (Mellen, 1981). The evolutionary logic of Bowlby's theoretical orientation is depicted in Figure 2.1. His basic argument is that the attachment and caregiving systems resulted in proximity between parents and children. Genes mutated at some time during the EEA and created attachment and caregiving behavioral control systems. These genes, under appropriate conditions of nutrition and social environment, laid down the neurons of the two systems (the biological growth arrows "a"). The attachment and caregiving systems created proximity between child and parent. Protection from predators and the survival of the child were results of this proximity (the outcome arrow "b"). By a process of natural selection, these behavioral control systems became prevalent because humans without these behavioral control systems would have disproportionately lost their children to predators and their genes would thus have been lost (arrow "c"). The surviving genes continued to produce in the next generation an attachment behavioral control system in the child and a caregiving behavioral control system in the parent. This type of account is called a "functional" argument because it "explains" behavior (caregiving and attachment behavior) by its consequences (survival of the child) (Stinchcombe, 1968). As we look at the evolution of parenting in Chapter 4, we will see that the evolutionary account can be extended back at least another 150 million years and perhaps another 90 million or so years before that.

Bowlby's concern in the 1930s with delinquent boys, in the 1940s with children separated from their families by the war, and later study of children in hospitals led to a focus on the child's fear of abandonment and loss (Bowlby, 1988; Karen, 1994; Kobak, 1999). Bowlby (1969/1982, 1988) introduced the concept of the attachment behavioral control system to help explain the anxiety that very young children exhibit upon separation from their parents or parent figures, the signs of joy they exhibit upon reunion, and the patterned deviations in these responses among children who had experienced prolonged separation from parents at a very early age. Bowlby took these regularities and patterned deviations as evidence that an innate internal system with autonomic components governs the reaction of children to parental separation. Reasoning from the ubiquity of such attachment behaviors across a number of species and the prominence of stereotyped actions in the attachment behavioral repertoire, Bowlby hypothesized that this system has a distinct evolutionary function. Bowlby's evolutionary arguments are consistent with current evolutionary theory with its emphasis on the "selfish gene" (Dawkins, 1976/1989; Tattersall, 1998). Protection of children is not the purpose of the attachment or caregiving systems—evolution does not have a goal (Dawkins, 1976/1989; Tattersall, 1998)—but protection is a nonpurposive consequence of the system. Bowlby rejected the Freudian assertion that this function centered on immature organisms' need for food or shelter, stating instead that it resulted from immature organisms' need for protection from predators. The attachment control system provides such protection because it predictably results in increasing the proximity of vulnerable immature organisms to mature organisms of the same species who are better able to fend off predators.

Bowlby and other attachment researchers have identified a number of behavioral control systems hypothesized to have been "selected" by evolution. Some of the control systems identified by attachment theorists are simple fixed action patterns, like rooting, grasping, crying, and smiling (Bowlby, 1969/1982, p. 66). Others are more complex cybernetic (goal-corrected) control systems, including a sexual system, a comforting system, an attacking system, an eating system, an exploratory system, and a learning system (Bowlby, 1969/1982, pp. 116, 119, 130, 137, 378; see also Ainsworth 1989), an affiliation system, a wariness system (Bretherton & Ainsworth, 1974; Sroufe & Waters, 1977), and resistant and avoidant systems (Ainsworth, 1982). Some of these systems deal with a general orientation to the environment; others take a specific other actor as object. However, Bowlby's main focus was on the complementary attachment and caregiving behavioral control systems. The behavioral control system of attachment takes a specific other actor as object and operates to maintain close proximity to the object. Close proximity has survival consequences for the young child and thus, by this logic, the genetically based attachment control system has been a result of evolutionary selection processes (Figure 2.1). The attachment behavioral control system enhances safety because it is able to activate a separate system, the caregiving behavioral control system, in a reliable partner (Solomon & George, 1996). The attachment and caregiving behavioral control systems are complementary (Hinde, 1976; Weiss, 1974). The child may cry when in danger (attachment behavior), but unless the parent comes (caregiving behavior), the child will not be protected.

Attachment theorists have uniformly avoided asking whether parents want to nurture or whether children want to be protected. Instead, some researchers have been content to argue that, because attachment and caregiving have positive consequences for the species, it has been enough to assert that systems to provide these consequences do arise and are activated (Buss, Haselton, Shackelford, Bleske, & Wakefield, 1998; Cassidy, 2000; Geary, 2000; Simpson & Rholes, 2000).

In fact, the order in which I have lettered the arrows in Figure 2.1 privileges the view that genes are the fundamental first cause in the process. It is important to remember that genetic change is not caused by natural selection. A new gene can only be preserved after it has autonomously come into existence. Natural selection does not produce genetic change; it only propagates it (Tooby & Cosmides, 1992).

Issues of terminology

There is some potential confusion in Bowlbian attachment terminology. The term "attachment" has sometimes been used to refer to the control system in the child and sometimes to the dyadic relationship between parent and child. In the context of adult relationships, "attachment" has often been used to label the overall relationship between two persons. Thus, "attachment" has been used to refer to both the dyadic system and to one of the two behavioral control systems that make up the dyadic system.

It is somewhat difficult to discuss a process that has differentiated roles. The usual solution has been to explain the logic in the context of a specific theory. This is what Bowlby and most attachment researchers have done, describing a caregiving process in parents and an attachment process in children. This choice of perspective and of terminology has had the advantage of being comfortable for readers by providing rich images. It has had the disadvantage of confounding the logics of caregiving and attachment with the social context of parents and children. When a theoretical logic is presented only within a specific context, such as an attachment theory of the parent-child relationship, it can be unclear which parts of the explanation apply in a theory that describes another context, such as an attachment theory of adult relationships. Does the adult relationship have to be unilateral, as parent-child relations appear to be? Do the adult partners have to be of unequal power?

Since the fundamental logic of the mental structures of caregiving and attachment is not inherently restricted to any single stage of life, generic terms are preferable to describe the two persons involved (and in nonhuman species, the two animals). In this chapter we will use the generic terms "ego" for one partner and "alter" for the second partner. This is a usage that has a long tradition in sociology, although other fields use other terms (such as "person" and "other" used by some psychologists, or as "A" and "B" or "P" and "O" used by other psychologists and economists). Another alternative would be to use the generic terms "caregiver" for one partner and "dependent" for the second partner. This usage would be consistent with the attachment literature, where "caregiver" is commonly used. However, this terminology implies a unidirectional relationship. Although this usage is consistent with Bowlby's original formulation of caregiving-attachment as an unvarying, biologically based, mother-child relationship, it has the unfortunate result of obscuring the reciprocal nature of many if not most "attachment" relationships. Perhaps for this reason there have been few if any attempts to develop an explicit theory of the child's efforts to protect, support, and comfort parents, although many authors have described empirical examples of this behavior (e.g., Apter, 1990; Bowlby, 1979; Justice & Justice, 1990), mostly considering it pathological.

We will see in subsequent chapters that the genetic program that creates the mother-child dyadic preference bond also creates the father-child, father-mother, mother-father, child-parent and other dyadic preference bonds. Although the neurobiological evidence has not yet verified that the caring motivation and caregiving behavioral control system is the same in all these relationships (see Chapter 4), this seems to be but a matter of time and more research. Because the process we are beginning to understand is multidirectional, it will not serve us well to use unidirectional terminology. To aid communication, I will usually refer to the caregiver as "ego" and the partner who receives nurturance as "alter." Often we would see the mother as "ego" in a parent-child pair, but sometimes the child would be "ego" and give nurturance to the mother. In a married couple, sometimes the wife is "ego" and the husband is "alter." At other times and even at the same time, the husband is "ego" and the wife is "alter." The terminology is chosen to emphasize that either partner and both partners in any pair can take the role of ego or alter or both simultaneously. When specifically discussing Bowlby's concept of caregiving, "ego" will be "the caregiver" and "alter" will be "the dependent."

THE ATTACHMENT BEHAVIORAL CONTROL SYSTEM

Attachment logic has taken several forms. Two primary forms will be referred to as the "proximity" attachment and "security" attachment.

A behavioral control system, as Bowlby uses the term, is a cybernetic functional system. It is described by the same logic as an evolutionary functional account except that the consequence of a cybernetic system is intentional instead of unintentional—the consequence is a *goal* of the system. A cybernetic process describes how a system, given a goal, makes comparisons of its current state (or its predicted state in the case of a feedforward process) and its goal state (the "set goal" of the system) and responds to discrepancies by regulating an effectors system which takes action to move the current state toward the goal state (see discussions in Bowlby, 1969/1982; Broderick, 1993; Buckley, 1967; Hill, 1971; Kantor & Lehr, 1975).

Comparison and regulation processes within a cybernetic process constitute a "feedback loop." In a simple thermostat, the set goal is the temperature to which the thermostat has been set. The comparison process uses a thermometer to measure the actual temperature and compares it with the goal temperature in order to send a message when the actual temperature and goal temperature are different. The regulator is a switch that sends a "start" or "stop" message to the mechanism, a heating or cooling unit. If it is working properly, the heating/cooling mechanism then operates to move the actual temperature toward the goal temperature until the goal is achieved, at which point the regulator sends a "stop" message. Cybernetic systems are most often described only as feedback systems. However, a distinction can be made between a feedback system and a feedforward system. A feedback system corrects for the discrepancy just detected in the set goal. A feedforward system attempts to *predict* the future discrepancy in the system and either avoid or correct for that predicted discrepancy. For example, a parent may hear a child's crying, detect a discrepancy from the child's goal of satiation, and through a feedback process continue feeding the child until the goal is reached. On the other hand, the parent may anticipate the child's hunger and through a feedforward process act to prepare food and begin to feed the child before the child is even aware of hunger. A cybernetic system is thus a goal-corrected feedback or feedforward system.

Cybernetic behavioral control systems have *three* different levels at which activation takes place. For a biological system, at the first level there is *genetic/developmental activation*. Biological activation is determined by genes which direct the body's hormonal system and central nervous system (CNS) development. The importance of hormones and the CNS emphasizes both the genetic and developmental contribution to biological activation. Second, there is *stimulus or operational activation*, which involves activation by a stimulus external to the behavioral control system, and often external to the organism, as when a signal from the environment turns the system on. Third, there is the *motivational activation* of specific behaviors within the behavioral control system by a comparison and regulation process (called the "regulator" by Bretherton, 1980) in order to achieve or maintain the set goal. Motivational motivation, or regulation, is governed by processes of comparison and planning. A comparable example from the world of technology is a thermostat. The manufacture of the thermostat corresponds to the "biological" activation of the thermostat. Stimulus activation is by the person who sets the thermostat to a desired temperature. Regulation (motivational activation) is performed by a temperature-sensitive mechanism inside the thermostat that turns the furnace or air conditioner on or off.

Alongside this cybernetic goal-corrected process is an internal working model in memory where the organism records previous successful behaviors. The organism can subsequently retrieve these memories as the basis for future operations of the behavioral control system.

Proximity attachment behavioral control system

"Proximity attachment" primarily refers to Bowlby's various articulations of attachment theory between 1954 and 1963, when he was working closely with ethologist Robert Hinde. Secondarily, it refers to later articulations of the theory that emphasize ethological explanation.

The genetic/developmental activator of attachment is more than genes for Bowlby. He recognizes that genes carry "a potential to develop . . . behavioral systems, both the nature and the form of which differ in some measure according to the particular environment in which development takes place" (Bowlby, 1969/1982, p. 45). Thus, the attachment behavioral control system is created through the gene-directed biological processes of hormone production and central nervous system development (Bowlby, 1969/1982). With appropriate nutrition and social interaction, the circuits of the attachment behavioral control system are created in the brain. For Bowlby, stimulus activation of a system once it has biologically developed is usually by external factors, but sometimes activation is caused by internal states such as fatigue or insecurity. Internal conflict between behavioral control systems is resolved by the biological inhibition of one system in favor of another (e.g., Bowlby, 1969/1982). For example, when a child is playing near the mother and the mother moves away, the "child's attachment behaviour is likely to be elicited and his exploratory behaviour inhibited" (1969/1982, p. 237).

The proximity attachment behavioral control system itself consists of a set goal of proximity, a generalized decision mechanism, an internal working model, and attachment behaviors physically expressed by movement toward the partner. The attachment behavioral control system also produces emotional signals. In the attachment literature, the cybernetic feedback (or feedforward) process and the activation mechanism are frequently described for both human and nonhuman species. The internal working model and emotional signals are usually described only for humans. Bowlby identified the attachment system's set goal as proximity between the caregiver (ego) and the dependent (alter). Within the logic of this theoretical orientation, the attachment behavioral control system is activated in alter by an internal or external threat condition. When the attachment behavioral control system has been activated, the generalized decision mechanism compares current conditions to the set goal of proximity and then selects attachment behaviors for alter to perform by the "effector" (in this case the physical body) until a terminating condition (indicating proximity to ego) is registered (Bretherton, 1980; Hinde, 1982). In other words, alter's attachment behavioral control system monitors proximity to ego and, through the cybernetic feedback process, regulates attachment behaviors to be more intense if distance increases, or reduces attachment behaviors as distance is decreased.

Note that at the time a predator is first detected (by sight, sound, or smell), the proximity attachment behavioral control system is not active according to Bowlby's original formulation. Later (1969/1982), he relaxed this assumption. Otherwise, some other system would have had to detect the danger and send a signal to activate the attachment behavioral control system.

Emotional feelings arise from the operation of the behavioral control system. As the attachment system operates, it sends signals to alter about its operation in the form of emotional feelings. These signals are often visible to observers as well as to alter. Happiness, for example, is a signal that the set goal is being achieved, while distress is a signal indicating to alter that the set goal is not being met. Emotional feelings are thus often associated with the detection of a discrepancy from the set goal. For this reason emotional feelings are considered by Bowlby to be associated with, but not part of, the behavioral control system.

In the proximity attachment theory of childhood, attachment behaviors at birth are largely limited to preprogrammed and inflexible "fixed action patterns," such as "rooting, grasping, crying, and smiling when [the caregivers] first appear" (Bowlby, 1969/1982, p. 66). In Bowlby's theory of childhood, the attachment behavioral control system does not appear until age six months (1969/1982). Before this age, attachment behaviors are enacted by a more primitive psychological organization (Ainsworth, 1989; Bowlby, 1969/1982). Later, the system begins to incorporate other behaviors that become part of the system's repertoire if they prove to be successful in achieving the set goal of proximity. Alter's successful behaviors and ego's responses are encoded in alter's memory in the form of an attachment internal working model, described as a cognitive mental representation (Bretherton, 1980). Depending on alter's development, the attachment behavioral control system will incorporate successful new behaviors into the working model. For example, as alter becomes mobile, alter will add locomotion toward ego as an attachment behavior. Ego's caregiving responses will also affect the working model. If alter learns that ego will not offer caregiving in response to crying, alter will gradually remove crying from the attachment behavior repertoire in alter's working model. If ego is nonresponsive to all of alter's attachment behaviors, alter will learn, and will incorporate in alter's working model, the suppression of all attachment behaviors. Alter's working model, consisting of alter's memory of attachment behaviors, ego's caregiving behaviors, and similar memories with other caregivers, if any, is maintained in memory and will be available years in the future when alter becomes a caregiver (Solomon & George, 1996; Sroufe & Fleeson, 1986).

Since attachment theory describes a dyadic process, it is important to consider how a dyadic partnership is formed. For attachment researchers, the attachment relationship depends on the formation of a bond. An attachment bond is formed when the dependent chooses the caregiver as an object for attachment behaviors. Bonding involves an imprinting process (Bowlby, 1969/1982, 1977; West & Sheldon-Keller, 1994) by which the dependent as a child, with a built-in bias to give attention to humans, selects an attachment partner from whom the child has received nurturance (Bowlby, 1969/1982, 1977). An attachment bond is thus a choice (Hinde, 1982; Sroufe & Waters, 1977). Events involving the bond, including the creation or loss of the bond, are said to give rise to emotional feelings and are thus emotional events (Bowlby, 1977). How changes in the status of a bond occur, and how these changes give rise to emotions, are questions that are not addressed by proximity attachment. We will address the issue of the bond and its evolutionary and neurochemical basis in Chapters 4 and 5.

Security attachment behavioral control system

Proximity is purely a behavioral goal. Later theorists, and Bowlby himself at a later time, expanded the view that proximity is the set goal of the attachment system. This expansion did not occur all at once, and did not take the form of a critique of the prominence of proximity in attachment theory. Instead, it occurred over the course of several decades, and took the form of an internalization of the set goal.

This key revision of attachment theory (henceforth referred to as security attachment) resulted from the shift in focus to relationships among adults. Investigators studying attachment in very young children have tended to be content with the logic (or at least the language) of proximity attachment. However, as investigators began to study attachment over the life course, they began to question the direct applicability of proximity attachment to the behavior of adults (Berman & Sperling, 1994). The study of attachment beyond infancy raised two important issues that influenced the transformation of proximity attachment into security attachment.

The first issue was the primacy of proximity as a set goal. Proximity seemed an overly simplistic goal when applied to adult relationships. In addition, in research on children, researchers observed that children who possessed a secure working model of attachment were *not* the children who were most likely to remain in close proximity to their primary caregivers. On the contrary, these children exhibited more exploratory behavior, were more willing to wander further from their attachment objects, and were less anxious when separated from them for short periods of time, than were insecurely attached children (Bowlby, 1988; Feeney & Noller, 1996; Sroufe & Waters, 1977). Without denying that attachment reinforces proximity to the caregiver in infants, theorists reasoned that securely attached toddlers are more able to decrease proximity because they are confident that their caregivers are available to them and competent to intervene should intervention be desired. Hence, as these theorists have developed it, the security version of attachment theory postulates subjective emotional security rather than physical proximity as the set goal of the attachment behavioral control system (Bartholomew, 1990; Sroufe & Fleeson, 1986; Sroufe & Waters, 1977; West & Sheldon-Keller, 1994).

Authoritative accounts of attachment (e.g., Mikulincer & Shaver, 2007) have come to argue that attachment is activated exclusively by fear. Thus, the goal of the attachment system is to reduce fear. "We assume that every event perceived by a person of any age as threatening tends to activate the attachment system" (Mikulincer & Shaver, 2007, p. 32). Most other attachment researchers follow this model (Ainsworth, 1989; Berman & Sperling, 1994; Cassidy, 1999; Simpson & Rholes, 2000; Sroufe & Waters, 1977). Bowlby (1969/1982, p. 351) notes that the child's goal is to "terminate his distress and . . . make him feel secure." In the context of this discussion of the association between attachment and fear, it is useful to note that Bowlby actually described two forms in which attachment is manifest. In addition to high intensity, distress-elicited attachment, Bowlby also described "low intensity" attachment characterized by "smiling, relaxed locomotion, watching, and touching" (Bowlby, 1969/1982, p. 250). When Bowlby describes the conditions that lead to increased attachment behavior, he lists hunger, fatigue, illness, unhappiness, pain, and alarm (Bowlby, 1969/1982, p. 203). Of these, only alarm seems related to evoking proximity for protection; all seem related to evoking comforting and other nurturing behaviors usually unrelated to protection from a predator. It seems to be low intensity attachment that is being described when attachment is seen as involving "comfort," (as opposed to "comforting") "depending," "closeness," and "love" (Mikulincer & Shaver, 2007, pp. 17, 19, 22, 27, 39), and as "being understood and accepted" (Rothbaum & Kakinuma, 2004, p. 36). For now I will leave off consideration of this nondistress form of attachment. I will address it again in Chapter 4.

Feeney and Noller (1996) have forged a kind of reconciliation between proximity and security versions of attachment theory by proposing that proximity is the set goal as seen by an observer, while felt security is the set goal as experienced by the dependent.[2] Physical proximity is then one of many routes by means of which the dependent can achieve the set goal of emotional security.

The second issue raised by the expansion of attachment research to adults was the stability of the adult attachment internal working model. The proximity attachment working model was conceptualized as relatively stable (Bowlby, 1973; Feeney & Noller, 1996). This emphasis on stability may have resulted from Bowlby's clinical experience in which childhood attachment styles proved difficult to modify in therapy. Within security attachment theory, investigators have developed a more flexible concept of the working model (Ainsworth, 1989; Bartholomew, 1990; Berman & Sperling, 1994; Feeney & Noller, 1996; Klaus, Kennell, & Klaus, 1995; Sroufe & Waters, 1977). The security attachment working model is seen as less rigid, encoding "the affectively charged relationship between self and other" (Diamond & Blatt, 1994, p. 73). This working model contains a cognitive encoding of past experiences with attachment objects, and also emotional appraisals of those relationships (Collins, 1996). Thus, the internal working model is a conservative but changeable generalization of concrete attachment relationships.

Within security attachment logic, the attachment object is selected from among a wide variety of potential partners, not simply imprinted from among the earliest caregivers. In the course of a lifespan, alter may form attachment bonds with many objects, few of whom function primarily as unidirectional caregivers (Sroufe & Waters, 1977; West & Sheldon-Keller, 1994). The criteria of selection are given by the individual's working model of attachment.

In addition to the differences in set goals (proximity vs. security) between the proximity and security attachment systems, another difference is in the conditions for activation of the system. According to a suggestion by Bretherton (1980) and ratified by Bowlby (1969/1982), the security attachment system is to be seen as always activated. Heard and Lake (1997) refer to this as "vigilant quiescence" so that the perception of threats to security is located within the attachment behavioral control system instead of external to it. The generalized decision mechanism of the attachment cybernetic system detects the discrepancy between the current situation (anxiety or insecurity) and the continuously active set goal (security) and begins to select attachment behaviors to reduce the discrepancy. The strategies (cybernetic algorithms) to achieve the goal are encoded in alter's attachment working model. These algorithms include representations of alter, ego, and the relationship between alter and ego. The generalized decision mechanism continues to select previously successful behaviors from the working model or innovates new behaviors if previously successful behaviors are not available or become unsuccessful.

The security version of attachment theory has given greater attention to the attachment internal working model. Ego's caregiving responses affect this working model. When ego responds by making alter feel secure, and when ego's nurturance is accurately interpreted, then alter's internal working model of attachment that records these experiences includes a felt sense of security. For a child with a secure attachment, the working model will have encoded such behaviors as crying, asking, hugging, and the like that were previously successful in achieving felt security. Unfortunately, not all early caregivers are reliable. Ego's failure to meet alter's attempts to achieve security, such as by ignoring alter's bids for proximity and contact, begets an internal working model of "insecure" attachment. If alter learns that ego will not offer caregiving in response to crying, alter not only will gradually remove crying from the attachment behavior repertoire in alter's working model, but will also form a generalized expectation that crying is ineffective. If ego is nonresponsive to all or most of alter's attachment behaviors, alter will learn, and will incorporate in alter's working model, the suppression of all or most attachment behaviors. If a child has learned that a caregiver is not available and not responsive, then the child will develop an internal working model of the self as unworthy of or unable to acquire nurturance, and of ego—and the world—as unreliable and unavailable.

Within security attachment logic, attachment bonds are *formed* rather than chosen or "imprinted." Although the attachment bond is an "affectional" bond in alter that predisposes alter to emit attachment behaviors toward ego, the emotional components of this bond are not described in much detail. Alter is said to form an attachment bond toward the caregiver. Subsequent to the establishment of the bond, the *organization* of the attachment behavioral control system depends on alter's experiences with the caregiver (Cassidy, 1999). The development of a security attachment bond in alter depends on ego's contingent responsiveness to alter's bids for proximity and contact (Ainsworth, et al., 1978; Hazan &

Shaver, 1994). It also depends on alter's responsiveness to ego's caregiving, which in turn depends on alter's working model (Ashton, 1978; Heard & Lake, 1997; Stern, 1985; Winnicott, 1965b). Thus if alter, having experienced inadequate care in the past, does not expect responsive caregiving, then even sincere caregiving attempts may not be perceived as such. Attitudes and beliefs about alter, ego, and their relationship are compared with the distilled content of previous attachment relationships as alter elects either to accept or resist an attachment bond with ego (Solomon & George, 1996; West & Sheldon-Keller, 1994). In infancy, an attachment bond is said to develop toward the best caregiver around (the one who provides the best subjectively felt security).

The evolutionary account of attachment has described how an attachment behavioral control system could provide survival advantages within the environment of evolutionary adaptedness. However, the evolutionary advantages of attachment can only be realized if there is a preexisting caregiving behavioral control system and an available caregiver. Bowlby assumed in his evolutionary accounts that mature organisms are reliably motivated to accept the proximity of immature organisms, and to ward off any predators who are threatening to attack immature organisms. Crying, one of the prototypical attachment behaviors, would be an evolutionary *disadvantage* if there were no caregiver to respond, because crying is likely to attract predators. Offspring do not cry in species where parents do not provide protection. Crying is only an advantage to the extent that it usually attracts the caregiver faster than it attracts the predator. Thus, for Bowlby and some of his followers, the evolutionary survival of "innate" attachment behavior assumes the prior existence of a naturally selected caregiving or "retrieval" control system that responds to an immature organism's bids for proximity and protection.

THE CAREGIVING BEHAVIORAL CONTROL SYSTEM

Attempts to delineate the mechanism by which parental caregiving is achieved have been rare within the attachment tradition (see Solomon & George, 1996, and Heard & Lake, 1997, for the major, if limited, exceptions). Ainsworth (1989, p. 712) notes that "remarkably little is known about the processes involved in the formation and maintenance of the bond" of mother to infant. For Bowlby, caregiving by mothers is so "readily understood" as to require little analysis: "When looked at in terms of evolutionary theory, the occurrence of altruistic nurturance of young is readily understood since it serves to promote the survival of offspring" (Bowlby, 1988, p. 165).

Proximity caregiving behavioral control system

The evolutionary functionality of the dependent's attachment control system depends on its articulation (or "meshing") with the caregiver's caregiving behavioral control system. The caregiving behavioral control system, as it can be discerned in the writing of attachment theorists, shares with the attachment behavioral control system the functional consequence of protecting dependent children from predators and thus facilitating the passing on of the parent-child genetic heritage.

Similar to the proximity attachment system, the proximity caregiving behavioral control system in ego is a cybernetic system with a set goal of proximity to alter, a generalized decision mechanism, and a caregiving internal working model that records successful and unsuccessful attempts to maintain proximity (Bowlby, 1969/1982). Among attachment theorists, the caregiving system is usually discussed as activated by alter's attachment behaviors. These attachment behaviors are emitted by alter's attachment behavioral control system, which is activated by alter's internal state (e.g., fatigue), the environment (danger), or the relationship (ego's absence or distance). Ego will also retrieve alter when ego perceives danger to alter (Cassidy, 1999). Thus, attachment theory usually describes the caregiving behavioral control system as mainly reactive, either to alter or to other environmental stimuli. In Bowlby's original formulation, until alter emits attachment behaviors or ego perceives danger to alter, the proximity caregiving behavioral control system is not activated and does not operate. The cybernetic process has a set goal of proximity. Ego enacts behaviors that, according to memories recorded in ego's caregiving working model, are expected to lead to retrieval of alter. Once activated, ego's caregiving behavioral control system monitors proximity to alter and, through a goal-corrected feedback process, retrieves alter when the distance becomes too great. As a goal-corrected system, the caregiving behavioral control system can be creative. If the behaviors encoded in the internal working model do not work, ego will enact alternate behaviors until the set goal of proximity is achieved.[3] The proximity caregiving behavioral control system continues to operate until a terminating condition (proximity to alter) occurs.

The proximity attachment view regards attachment and caregiving behavioral control systems as distinct systems. Caregiving and attachment internal working models are outcomes (only) of their respective behavioral control systems. Nevertheless, attachment researchers routinely assume that the child's attachment behaviors recorded in an attachment internal working model are routinely transferred to the caregiving internal working model later when the person engages in adult caregiving (Solomon & George, 1996; Sroufe & Fleeson, 1986).

In the proximity attachment view, both the proximity attachment and proximity caregiving systems have the same set goals: proximity of alter and ego (Bowlby, 1969/1982; Solomon & George, 1996). The identity of set goals creates a strict complementarity between the caregiving system and the attachment behavioral control system. This strict complementarity results, however, in an inadvertent trivialization of caregiving behavior. The goal of proximity can explain why ego might initiate retrieval behaviors when alter strays beyond a certain proximity threshold, but cannot explain the broad spectrum of caregiving activities, including feeding and grooming, teaching and praising and rescuing, that characterize the relationships Bowlby describes between immature organisms and their attachment objects. Bowlby does not explicitly address this objection. Instead, he observes that "maternal behavior is of more than one kind," and that "retrieving" is the behavior that most often articulates with the attachment behavioral control system (Bowlby, 1969/1982, p. 239). Although retrieval behavior "has been included under many heads" such as mothering, maternal care, caregiving, and nurturance, Bowlby argues that "it is useful to distinguish" between retrieval and other kinds of behaviors grouped under these general categories (1969/1982, p. 238). In evolutionary terms, we find retrieval in most mammalian species (although not apparently in rabbits). This is a weak argument for excluding all behaviors but proximity seeking and retrieval from caregiving. However, we need not belabor it as Bowlby himself eventually moved from the proximity version of caregiving. Although he uses the term "retrieval" to name the system in the section on maternal caregiving in *Attachment* (Bowlby, 1969/1982), his more frequent choice is the term "caregiving," which clearly implies a broader set of behaviors.

Safety and security caregiving behavioral control systems

Bowlby's explicit theoretical analysis of caregiving is limited to describing caregiving as complementary to attachment (1969/1982, pp. 141, 182, 237), and describing mothers who retrieve children (1969/1982, pp. 236, 239-243, 251). It is clear, however, that Bowlby's implicit idea of caregiving is much broader than proximity and retrieval. Entries listed for caregiving in the index of *Attachment* describe "care of babies and young children" (1969/1982, p. 39), a "sheep brought up by the farmer's daughter" (1969/1982, p. 45), birds feeding young (1969/1982, pp. 50, 125), male primates protecting mothers and children from predators (1969/1982, pp. 62, 166), a goose returning its egg to the nest (1969/1982, pp. 67-68), nest building (1969/1982, pp. 76, 79), "feminine behavior" (1969/1982, p. 87), nest building of the canary and "maternal" behavior of the rat (1969/1982, pp. 90-94), parental behavior (1969/1982, pp. 130, 166, 181, 233), "maternal" behavior of young children (1969/1982, p. 159), "maternal" behavior of mothers (1969/1982, pp. 163-164, 239-247, 260-261, 273, 306, 341-346), mothers keeping infants close (1969/1982, pp. 184-194, 199), breast feeding (1969/1982, p. 249), mother's attention (1969/1982, p. 254), maternal talking (1969/1982, p. 274), maternal interactions "in a loving way" (1969/1982, p. 280), responding "in a sociable way," picking up, cuddling (1969/1982, pp. 287-288), social interaction (1969/1982, pp. 342, 344, 348, 349), and in general, how parents treat children (1969/1982, pp. 366, 367). In *Secure bond*, Bowlby (1988) occasionally replaces the "caregiving behavior" terminology with "parenting behavior."

Safety caregiving behavioral control system. All of this evidence suggests that the caregiving set goal is broader than simple proximity. In one attempt to broaden caregiving, Solomon and George (1996, p. 186) described the caregiving set goal as: "to keep the infant or child close to ego under conditions of threat or danger, (i.e., keep the child safe)." They subsequently updated this goal: "the behavioral goal of the caregiving system is to provide protection to the child" (George & Solomon, 1999, p. 652). George and Solomon are careful to restrict the caregiving set goal to alter's physical safety: "Do what is needed to protect this child, but no more" (George & Solomon, 1999, p. 187). Cassidy (1999:10) describes the set goal as "to promote proximity and comfort when the parent perceives that the child is in real or potential danger." Keeping alter safe is a useful expansion of the proximity caregiving set goal because it accounts for why parents permit and encourage their children to explore, which usually increases the parent-child distance under conditions of safety. The proximity attachment view accounted for this behavior by arguing that the caregiving behavioral control system was inactive except in the presence of danger. The safety caregiving behavioral control system, on the other hand, is always activated, and exploration is accounted for by redefining alter's safety from an activator (within proximity caregiving) to a set goal (within safety caregiving). The safety caregiving set goal is consistent with the system's functional outcome of the survival of offspring. The safety caregiving set goal has a greater verisimilitude in describing the goals of parenting than the proximity caregiving set goal. Human parents are usually consciously aware of the safety of their children. Human parents, as well as primates, dogs and cats, and hoofed mammals protect their offspring, including as necessary placing themselves between their offspring and predators. For example, a giraffe mother will stand over her calf and face a lion when the calf is too slow to run away (Masson & McCarthy, 1995). A cat who has never gone in the water will jump in to rescue her kitten. Squirrels and rabbits, while apparently not providing active protection against predators, provide passive protection in the form of general warning about the presence of predators.

Security caregiving behavioral control system. For Heard and Lake (1997, p. 54), "The goal of the caregiver . . . is reached when the caregiver considers the [dependent] is now able to cope without endangering themselves or desiring [an attachment] interaction." Heard and Lake are describing a terminating condition rather than the set goal itself, but we can infer that the security caregiving set goal involves encouraging and facilitating alter's ability to cope (presumably with "the world") in safety (physical and perhaps also emotional). It is clear that Heard and Lake intend to include felt security within "safety" because it is alter's degree of felt security that determines their attachment behaviors. Thus the caregiver's set goal is to encourage and facilitate alter's ability to act in the world with both physical safety and emotional security.

The security caregiving set goal of maintaining alter's felt security articulates well with the security attachment set goal of own felt security. As we will consider below, this may be a deceptively simple complementarity. The evolutionary evidence suggests that a security set goal of caregiving evolved after the proximity and safety set goals had evolved. Rabbits, rats and hoofed mammals seem to give no attention to anything that ethologists have identified as the feelings of the offspring. This is certainly partially a matter of the level of development of the caregiving behavioral control system and partially a matter that feelings are less fully experienced in these mammalian species than in species that emerged later. In dogs, cats, primates and humans, caregivers are oriented toward the felt emotions of their offspring. Neither Solomon and George, nor Heard and Lake have proposed an evolutionary account of the origin of the expanded caregiving set goal. An evolutionary analysis will be discussed in Chapter 4.

Since the safety and security caregiving behavioral control systems are continuously activated, then any information relevant to alter's safety or felt security can lead to the production of caregiving behaviors. The relevant information can include alter's attachment behaviors, but can also include perception of dangers to alter (cybernetic feedback) or anticipation of danger (cybernetic feedforward) or perception or anticipation of insecurity.

The safety and security caregiving behavioral control systems have been a significant advance over the proximity caregiving behavioral control system. These conceptions expanded a rather trivial meaning for caregiving (physical proximity, which is trivial in a psychological sense, although not at all trivial in the evolutionary sense of a consequence leading to survival) into a more satisfying meaning (providing safety and security). However, there are some as yet unresolved complications to the new focus on emotional security as a set goal. The security attachment logic has identified a plausible, if limited, account of parental altruism and relationship altruism that is not based on self interest. It has expanded the content of the attachment and caregiving set goals to include alter's emotional states of security and insecurity. In so doing it has also made the caregiving set goal distinct from the attachment set goal. Instead of the same goal (proximity) for both, now the attachment goal is own felt security while the caregiving set goal is the partner's safety and felt security. However, this creates a problem for both the psychological logic and the evolutionary logic of Bowlby's scheme. If the caregiving set goal is different from the attachment set goal, then it is no longer possible to claim that the adult's caregiving set goal psychologically grows out of the child's attachment set goal. A full discussion of the psychological emergence of caregiving is needed and will be the subject of much of the rest of this book. In addition, it becomes more important to account for the unique evolutionary background of caregiving. The evolution of caregiving will be considered in the next chapter.

ISSUES IN THE PSYCHOLOGY OF CAREGIVING

There have been a number of underdeveloped areas in attachment logic:

- The lack of a place for emotion within the cybernetic caregiving and attachment behavioral control systems (emotions are viewed as a consequence outside the systems);
- The lack of a motivation for safety and security caregiving;

- A limited account of the meaning of the attachment and caregiving bonds; and
- The lack of an explanation for responsiveness and sensitivity within the caregiving behavioral control system.

An account of the psychology of caregiving needs to deal with problems of intention and choice among caregivers.

The role of emotion

By expanding the set goal of caregiving to safety and security, a more general and more plausible set goal of caregiving has been advanced. The set goal of the partner's safety and security is more nearly consistent with our commonsense understanding of caregiving. This development means that the theoretical importance of emotion is increased. In line with the focus on security, some authors have described attachment as an "affect regulation" system (Bartholomew, 1990; Feeney & Noller, 1996; Sroufe & Waters, 1977; West & Sheldon-Keller, 1994). This may be a somewhat optimistic characterization, given that the only emotion (affect) explicitly regulated in Bowlby's cybernetic model of the attachment system is security. One may note that when a dependent detects a discrepancy between desired proximity and actual proximity, alter may feel a number of associated emotions, such as anxiety and fear. Attachment researchers and others have noted these associated emotions. There is no consensus on the emotions associated with caregiving. While Berman & Sperling (1994) claim that attachment and caregiving produce the same emotional feelings, Heard and Lake (1997) distinguish the satisfaction and relief of attachment from the comfort of caregiving. George and Solomon (1999) describe the mother's pleasure and satisfaction from protecting the child and anger, sadness, anxiety, and despair when protection is threatened or blocked. However, these emotions are not regulated by the attachment behavioral control system. Only proximity and security are directly regulated. Other emotions are conceptualized as consequences outside the caregiving and attachment systems.

One attempt to broaden the use of emotion within attachment was offered by Shaver and colleagues (Shaver, Hazen, & Bradshaw, 1988). These authors attempted to integrate love with attachment and caregiving in adult relationships. Their conclusion was that romantic love is defined by the integration of the attachment behavioral control system, the caregiving behavioral control system, and a sexuality behavioral control system. This was a very important contribution, but, by placing love conceptually above attachment, caregiving and sexuality, it had the unfortunate result of placing love (at least "romantic" love) *outside* of attachment and caregiving. In another attempt to broaden the use of emotion, Feeney and Noller (1996) located emotion within security attachment in two ways. First they said that attachment is "a theory of affect regulation; that is, a theory about how people handle negative emotions" (1996, p. 36). The negative emotion is alter's distress at ego's unavailability or nonresponsiveness. Second, Feeney and Noller followed Shaver & Hazan to relate love to attachment. However, given the failure to find a theoretical role for affection within either the attachment or caregiving behavioral control systems, Feeney and Noller were being unduly optimistic when they characterized affection in terms of its "centrality to attachment theory, which deals with the formation and expression of bonds of affection" (1996, p. 42).

Bowlby was very clear that, to him, whatever the role of emotion, emotions were not to be taken as causes of attachment or caregiving. He explicitly argues that attachment is not driven by emotion: emotions are "phases of an individual's intuitive appraisal" (1969/1982, p. 104). While this characterization was consistent with thinking in his time, I will suggest below that this is not a useful characterization today. Neurobiological research has suggested that fear can cause one to run from a bear even before one has cognitively appraised the bear as dangerous (Damasio, 1994). Furthermore, rather than tracing both caregiving and attachment to largely cognitive decision processes with perhaps an associated emotional tone, I will show the usefulness of conceptualizing emotional motivations as the foundations of both caregiving and attachment.

A motivation for caregiving

A major and critical issue for attachment theory is a motivation for caregiving. A motivation for attachment appears to be unproblematic—it is easy to think of attachment as motivated by self preservation or self interest. Attachment researchers have attempted to derive the motivation for caregiving from the attachment internal working model (Heard & Lake, 1997; Solomon & George, 1996). Sroufe and Fleeson (1986) make a social learning argument that children learn both caregiving and attachment sides of the relationship by observation. Research has shown that there is an empirical association between a person's childhood attachment working model style and adult caregiving (Feeney & Noller, 1996). However, attachment theory has not yet given a clear theoretical account showing how an attachment working model develops into a working model for caregiving. The transformation is plausible within proximity attachment because both the attachment behavioral control system and the caregiving behavioral control system have the same set goal: proximity of alter and ego. Yet proximity attachment logic only accounts for a highly restricted set of caregiving behaviors.

Compared to proximity attachment and caregiving, the processes of security attachment and security caregiving have more nuanced and more emotional set goals. Yet its very increased emotional content makes the transition from the attachment internal working model to the caregiving working model more problematic. The attachment internal working model provides an experiential basis (based on memories of past experiences) for alter to achieve the attachment set goal of own felt security. The caregiving internal working model similarly provides an experiential basis to achieve the caregiving set goal of the partner's felt security. There is, however, no mechanism in security attachment logic for an actor's set goal of *own* sense of security in an attachment behavioral control system to be transformed into the actor's set goal of the *partner's* sense of security in a caregiving behavioral control system. The transition from one's security attachment set goal (focused on self) to one's caregiving set goal (focused on other) is a crucial underdeveloped area of attachment-caregiving theory. These two weaknesses—the absence of an explanation of how an attachment internal working model transforms into a caregiving working model over time, and the absence of a narrative account for alter's ability to "become" the caregiver for another dependent—are connected. Both ask how an actor becomes a caregiver, and both weaknesses can be attributed to the absence of theoretical development of processes within the caregiving behavioral control system. Most of the theoretical development of attachment theory since Bowlby's original foundation has focused on the working model rather than on the goal-corrected cybernetic processes of attachment. Unfortunately, this direction of development, while beneficial in terms of measurement and research (Feeney & Noller, 1996; Van IJzendoorn & Tavecchio, 1987), has yielded limited theoretical understanding of caregiving processes.

Missing in the proximity and security accounts of caregiving is a plausible motivation for caregiving, a reason why ego should choose to nurture alter. In the proximity account, developed in the 1950s, ego was assumed to be a mother, based on cultural patterns in Britain and the United States. We saw in Chapter 1 how maternal behavior had been considered unproblematic and theoretically uninteresting. When Cassidy (1999) considers a motivation for caregiving, she declares it an "inherent motivation" but then does not say what this means. In the 1970s and 80s, attention turned to adult relationships where men and women were in relatively equal, mutual relationships. Security attachment privileged the "male" explanation of self interest by focusing on attachment's self-interested set goal of own security. This even led to the proposal that caregiving be dropped as a separate system (Berman & Sperling, 1994). Thus both men and women (emphasizing always heterosexual adult relationships) were assumed to be motivated by the self interest attachment set goal of own felt security. It was tacitly assumed that caregiving would occur as some kind of implicit exchange in service of their own felt security—each partner giving nurturance because each wanted to receive the other's nurturance.

In the 1990s, theory about parental caregiving was challenged by research addressing the issues of paternal parenting and adoption. Research has shown that adoptive parents show similar caregiving behaviors to biological parents. Furthermore, research has pushed the study of parents as caregivers beyond the original focus on mothers to fathers (Dollahite, 1998; LaRossa & LaRossa, 1981; Pleck, 1985; Pruett, 1987). A secure attachment bond between children and fathers has been found to depend on the fathers' amount of caregiving behaviors (Kotelchuck, 1976; Lester & Klein, 1974; Molinaro, Woolfolk, & Palkovitz, 1997; Ross, Zelazo, & Kotelchuck, 1975). Because biological accounts of caregiving had never been intended to apply to fathering, attempts have been made to discover the motivation of men who have undertaken caregiving of children (Doherty, 1997; Marsiglio, 1991; Pruett, 1987; Snarey, 1993). A number of commonalities are seen in the reports of caregiving fathers. In these reports, fathers begin by being very unsure of their caregiving ability, their feelings grow over time with contact with the child, and most of their caregiving skills develop by learning from the child. Noteworthy in these reports is the lack of evidence that boys' attachment experiences are the basis of paternal caregiving. It is from the father's attention to the child and readiness to learn from the child what works that appears to be the hallmark of active fathering. The same patterns had previously been described for mothers, but attachment researchers had not applied these findings to caregiving. Robson and Moss (1970) had reported that fully 41 percent of first time mothers claimed that at birth they had no positive feelings toward the newborn (see also Pruett, 1987; Rapoport, Rapoport, & Strelitz, 1977). Mothers were often initially insecure and their feelings grew slowly (Cowan & Cowan, 1992). Mothers and all parents don't just affect their children; parents are also affected by their children (Bell, 1974). What is needed is an account of caregiving that can identify a motivation for caregiving, and describe the emergent feelings toward the child as well as emergent feelings of competence.

Instead of motivation, Bowlby asserts that caregiving is the result of appraisal. That is, the parent perceives the child and selects a class of behavior "appropriate" to the child, for example "appraising the baby as something to be comforted" (Bowlby, 1969/1982, p. 116). There is no emotion involved in this appraisal, although after the appraisal, "sympathy for the baby may well be experienced (in contrast, say, to irritation or anger) at the moment the baby is appraised as 'fit to be comforted'" (Bowlby, 1969/1982, p. 117).

While security attachment logic captures important aspects of alter's relationship to a caregiver—including a set goal of felt security, an internal working model (which allows feedforward processes based on anticipating the caregiver's behaviors), an internal security monitor, and a cognitive decision mechanism—it contains a serious omission. The theory of childhood attachment *describes* a hierarchy of attachment figures, but does not fully *explain* the hierarchy. In so doing it de-emphasizes the volitional component of attachment. Bowlby's conception of both proximity and security attachment emphasizes that the attachment behavioral control system is "elicited" or is "inhibited." Most human activity, however, particularly adult activity of interest to social scientists, is volitional (Aune, 1977; Borgatta & Borgatta, 1992; Giddens, 1979; Habermas, 1981). Human beings perform some nonvolitional activities. We are startled and we feel fear in ways that we do not choose, and in such cases sometimes we run before we have decided where. Yet in most cases we choose where to run. Fear of a predator is nonvolitional, but running is usually volitional. The child's locomotion toward a caregiver is generally by choice. Thus it is important to recognize that the child is the author of most attachment behaviors, rather than simply being the passive object of the attachment behavioral control system.

It is equally important to recognize that parents are authors of their caregiving behaviors. One might simply argue that parenting is a level one (developmental) activator of caregiving. This logic is often described in terms of "parental investment" (Clutton-Brock, 1991; Trivers, 1985). By this logic, parents, especially mothers, nurture children because of their "investment" in terms of time and energy in giving birth. All this time and energy would be "wasted" if children do not survive and thrive. And yet this continues to beg the question of what is the return on investment for the parent. Parents who have a genetically-based motivation to nurture the child will exist to "invest" because their own parents "invested" in them. But what is the motivation in all of these generations of parents to provide nurturance to their children?

Persuasive accounts of attachment and caregiving need to deal with the issue of choice and to identify volitional motivations for attachment and caregiving. For human activity, the activator will have to be a motivation within the person that leads to or directs behavior. A sex drive serves as a motivation within an organism to engage in mating behaviors, the predictable functional outcome of which is the reproduction of the species. Whatever it may be in other species, for humans there is a volitional component. If sex were nonvolitionally activated in humans, people would couple whenever they were attracted. Instead, humans make choices about sex, hard ones and easy ones, conflictual ones and cooperative ones, "smart" ones and "stupid" ones. People may be seen as motivated to pursue sex, but they make choices among competing motivations, internal and external conflicts, morality, opportunity, and constraint. Thus, even when a behavior like sex has a clear functional consequence, an explanation of sexual behavior requires that we identify a volitional motivation (Conway & Schaller, 2002). A motivation of love for other species members (or alternate motivations like pride or fear or shame) can lead to a mechanism of attacking a dangerous predator (and risking death). Such a mechanism can be evolutionarily successful, in spite of the risk to the individual. Even if death occurs for the individual, the survival of others with the same genetically based motivation will lead to species success and "success" for the genes. Conceptualization of volitional motivations for caregiving and attachment would strengthen attachment theory and increase its usefulness.

Attachment and caregiving bonds

Attachment and caregiving bonds are particular kinds of "affectional bonds." Bowlby defines attachment as "the propensity of human beings to make strong affectional bonds to particular others" (Bowlby, 1969/1982, p. 201). According to Ainsworth, attachment is the bond itself: "the affectional bond or tie an infant forms between himself and his mother" (Ainsworth, et al., 1978, p. 302); "attachment refers to an enduring affective bond between particular individuals" (Bartholomew, 1990, p. 149). Affectional bonds (1) are persistent, (2) are directed toward a specific partner, (3) are emotionally significant, (4) motivate the person to maintain proximity or contact with the partner, and (5) generate feelings of distress at involuntary separation (Ainsworth, 1989). An attachment bond is an affectional bond that leads one to seek "security and comfort in the relationship" (Cassidy, 1999, p. 12). Some attachment theorists treat the "bond" between parent and child as an evaluation-based cognitive decision (Bowlby, 1977; Hinde, 1982; Sroufe & Waters, 1977) or as a computer program (Bretherton, 1980).

In attachment logic, the attachment bond and caregiving bond are different and separate from the attachment and caregiving behavioral control systems. According to a number of attachment researchers, attachment and caregiving bonds do not vary in terms of strength. (Ainsworth, 1972; Cassidy, 1999; Main, 1999; Sroufe & Waters, 1977; Weiss, 1982). Within this conceptualization, the term "attachment" should only be applied to the most enduring and irreplaceable bonds (Ainsworth, 1989; Berman & Sperling, 1994; Bowlby, 1969/1982; Main, 1999; Simpson & Rholes, 2000). If two people have attachment bonds (to their respective partners), the strengths of their bonds are the same (they both have a "1" instead of a "0"). All children who have the requisite genetic constitution, if they are attached at all, are said to be equally and fully "attached." In this view, there are no *levels* of attachment, but there are *types* of attachment. Thus persons are seen as having secure, anxious, or avoidant styles of attachment (in the three-style formulation: Ainsworth, et al., 1978) or fearful style (in the four-style fear-attachment formulation: Bartholomew, 1990; Bartholomew & Horowitz, 1991).

This restriction can create difficulties for theorists. For example, some attachment researchers agree that seeking comfort from a stranger (in the obvious lack of an "enduring and irreplaceable" attachment bond) is still governed by the attachment system (Ainsworth, et al., 1978; Bretherton, 1978; Rheingold, 1969). Thus, the claim that an attachment bond must exist before attachment behaviors are possible may be useful for some purposes because it helps focus research on the dynamics of existing attachment relationships, but at the same time it makes it much more difficult to understand episodic attachment behaviors toward strangers, as well as understanding how attachment relationships come into being in the first place. Main (1999) gives an example of a child waiting in Main's office with Main and the mother before the Strange Situation. Thunder is heard, and the child goes to Main in her fear. In the Strange Situation, this child was coded as extremely avoidant attached to the mother. However, the actions in Main's office give evidence that the child was more trusting of Main, a complete stranger, than of her own mother. It may well be that many avoidant persons (such as this child) are pursuing a "deactivation strategy," suppressing a previously developed attachment system. But at least some avoidant persons may never have developed an attachment bond with the caregiver in the first place.

Given a nominal type of attachment, the constant attachment system may be *activated* at different levels, so "attachment behaviors" may vary in intensity even though attachment per se is not considered to vary in level (Ainsworth, 1982; Ainsworth, et al., 1978; Cassidy, 1999; Sroufe & Waters, 1977). In this view, if an attachment relationship exists, one may measure its attachment style, and one may measure its momentary level of activation. If the relationship is not an attachment relationship, there is in this view no style or activation to measure. Most tests of attachment style and dimensions assume that an attachment relationship already exists before measurement (Zeanah, Smyke, Koga, & Carlson, 2005). Because most fear-attachment researchers have not been interested in levels of attachment there have been no widely used diagnostic tests developed for the existence of an attachment system.[4] As a result, measurement paradigms like the Strange Situation for children lump unattached children with those experiencing deactivated attachment and call both "avoidant attached."

For many attachment researchers, although the attachment bond is a constant, the attachment system has a variable intensity of activation (Ainsworth, 1982; Ainsworth, et al., 1978; Cassidy, 1999). Still other researchers, however, assert that attachment itself can vary in intensity (Berman & Sperling, 1994; Kahn & Antonucci, 1980; Levitt, Coffman, Guacci-Franco, & Loveless, 1994; Troll & Smith, 1976). But in general, variations across relationships are seen to depend on different *organizations* of the behavioral control system, not on strength of the bond (Sroufe & Waters, 1977). According to Ainsworth's description, the bond is emotional, dyadic and persistent. And yet it is not clear what the bond *is*. In other usage, a "bond" can refer to a chemical force that keeps atoms together in a molecule, a glue that keeps other objects together, or a promise of future performance. Since attachment researchers often use "tie" as a synonym for "bond," they probably mean a force or glue that keeps people together. An affectional bond is "emotional," but within published attachment theory the only emotion seems to come when the bond is lost. Attachment behavior involves "seeking" security and comfort, but these emotions are outcomes of the caregiving system, not part of the bond itself. Bonds are persistent but it is not clear why they persist. Ainsworth's definition describes something very much like an addiction. It isn't clear what the person gets out of the bond, but there is a pain of withdrawal when the bond is lost, so the person is motivated to maintain contact. Of course, it may be that attachment bonds are just "metaphorical" (Shaver & Fraley, 2000), and this may be why attachment researchers haven't given much theoretical consideration to how bonds form and what they are made of.

Ainsworth's definition of affectional bond is peculiar in that it asserts that proximity is an outcome of all affectional bonds, not just the attachment bond and the attachment behavioral control system. Perhaps this is a residue of the superseding of the proximity attachment behavioral control system by the security attachment behavioral control system. This is an important theoretical development nevertheless, because it moves beyond the functional evolutionary "explanation" of caregiving by suggesting that there is something emotional (an "affectional" bond) about proximity behaviors. However, the rather casual remark that an affectional bond is "emotional" is not sufficient to explain why this bond should be permanent. It is important to identify what the emotion is that makes the bond endure.

An attachment bond is said to be formed between alter and ego when alter chooses ego (called an "attachment object") as a target for attachment behaviors. In the proximity version of attachment, the child chooses a caregiver who has previously nurtured the child. Within security attachment logic, ego is selected during the life cycle from many potential caregivers, not simply imprinted from among the earliest caregivers. An attachment bond is thus a choice (Hinde, 1982; Sroufe & Waters, 1977). A caregiver is selected depending on what they offer in exchange (Heard & Lake, 1997). The caregiver is said to be selected from those who provide nurturance (Bowlby, 1969/1982; Hinde, 1982; Sroufe & Waters, 1977; Zeifman & Hazan, 1997). The caregiver is selected because "preferred" (Ainsworth, et al., 1978, p. 25), because the person believes the caregiver has the potential to provide felt security (Berman & Sperling, 1994). A consistent element in all these accounts is that a precondition for the formation of an attachment bond in alter is prior caregiving behaviors from ego. This implies that attachment is dyadically derivative of caregiving.

Events involving the bond, including the creation or loss of the bond, are said to give rise to emotions and are thus emotional events (Bowlby, 1977). Thus it is not the bond itself that is described as an emotion—only the consequences of changes in the status of a bond are named as emotions: emotions are a "reflection of the bond" (Bowlby, 1979). According to Bowlby, the caregiving bond is formed in "the same way" as the attachment bond (1969/1982, p. 241). This is a reasonable statement in the proximity version of attachment, where it means that ego imprints alter. However, if this is what is intended, it further treats ego as a nonvolitional participant in caregiving. On the other hand, perhaps Bowlby is referring to the security version of attachment. Even then, it is not clear what it means to form a caregiving bond in "the same way" as an attachment bond, since alter chooses an attachment bond on the basis of an experience of receiving nurturance. Given that the object of an attachment bond is someone who has *already* provided nurturance, this curious statement seems to say, paradoxically, that a parent chooses to give nurturance to a child from whom the parent has already *received* nurturance. It requires some theoretical justification to assert that ego will choose a specific caregiving bond (for the purpose of *giving* nurturance) on the basis of experiences of *receiving* nurturance from the partner. Feeney and Noller have claimed that attachment bonds are "bonds of affection" (1996, p. 42), but aside from asserting a correlation between attachment and affection, they have not described a theoretical connection between the two. Further attention needs to be given to the origin and nature of the caregiving bond.

An explanation of responsiveness and sensitivity

Attachment researchers have given a consistent empirical description of "quality" caregivers. Quality caregivers are "responsive" to the dependent (Ainsworth, et al., 1978; Feeney & Noller, 1996; Isabella, 1993; Solomon & George, 1996; Sroufe, 1988) and they show "sensitivity" toward the dependent (Ainsworth, et al., 1978; Feeney & Noller, 1996; Heard & Lake, 1997; Solomon & George, 1996). Attachment researchers have concluded on the basis of empirical research that the parents of secure children can be characterized as "sensitive" and "responsive." While attachment researchers have made a strong case for the empirical association of sensitivity and responsiveness with "good" caregiving, they have not attempted to explain theoretically how these attributes arise in the caregiving behavioral control system. Unfortunately, even though many authors agree about the nature of quality caregiving, empirical generalization and moral exhortation are not substitutes for a theoretical explanation of how sensitivity and responsiveness are produced. Attachment logic has suggested why sensitivity and responsiveness might be important for the child, but it has not been able to explain why they are important to the parent.

The failure to give a theoretical explanation for responsiveness and sensitivity can probably be traced to the origins of attachment theory in ethology. In ethology, description of humans and other animals have always focused on observable behaviors. Ethologists have been largely reluctant (for good reason, given the resistance of critics: Crist, 1999) to ascribe motivation to nonhuman animals. As a result of this background, attachment researchers have simply assumed that the behaviors of "quality" parents are observed by the child and recorded in the child's attachment internal working model. In adulthood these recorded behaviors are then assumed to be transferred, apparently without modification, to the adult's caregiving internal working model and then automatically enacted in caregiving behaviors to the adult's children (Berman & Sperling, 1994). By asserting that adults produce these unmotivated behaviors by a kind of intergenerational contagion, the attachment theory of parenting oversimplifies and further trivializes the process of caregiving. To be clear, I do not claim that trivialization of caregiving is characteristic of attachment *researchers*, who have been quite attentive to the conflict and choices of parents. My criticism is directed at attachment theory: attachment researchers have not built their insights about parental experience into their published explanations of the cybernetic caregiving behavioral control system.

In order to provide solutions to the limitations we have identified in attachment logic, we need to consider the evolution of mammals (Chapter 3) and the psychobiology of the brain (Chapter 4). Then we will be ready to offer a complementary account of caregiving and attachment, an account which acknowledges the integrity of caregiving logic and specifies the process through which caregiving and attachment bonds are initiated and sustained. These extensions to attachment and caregiving logic will provide an account of the place of emotion in both caregiving and attachment—not as an epiphenomenal consequence of caregiving and attachment, but as a fundamental motivation for each. These motivations will also help us to account for the qualities of a "good" caregiver and a "good" dependent.

Notes

* A portion of this chapter was published as Bell & Richard (2000a, 2000b).

1. The terminology of the "behavioral control system" is taken from ethology and the study of animal behavior. There is a tradition in ethology to avoid any discussion of unobservable mental states (Crist, 1999). However, neurobiological research has shown that the brains of "lower" animals are quite similar to the brains of humans (MacLean, 1990; Panksepp, 1998), so that there is little reason to be so reticent about motivations. In subsequent chapters, I will change terminology from Bowlby's "behavioral control systems" to a more appropriate "motivation systems."

Evolution, of course, occurs through genes. The metaphor of competing genes is illuminating but, as far as we know, genes do not take an active part in their survival, notwithstanding the anthropomorphic survival "strategies" and "design" described by some authors (Axelrod, 1984; Clutton-Brock, 1991; Dawkins, 1976/1989; Williams, 1966; Zeifman & Hazan, 1997; see also Chapter 4). What genes do is to produce structures or behavioral mechanisms that determine the relative probability of survival of individual organisms within a particular environmental context (Caporael, 1997). Therefore, the focus here and in the next chapter will be on the behavioral mechanisms of individuals within species and not specifically on the genes that enable the mechanisms.

2. This is perhaps a somewhat disingenuous solution, since Bowlby's evolutionary account was based on the anti-predator behavioral effects of proximity, rather than the dependent's perception of proximity. It could be argued that the secure dependent may be less vigilant than a less secure person, so that security might *increase* the risk of predation in dangerous environments, in the absence of active parental caregiving.

3. Bowlby—anticipating criticism that Harris (1998) would make 40 years later—recognized that studying specific behaviors would not be productive: the set goal is not a behavioral one—it is related to an outcome (proximity, safety, felt security) that may be achieved through a large variety of alternative behaviors. The behaviors one chooses to make a 6-month-old feel secure are different from the behaviors to make a 5-year-old secure. And the behaviors that make one 5-year-old secure are often different from those that make another 5-year-old secure.

4. The conceptual foundation for such a test has been described by Ainsworth. All attachment bonds are said to be affectional bonds, and affectional bonds (1) are persistent, (2) are directed toward a specific partner, (3) are emotionally significant, (4) motivate the person to maintain proximity or contact with the partner, and (5) generate feelings of distress at involuntary separation (Ainsworth, 1989).

Chapter 3. The Evolution of Caregiving and Attachment*

The evolution of caregiving begins with the premammalian reptiles. Reptiles and mammals have an automatic fear and rejection of strangers. This chapter presents evidence for the evolution of a mechanism that inhibited stranger rejection, and the subsequent development of a dyadic preference that evolved prior to the emergence of mammalian species. Subsequently the dyadic preference evolved among mammals, reaching its expression in humans as the emotion of caring (nonsexual love). The caring emotion motivates the caregiving system.

In this chapter we turn to a consideration of where attachment and caregiving may have come from, how they may have evolved. Evolution is not an easy topic to explore. It requires making inferences based on fragmentary and disparate data. This is not, of course, a problem unique to evolution. Astronomers make inferences about the origin of the universe from the light of stars they believe has taken millions of years to arrive here. Archeologists make inferences about prehistoric peoples and cultures from the contents of their trash heaps. Evolutionary scientists make inferences from the incomplete fossil record and from behavioral and genetic comparisons among existing species.

Evolution occurs because of genetic changes that affect physical structures. The brain is one of these structures, so that psychological and social processes also undergo evolutionary change (Deacon, 1990; Tooby & Cosmides, 1992). Evolution is the cumulative effect of small mutations that increase the probability that an organism will survive to pass on the underlying genes.

Many evolutionary accounts of biological structures and social behaviors focus on functional design. A mechanism (a behavior or biological structure) is identified and then an argument is formulated that the mechanism would have provided net survival advantages to the genes that created it, and thus it is concluded that genes must logically exist to produce the behavior (see Chapter 2 for a discussion of functional logic). This approach treats the mechanism as a "black box" whose actual content is considered unimportant. The fact that the mechanism provides survival advantages is considered enough of an "explanation."

Because a given behavior could potentially fulfill many functions, evolutionary scientists have insisted on relatively stringent criteria for an evolutionary argument. Some have chosen optimality as the criterion. In order to show that a given mechanism was chosen by natural selection, by this logic, one must identify a function (consequence) of the mechanism and show how that mechanism is complex, economical, efficient, reliable, and precise in achieving the consequence (Buss, et al., 1998; Williams, 1966; Wright, 1994). For example, one identifies the function of the telephone as transmitting voices by showing that the telephone is a complex and unusual mechanism, that it is economical and precise in turning voice into electrical current and back into voice, that it is efficiently constructed to transmit human voices rather than other sounds, and that it reliably transmits voices (Roney, 1999). Thus, because the telephone so well achieves the identified function of human communication, one is justified in concluding that the mechanism was *designed* for the functional consequence of human communication.

I am extremely uncomfortable with this approach when applied to biology; it is not the approach I will take. There are three problems with it. The first problem with the design approach is that it assumes efficiency; the second is that it implies a designer; the third is that, even if the idea of design is only a metaphor, it is an inappropriate metaphor (Blumberg & Wasserman, 1995). The functional approach works with the telephone because the telephone was literally designed by identifiable human engineers to fulfill its one function. Natural selection as design only works when one assumes a designer. In addition, the design metaphor leads to the labeling of "inefficient" behavior as a "mistake" or "malfunction" (Bowlby, 1969/1982; Clutton-Brock, 1991; Williams, 1966) or "bad" (Daly & Wilson, 1983). For example, some behavior may be labeled efficient by the theorist who assumes that an emotion is designed for procreation (e.g., emotion directed toward an opposite sex partner) and thus used as evidence for design, while the identical behavior is labeled inefficient in another case (e.g., emotion directed toward a same sex partner). Efficiency in these instances is used to reject evidence rather than to reject theory. Efficiency is a property of the *metaphor*; it is not a property of nature (see, for example, Schachter, 1999, for a discussion of the inefficiency of memory). There is no reason to require an adaptation to be "efficient." Williams (1966) and Bowlby (1969/1982) may consider it a "mistake" for a mother to nurture an adoptee or a spouse because they do not share an "efficient" number of genes, but it is not clear whose "mistake" it is. It is not clear whether Williams, Bowlby, and others are claiming that Nature made the "mistake" when it did not "select" a mechanism that made decisions based on comparison of genetic similarity or that adoptive parents and spouses are making a "mistake" if they ignore genes when they love.

Evolutionary scientists have made it clear that mechanisms do not evolve full blown. They emerge in a long series of very small steps, each of which is built not only on top of but also mingled in with all the other currently existing mechanisms (Dawkins, 1987). Each change occurs within a network of preexisting structures, so that a change may affect and be affected by a plethora of other structures and their interrelations.

> Few if any brain structures initially evolved their present form precisely for the purposes they now serve. . . . Because the brain was not predesigned for its current adaptations the strategies employed in its operation will not likely yield to a purely functional physiological analysis (Deacon, 1990, p. 698).

Some authors who have no patience with a divine interpretation of evolution still use the design metaphor. If there is an appropriate metaphor for natural selection, it is not the metaphor of the engineer or the designer. Nor, I think, is it the metaphor of the "tinkerer" or "handyman," who tinkers with existing mechanisms to make them work a little better (Damasio, 1994; Dawkins, 1987; Jacob, 1977). Neither metaphor is appropriate because each postulates some kind of intention prior to evolutionary change.

Using the design metaphor, one can talk about natural selection as "ultimate causation" (Daly & Wilson, 1983). However, any claim that "behavior X" *is caused* by natural selection is logically incorrect, because the selection of a behavior (or the gene that produces it) can only occur after the behavior (and gene) comes to exist. Once a gene has caused the behavior, the processes of differential survival (natural selection) can occur so that we may say that natural selection caused the behavior to persist (but not to occur in the first place). The causal focus needs to be on the biopsychosocial mechanism by which the behavior is produced.

Natural selection means that every ancestor of mine, back to whenever we want to start counting, did not die until they had passed on some of their genes to my next ancestor in line. That is, the bundle of characteristics of each of my ancestors was appropriate enough for each of the environments in which they lived that they *did not die* until they had passed on that bundle of characteristics (plus a mutated gene or two). The bundle of characteristics that have been passed on down for me are my natural selection heritage. They are what makes me (and my genes) successful in our current ecological niche in the current environment. We usually think of natural selection in terms of hundreds and thousands of generations of not dying.

In addition to avoiding the metaphor of design, I am also going to avoid the metaphor of strategy. It is often said, for example, that human males use a "strategy" of maximizing female sex partners because such a "strategy" maximizes their chances of having their genes passed on (Daly & Wilson, 1983; Williams, 1966; Wright, 1994). Human females, on the other hand, are said to follow a "strategy" of quality over quantity because of their greater investment of body energy and time, so they want a mate who can provide for them and the child and thus maximize the survival of their genes in their child (Clutton-Brock, 1991). "Parental love itself is actually but an evolutionary strategy whereby genes replicate themselves" (Barash, 1979, p. 25). The problem with the strategy metaphor is that it is factually wrong. Strategies (like a military strategy, or a candidate's political strategy, or a game player's strategy, or a marketer's strategy) are goal-directed outcomes of conscious thought. None of the authors above claims that males and females consciously plan to maximize the survival of their genes.

Another problem with the strategy metaphor is that it leads to the use of moral language. Authors who write about strategies find themselves using the language of "should" and "must" (Clutton-Brock, 1991; Daly & Wilson, 1983; Williams, 1966). If the organism has a functional goal of inclusive fitness, then the organism "should" perform action X to achieve the goal. An organism whose genes are to be transmitted "must" perform action Y. Moral statements are not the intent for these authors. "Evolutionary psychology is a science that describes and explains: it does not prescribe" (Buss & Wakefield, 1999, p. 444). I am convinced that the authors who use "must" and "should" statements intend to be descriptive and not prescriptive. One may say, quite disingenuously, with Wright (1994, pp. 26n, 31) that "natural selection's 'values'" are "just metaphors," but readers have to process the author's metaphor through language apparatus that takes "value" to mean "good." It is better to avoid such metaphorical language entirely. The real issue is how men come to act in ways that often achieve quantity consequences, how women come to act in ways that often achieve quality consequences, and how parents come to nurture their biological and adopted children and one another. Since both the design metaphor and the strategy metaphor are misleading, these metaphors must be avoided if we are to increase our understanding of the causes of such behaviors.

Another reason to avoid the activist language of design and strategy is that it assigns "choices" to genes and not to animals. As Crist points out, the language of genes and ethological behaviorism

> ends up representing animals as blind to the upshot of their behaviors, and without command over their expression. Thus animals' behaviors emerge as involuntary—not in the sense of being forcefully coerced or more subtly obliged, but rather compulsively steered by (interior-physiological and/or exterior-environmental) stimuli beyond their control and comprehension (Crist, 1999, p. 9).

It not enough to assert that it was functionally useful to mammals (or their genes) for parents to protect their offspring and then assume that the genes then "made it happen." Parents did not "have to" provide protection to young. There was no mandate to parents to change genetically. No genes started to think, "Hey, we have to start protecting the young." And yet the descendents of those parents who did somehow develop mechanisms for providing protection to young would have slowly displaced the descendents of nonprotecting parents as the unprotected young were disproportionately harvested by predators and accidents. It is necessary to try to identify the mechanisms through which such protection was motivated.

The issue addressed in this chapter, then, is how mechanisms like attachment and caregiving came to work, not why they increased fitness. Thus, the approach used here will be the passive view of Darwin that whatever works is represented in later generations, rather than an active (or activist) view that postulates "competition" among genes (Caporael, 1997). It was not survival that created genetic changes. Instead, it was the changes in mammals and simians and humans that motivated parental nurturance through some physiological and emotional processes that led to survival-related consequences. This is in fact logically required, because the changes occurred *before* their functional consequence, so they cannot be explained by the consequence. The important issue is what biological and psychosocial processes the new genes produced and how these biological and psychosocial processes generated social actions that turned out to be useful.

Below I will propose an evolutionary model of caregiving in which the proximity, safety, and security versions of caregiving will be explained in terms of sequentially evolving neural structures. The evolutionary model will illuminate the emotional bases of parenting. The model will show how an unconscious emotional preference associated with sex in lizards was modified first into a limited mother-child bond and then became generalized into a caregiving bond as identified by attachment researchers. I will suggest that a dyadic bonding system (similar to the proximity caregiving system) evolved before the appearance of the first mammals as much as 240 million years ago and that something like the security caregiving system did not emerge until considerably later.

EVOLUTION OF THE BRAIN

New motivation systems are differentiated out of old systems. The old systems still exist, even though the new systems may have new and greater capabilities. It may take a human with a disproportionately large cortex in the animal kingdom to feel the full feelings of attachment and caregiving, but rats and rabbits, while having less ability to experience the underlying emotions as conscious feelings, have approximately the same brain structures for motivation systems in the areas under the neocortex. As will be discussed in detail in the next chapter, I make the distinction between an emotion (an unconscious motivation) and a feeling (the conscious awareness of an emotion) (Damasio, 1994; LeDoux, 1996). Feelings and emotions, while usually connected, are independent events. Emotions can occur without feelings (without conscious awareness), as seen in some advertising where a consumer is moved to prefer a product (e.g., deodorant, a candidate for office) without being aware of the emotions that have been activated. Feelings can also occur without emotions, as when a person feels aroused and constructs a fictitious emotional explanation for the arousal (Schachter, 1999; Schachter & Singer, 1962).

Blumberg and Wasserman (1995) point out the dangers of anthropomorphism that can occur if one assigns human consciousness to nonhuman animals. On the other hand, as Crist (1999) points out, charges of anthropomorphism often involve an implicit denial of the continuity between humans and other animals. While it is important to realize that nonhuman animals do not have human consciousness, it is important also to realize that consciousness, like all other brain mechanisms, lies on a continuum from zero. While a rabbit or lizard cannot plan a board meeting, rabbits and lizards can search their environment for dangers and learn to avoid previously threatening settings. The human is probably using much the same brain mechanisms as she surveys the board meeting for social rather than (we hope) physical threats and avoids previously threatening language and settings. The human certainly has, with her large neocortex and more differentiated limbic system, greater ability to process signals, to remember previous settings, to plan strategies, and to construct explanations of behavior. Nevertheless, fundamental brain structures exist on an evolutionary continuum. The human father who feeds, bathes, changes, rocks, and holds his infant is "further along" on the same evolutionary continuum as the male rat who nuzzles his pup.

Evolution is conservative. Instead of the emergence of brand new systems, most evolutionary changes involve the differentiation of a current system to produce a new outcome (Bowlby, 1969/1982; Damasio, 1994; Dawkins, 1987; LeDoux, 1996; Plutchik, 1980). New systems develop from pre-existing structures (Gould, 1991; Lavorgna, Patthy, & Boncinelli, 2001; LeDoux, 1996). However, these new systems do not replace old systems or add distinct new systems, but develop as differentiated but overlapping systems: each new system increases the complexity of the organism (Deacon, 1990).

Let us now begin to examine to evidence on the evolutionary developments that eventually led to the caregiving system. To do this, we must go back before humans, and in fact before mammals.

At this point I will switch from the vocabulary of "behavioral control system" used by Bowlby to the vocabulary of "motivation system." In so doing, I will switch focus from where behavior is going (its set goal) to where the behavior is coming from (its motivation). The motivations I will describe are emotions, so I will often emphasize that they are emotional motivations. In the discussion of the evolution, neurobiology, and psychology of attachment and caregiving, I will use the term "system," as Bowlby does, to refer to coordinated emotions, goals, and behaviors, and I will use "circuit" to refer to the biological source of the system in the brain. Thus, in the terminology that I will use, the "attachment circuit" refers to the brain's neurons that are consolidated to produce the motivation to seek security and comfort from a particular partner. I will often refer to the number or density of neurons that constitute a given motivation system. I use this terminology to give a conceptual metric to the "strength" of a motivation system. I do not propose that counting neurons is a good, or even possible, way to measure strength of a motivation system.

Motivation Systems in Reptiles

To look at the premammalian origins of parental caregiving, we need to look at the reptiles from which mammals evolved. We cannot of course observe the parental behavior of those reptiles because they have been dead for a few hundred million years. From the original "stem reptiles" (cotylosaurs), the mammal-like reptiles (therapsids) evolved around 240 million years ago. This was back on the supercontinent of Pangaea (Fortey, 1997). From therapsids, the precursors to the mammals (pantotheres) emerged (MacLean, 1990). To get insight into the stem reptiles and mammal-like reptiles, contemporary students of evolution occasionally have turned to lizards. Contemporary lizards have of course evolved over the intervening years (the same intervening years during which mammals and humans evolved). Yet they are probably the closest contemporary models to those early reptiles (MacLean, 1990).

Lizards are born knowing how to do just about all they will need to do (MacLean, 1990). A lizard's day is organized into relatively unvarying routines. Lizards emerge in the morning from their shelter to follow a master daily routine described by several motivation systems. Some lizard behavior can be described, for example, by a temperature regulation system. Being exothermic (cold blooded), lizard activity is dependent on the temperature of their surroundings. The temperature regulation system is one of the first systems operationally activated by the lizard's master routine. First thing in the morning, the regulator detects a heat deficit and (level three motivational activation)[1] executes behaviors to move the lizard to bask in a spot in the sunlight. Memories of good basking spots are retrieved from the internal working model, or map of the environment. As the day heats up and the lizard's internal temperature begins to move beyond the set goal, the lizard moves to a cooler location. Lizards drink and feed during the day using other motivation systems. In reptiles, the link between an urge and an action is relatively direct, often "hardwired" in the contemporary computer metaphor. A thirsty reptile (with an "urge" to drink) goes directly to drink. For drinking, the lizard has an internal working model that has recorded where water is likely to be available. Moving to that location when thirst signals (when there is a large discrepancy from the set goal of enough water), the lizard continues to drink until the set goal is achieved.[2]

Lizard behavior is sometimes described in terms of daily routines composed of relatively unvarying subroutines and motivation systems. These routines and subroutines are described as "relatively unvarying" because they show a great deal of continuity. However, lizards do learn. They learn where food is available and change routines when food availability changes; they learn about one another and their relationships, both hierarchical and sexual, and change routines as relationships change. Lizard learning is both individual, as in learning where food or water can be found, and social, as when one lizard finds a new pathway to food and the other lizards begin to follow that new path (MacLean, 1990).

In addition to strictly physiological systems like temperature and water regulation systems, there are a number of what may be thought of as "psychological" motivation systems that have been identified. Neural circuits of four of these "psychological" motivation systems have been identified in the brains of reptiles (they have all been identified in the brains of mammals as well). These are the seeking, fear, anger, and lust motivation systems.

The Seeking Motivation system. It is speculative but probable that the motivation circuit that evolved first was what has been called the "seeking" motivation system (Heckhausen, 2000). Centered in the lateral hypothalamic corridor, running from the ventral tegmental area to the nucleus accumbens, the seeking system at first controlled the search of the environment to find food (Panksepp, 1998). As the neural circuits of the seeking system differentiated over evolutionary time, a generalized exploratory component was added to seeking processes. Thus, as new species evolved, they began to explore their environments during times when they were not seeking food, storing information for later use. Here we see an example of how an expansion of the motivation circuit occurred along with an expansion in cognitive resources, in this case memory. Later differentiations of the seeking system created more complex appetites (Panksepp, 1998).

What appears to have made the seeking system particularly efficient as a motivation system was the eventual accretion onto the basic system of an incentive system based on dopamine. When the seeking system succeeded in achieving an appetitive goal, dopamine came to be released, producing feelings we now call "happiness" in humans. At the same time and even more important, the dopamine system induced a reorganization of seeking system neurons. In the simpler animals this process meant that when an organism performed an action in a certain situation that produced a dopamine reward, the seeking neural circuits associating that action with that situation became better organized. In later occasions in the same situation, the seeking system became more quickly aroused than before, and was more likely to perform the same action again. This system did not require a great deal of cognitive processing ability. Similar situations would present similar perceptual patterns and the neural association would likely produce the same action that was reinforced before. This incentive system enabled the seeking system to learn about the environment through reinforcement (Panksepp, 1998; Pavlov, 1960). With the operation of the incentive system, the efficiency of the seeking system of a given organism was able to increase over the lifetime of that organism through reinforcement and learning.

The Fear Motivation system. Next to evolve after the seeking system was probably the fear system (Damasio, 1994). Whereas the seeking system was centered in the hypothalamus, the fear system was centered in a new organ, the amygdala. Fear was an emotional motivation that energized the organism to protect itself from danger. The primitive fear system initially functioned as a defense mechanism against other organism's primitive seeking systems. The fear system was early on connected to the sense of smell, so it initially functioned to identify, and motivate the avoidance of, strange smells. Thus fear emerged in rudimentary form as an aversion to stimuli associated in the environment with danger. As the fear system differentiated, it became associated with a developing memory system in the amygdala (LeDoux, 1996), so that the organism could remember when the fear system had previously been activated. An organism that remembered to avoid places where predators lurked had a survival advantage.

Whereas the seeking system, as it evolved and differentiated, became organized in a manner that provided for efficiency and conservation of energy, the fear system became organized differently. The fear system did not need to be efficient. It needed to be fast and decisive. The fear system, like the seeking system, was a motivation system in which future actions were modified by current experiences. The fear system did not use the dopamine happiness circuits as a basis for changing probabilities of action, but instead had its own internal memory system, not as detailed as in cognitive memory but faster to respond (LeDoux, 1996). In fact, the fear system's memory system may predate the more complex memory systems in the hippocampus and the neocortex. In addition, the fear system, biologically centered in the lateral and central amygdala, connects to most major body systems. When fear is activated, the endocrine system produces adrenaline, which increases alertness and energy. Muscles tense, which protects against attack. At low levels of arousal, the fear circuit leads to freezing and immobilization behaviors; at higher levels of arousal, it leads to flight responses (Panksepp, 1998; Porges, 1999). The fear system, because it is organized around situations of immediate survival, is much more energy intensive, with much longer arousal than the seeking system. If an organism forgets where a meal can be found, it might take longer to feed, but the organism is still likely to survive. But if the organism forgets the location of a predator, the negative consequences could be permanent.

The Anger Motivation system. Next to evolve was the anger system. The anger system appears to have evolved initially in the form of a reaction to being physically restricted, for example, as an animal is seized by a predator. When an organism is captured by the jaws or paws of a predator, the anger circuit in the brain instigates a violent attempt to escape from being restricted, a behavior with obvious survival value (Panksepp, 1998). Initially, the anger motivation system was probably a simple differentiation of the fear system. The anger system further differentiated in subsequent species, developed its own complications, and eventually became separate from (although still highly interconnected to) the fear system. Initially evolving as a protection against physical restraint, it eventually evolved into a reaction against social restraints and then eventually among "higher" vertebrates into a more general circuit "to motivate individuals to compete effectively for environmental resources" (Panksepp, 1998, p. 197). Thus, dominance displays are produced by the anger motivation system.

The Lust Motivation system. Lust evolved as a motivation aroused by "copulative opportunities." That is, a male confronted by an available female was motivated to achieve copulation. The earliest lust motivation system was presumably relatively indiscriminate, but eventually the lust system began to recognize the lust motivation in other animals of the same species so that two or more animals might compete for a copulation opportunity, establishing hierarchy, or make choices among competing partners.

The four motivation systems just examined are not socially proactive motivation systems. In general, lizards live alone. Lizards establish a home site, a shelter where the lizard rests and sleeps. Individual lizards have territories, which they defend against other lizards. Sometimes a male-female pair will jointly occupy a territory. When food is plentiful in an area, lizards and other reptiles may live together in "colonies," but their actions remain essentially solitary. Lizards never help one another (Eibl-Eibesfeldt, 1996).

The reptiles that were precursors to mammals were oviparous; that is, they laid eggs (Clutton-Brock, 1991). In general, reptile mothers laid their eggs in out-of-the-way places, usually burying them, and then went away. Once the eggs hatched, reptile offspring fended for themselves; they did not call to their parents for help. In fact, an infant reptile who hatched from an egg had to crawl into the underbrush to avoid being killed by adults, including its own parents (MacLean, 1990). Reptiles found the smell of their offspring to be "strange," and they tended to react aggressively, often killing the young if they wandered too close to an adult (Panksepp, 1998).

EVOLUTION OF PARENTAL CAREGIVING

Primitive or elaborate forms of caregiving and attachment are characteristic of all mammals. To find the evolutionary origins of caregiving and attachment, we must go back at least 180 million years to the emergence of mammals and before that to the emergence of the mammal-like reptiles about 240 million years ago during the Triassic period before the supercontinent of Pangaea began to break up (MacLean, 1990). The earliest mammals were small, hairy, and warm-blooded. They had motivation systems that operated much like the motivation systems that operated in reptiles. For example, the fear reaction in mammals is quite like that of reptiles. Adrenaline is pumped, the heart beats faster, blood pressure increases, muscles tense in a "freeze" response, and attention is sharpened. However, one thing mammals do that is not done by reptiles is to nurture their young.

The tendency of mammals to give attention and nurturance to their young for some time after birth turned out to have a tremendous impact on evolutionary development. Following the die off of the dinosaurs about sixty-five million years ago, it was the mammals and birds (both warm-blooded and insulated by fur or feather) who emerged to fill the ecological vacuum left by the disappearance of the dinosaurs. I will have little to say about the evolution of birds, because their ability to fly and lay eggs in inaccessible locations freed them from some evolutionary "pressure" to provide direct protection to their young (besides, it didn't lead to humans). The evolution of mammals, however, tells a fascinating tale. This tale involves the development of caregiving by parents directed toward offspring.

As a preliminary account of the evolution of mammalian caregiving, I propose a model that traces the evolution of mammalian caregiving from the infant-rejecting systems of reptiles by means of four relatively discrete sets of genetic changes. The changes were (1) the partial inhibition of the mechanism for rejecting strangers; (2) the development of emotional bonding (corresponding approximately to the affectional bond identified by Bowlby); (3) the development of mammary glands and vivaparity (live births); and (4) the development of a nurturant caregiving system directed toward the needs of the infant (involving first what may have been a "passive protection" caregiving system involving warning of danger, then a proximity caregiving system aimed at retrieving the young, even later a security caregiving system that added active protection and encouragement of the young, and finally a more general caregiving system aimed at meeting multiple needs of the young).

Inhibition of stranger rejection

Reptile adults will reject and kill their young. Many mammals will also attack and kill young of the same species under certain conditions. It is usually unrelated young who are at risk (Clutton-Brock, 1991). Male lions who displace the previous leaders of a pride will kill the cubs of the displaced males (Daly & Wilson, 1983). Captive gorilla and chimpanzee mothers will frequently kill or avoid their firstborn (Keverne, Nevison, & Martel, 1999). Daly & Wilson (1999) describe the related problem of the abuse of human children by unrelated adults.

This rejection of the young can be seen as a continuation of the reptile stranger rejection system. As long as this stranger rejection system continued to dominate, mammalian parental caregiving was impossible. The proposed caregiving evolutionary model suggests that two changes occurred that enabled the emergence of mammals from the reptilian precursors. The first change was the emergence of a system to inhibit the rejection of offspring; the second change was the emergence of a system to keep them near. We do not as yet know for sure how the first change was effected.

Mammals, like reptiles, have a smell-based system to detect strangers. It exists in the lowest, most primitive parts of the brain. Although the system is primitive, it is not simple: by the time of the reptiles, there were two separate smell systems, a main olfactory system for detecting "light" smells such as given off by food, and an auxiliary system for detecting "heavy" smells, like pheromones. These systems became highly developed, and they allowed an animal to locate food and water and to detect strange animals who might be predators. For animals who were predators, this system also supported the seeking system. These were unconscious systems located in the "emotional" part of the brain, achieving quick decisions whose consequences were often survival. While it was beneficial to reptiles to detect and avoid strange animals who might be predators, the smell-based emotional systems did not distinguish between a strange smelling animal who might be a predator and a strange-smelling animal who was an offspring.

A mechanism emerged in some reptiles to modify (and partially turn off) the stranger rejection system. The neurochemistry and brain structure of the inhibiting system will be described in the next chapter, but for now, it is enough to recognize that this evolutionary change appears to have occurred in reptiles who were ancestors to both birds and mammals. Once an allele (a particular form of a gene: e.g., one allele of the gene for eye color produces brown eyes; another allele gives blue eyes) to inhibit rejection of a similarly smelling animal came into being, mothers with the allele were not inclined to attack and destroy their own offspring at the time of birth (Maestripieri, 1999). Originally this inhibiting system was activated by hormones produced in reptile mothers during the egg-laying process. The result was that when the eggs hatched, the mothers did not reject their offspring and did not kill them.

The evolution of a dyadic preference

However, not killing one's children is not the same thing as caregiving. The caregiving evolutionary model presented here proposes that the second evolutionary change that predated the emergence of mammals from reptile precursors was the creation of an emotional dyadic preference in the parent toward the child. This unconscious preference is relatively automatic in its operation. As Shaver and Hazan have it, "it just happens" (1988). This affectional dyadic preference is the precursor to the caregiving bond described in attachment theory.

In evolutionary terms, the dyadic preference almost certainly developed initially in mothers, produced by neurochemicals associated with pregnancy and egglaying. Thus, as I will discuss in detail in the next chapter, the dyadic preference can be seen to be embodied in brain neurons. The preference appears to be induced by the same or related neurochemicals involved in inhibiting stranger rejection, but acting in different parts of the brain. While inhibiting stranger rejection meant that mothers did not kill their infants, the emotional preference meant that mothers actively tolerated and preferred their infants. The neurotransmitter most implicated in the dyadic preference toward the child, oxytocin, is the same neurotransmitter released during mating (Panksepp, 1998) and thus related to both the pair bond and the parent-child bond. At first, the new weak olfactory-based system probably meant that the mother was more "comfortable" with her own eggs and then with her own children (they smelled "right").

Not being afraid of infants, not committing aggression against infants, and tolerating their presence were certainly the first steps toward caregiving. They were small steps, and steps likely to have maximum survival advantages only in relatively solitary reptile or transitional species, as the mother's tolerance of her offspring was unlikely to improve the offspring's inclusive fitness if the mother was surrounded by other adults with no such tolerance. The dyadic preference came to prove evolutionarily successful as preferred offspring were more likely to survive. Over generations, the preference became stronger and came to be activated by physical contact and interaction. Since physical contact and interaction—unlike pregnancy and egglaying—were not sex-linked phenomena, mammalian males as well as females came to exhibit dyadic preference.

The emotional process of dyadic preference as modeled here corresponds in many ways to the process that Bowlby described as the affectional bond. Dyadic preference leads to proximity as the simplest behavioral expression of preference. The earliest forms of this dyadic preference did not involve the feelings that Bowlby described for later forms of an affectional bond in humans. It is reasonably certain that premammalian reptile mothers did not experience discernible grief at the loss of a child, for example. Even in some primates, a dyadic preference appears to be established in which anxiety and grief do not follow on separation from the infant (Mason & Mendoza, 1998). Nevertheless, this early primitive dyadic preference bond was enough to allow the emergence of the first mammals.

The emergence of mammals

In the evolutionary model proposed here, a primitive emotional preference probably evolved in the mammal-like reptiles, the therapsids, or in the direct precursors to the mammals, the pantotheres. This preference had to have evolved before the lactation that defines mammals, because lactation could not have plausibly evolved as long as mothers were still rejecting and killing their offspring. But once mothers stopped killing their offspring, and in fact began to prefer being in their presence, the opportunity presented itself for the hypothesized third set of genetic changes leading to the evolution of mammals.

Vivaparity (live births) has independently evolved in a number of reptile species since the emergence of mammals, which suggests that there is some competitive advantage to live birth (Clutton-Brock, 1991). In very few oviparous reptile species is there any postlaying care of eggs: all crocodilians protect their eggs, but only about 3 percent of oviparous snakes and 1 percent of oviparous lizards do (Clutton-Brock, 1991). Protection of the nest (and thus incidentally of offspring) among oviparous species seems to be restricted to predators (crocodiles and pythons, for example), where the parents have the physical wherewithal to protect against most dangers.

Clutton-Brock (1991) notes that warm-bloodedness and lactation probably developed before vivaparity. Early mammals and pre-mammals who resulted from genetic changes that made them more endothermic (warm-blooded) could more easily hide under cover while their ectothermic relatives were harvested by predators when basking in the sun. Pre-mammalian young, hatched from eggs, who sucked the sweat from their emotionally bonded mothers would have been less exposed to predators because they needed to make fewer trips to a watering place. Random genetic mutations that produced specialized sweat glands would have further contributed to the survival of offspring (Fortey, 1997), although Tudge (2000) suggests that mammary glands may have evolved from scent glands instead. Other mutations that added nutrients to the modified sweat or scent glands (now mammary glands) would have promoted the survival of mammal young. It was only after these early mammalian or pre-mammalian mothers began feeding their egg-borne offspring that there was likely to be a survival advantage in live births. "Parental provisioning may have allowed reduction in egg size, resulting in the development of egg retention and eventually in vivaparity" (Clutton-Brock, 1991, p. 257).

The development of the mammary gland had far-reaching consequences. The first consequence was direct—offspring of a mother who preferred them and also fed them were doubly removed from predators. Being close to mother and not having to leave her to procure food or drink would have significantly increased survival chances. We do not know if the pleasure-producing dopamine system that is now associated with dyadic preference was part of the original caregiving system, although it is plausible that it was. Without dopamine, the parent or other caregiver might tolerate the infant and "let" the infant be near. With dopamine, the parent would actively enjoy the infant and would have an incentive to be close to the infant.

The second consequence of the mammary gland was more indirect than the first. The infant's touch of the breast caused the secretion of the neurotransmitter hormone oxytocin, which in turn caused the breast to release milk. This was the same neurotransmitter involved in the sexual pair bond and dyadic preference. Thus nursing the infant led to a deepening dyadic preference in the mother. Furthermore, the oxytocin was secreted into the milk, which facilitated the formation of a dyadic preference in the infant toward the mother. Over time, the oxytocin releasing mechanism in the breast became generalized and associated with all of the skin. Unlike the release of oxytocin at birth and at the breast, the generalized skin release mechanism was not restricted to females. This touching-induced oxytocin release became associated with the skin of male and female both. We do not know how soon this skin-touch mechanism developed, but it appears to exist in a variety of mammals: aside from primates, it has been found in sheep and rodents (Carter, 1998a; Insel, Young, & Wang, 1999; Keverne, et al., 1999; Maestripieri, 1999; Nelson & Panksepp, 1998; Panksepp, 1998; Young & Wang, 2004).

The development of the skin-touch mechanism for activating dyadic preference meant that all members of a species, male and female, could form dyadic preferences. There were still inequalities in the underlying neurological structures in males and females, but in mammals the differences became quantitative rather than qualitative. Males were on average slower to form dyadic preferences, but they could and did form them.

The Evolution of the Caregiving Motivation System

The survival advantages of mechanisms for tolerating infants, forming an emotional preference, and feeding the infant directly supported the success of mammals. They provide the primitive foundation for what we think of in humans as caregiving behaviors. However, there is nothing in this early system that would lead to such advanced behaviors as the *defense* of an offspring against a predator, or the purposive teaching of offspring. Nor for that matter is there anything in the early systems that would have led the mother to consistently *retrieve* her young if they wandered off. However, according to the evolutionary model proposed here, eventually a fourth set of genetic changes occurred and a caregiving motivation system emerged from dyadic preference. Neurobiological evidence discussed in the next chapter will show that the caregiving motivation system, while clearly related to dyadic preference, became at least partially differentiated from it.

An emotional motivation system developed around the dyadic preference. When we examine the dyadic preference within the caregiving motivation system, we see that the preference becomes the "engine" that energizes the motivation system. To capture this change in perspective, I now change from the passive vocabulary of preference to the active vocabulary of emotion.

Going forward, I will refer to the dyadic preference as the emotion of caring. The emotion of caring is the motivation that drives the caregiving motivation system. When it first evolved, it was a very simple system, but after a hundred million years or so, it began to show characteristics associated with the feelings of affection that we recognize in humans. The caregiving motivation system and its emotion of caring were initially laid down in some of the oldest parts of the brain. Being in the oldest parts of the brain, however, did not mean that this motivation system would have to remain "primitive" or "simple," because almost immediately (in evolutionary time) this part of the brain began to differentiate and reorganize.

Initially, of course, in the first mammals, the caregiving motivation system and the caring emotion bore no resemblance to their appearance today in humans. The caring emotion (dyadic preference) was presumably very weak. It is unlikely that proximity per se was a set goal of the early caring emotion. Instead the original caring emotion was more likely a relatively diffuse preference, one of whose unintended consequences was proximity. Nevertheless, eventually changes occurred in the caring emotion as the underlying brain structures differentiated and reorganized. Over generations, random genetic changes that led to sharper forms of the caring emotion would have led to greater survival of children.

Looking backwards up the line of evolutionary descent from the first mammals, one of the obvious changes has been the increasing complexity of the brain. This increase in complexity occurs throughout the brain, including an increasing size of the neocortex where memories are stored, perceptions are analyzed, and plans are formulated (LeDoux, 1996; MacLean, 1990). Reptiles have very little neocortex, while rabbits, rats, cats, and humans have progressively larger neocortical areas. This implies that the caregiving internal working model, which is primarily a neocortical function, is increasingly elaborated in mammals and humans. Attempts to explain parental caregiving by Bowlby and other attachment researchers have primarily focused on the neocortex and a caregiving internal working model that develops out of childhood experiences and memories (e.g., Bell & Richard, 2000a; Berman & Sperling, 1994). However, parental caregiving is something that happens in mice and rabbits with a small neocortex as well as in humans with a very large neocortex. Rabbits with a minimal cortex feed their offspring and huddle with them, but will not retrieve them when they wander from the burrow (MacLean, 1990). In the rat, caregiving probably does not include the protection of offspring from danger other than retrieving them to the nest, although I am unaware of attempts to measure protection from predators. In the cat, the caregiving system includes protection of offspring from danger and adds some teaching of the skills of the hunt. In humans, caregiving adds a host of other behaviors, from teaching a wide variety of skills to maintaining the emotional security of the partner. And somewhere along the evolutionary line, as consciousness developed, we begin to see feeling, the conscious awareness of emotions. Feelings first appeared in rudimentary forms (perhaps like the joy, loneliness and grief perceived in dogs and primates) and eventually reached an elaborated human version.

The neocortex is not the only part of the brain that has increased in complexity. Increasing differentiation has also occurred in the limbic areas of the brain associated with emotions (Altman & Bayer, 1997; Berscheid, 1999; Deacon, 1990). For example, the human cerebellum contains about fourteen times as many folds as the rat cerebellum, each fold suggested to be a distinct structural and functional entity (Altman & Bayer, 1997). It is clear that one of the consequences of the differentiation of the emotional parts of the brain among mammals has been an increasing complexity in the goals of the dyadic caregiving motivation that grew out of dyadic preference. The origin of caregiving lies in the older limbic (or medial) cortex, where the hypothalamus and amygdala are located, where emotions (but not feelings) operate. This invites the fascinating speculation that there was some development in the limbic cortex of mammals that enabled and induced them to begin providing caregiving to their offspring. We do not know much about this newly evolved emotion of caring that underlies mammalian caregiving. It is not on the lists that most emotion researchers have developed.[3]

The evolution of the caring emotion from dyadic preference can be seen in the gradual enlargement of the scope of caregiving behaviors among mammals. When discussing the levels of development of the caregiving system, I am not claiming that humans are "more evolved" than, say, rabbits. In arranging mammals in terms of development of the caregiving system, then, I am pointing out what appear to be different levels of development rather than different amounts of evolution (all contemporary mammals have experienced exactly the same amounts of evolution and exactly the same amounts—in number of years—of natural selection). One could even argue that rabbits have experienced *more* evolution than humans because their generations are shorter. Nevertheless, it is reasonable to say that caregiving is less *developed* in rabbits. Rabbits have less differentiated brains with less neocortex than most other mammals.

Minimal caregiving motivation system. Rabbits, with about the smallest neocortex and about the least differentiated limbic cortex and hypothalamus among studied mammals, have a very limited caregiving system (and thus are hypothesized to have a caring emotion that is hardly distinguishable from the passive dyadic preference). Rabbits form dyadic preferences toward offspring and toward other adults, but these preferences are weaker than preferences for location. Males and females bond and stay together for long periods of time. Lockley (1965) describes how one male rival displaced the dominant "king" male and moved into the desirable "king's" warren with the "queens." The deposed dominant male then moved into the rival's former warren with the rival's former mate. Each of the females chose to remain in their accustomed place, including the rival's former mate, who lived alone for some time until the former "king" moved into the warren.

A minimal caring emotion leads to minimal caregiving behaviors in rabbits. Rabbits feed their offspring and huddle with them, but will not retrieve them when they wander from the burrow (MacLean, 1990; Ross, Sawin, Zarrow, & Denenberg, 1963). Although rabbits do not retrieve their kittens, they do perform a generalized kind of protection. When one rabbit perceives danger, she will let out a cry of warning (a cry that probably rarely puts her at much risk, as healthy adult rabbits, with sharp teeth and strong hind legs, are a match for most predators of the size of birds or cats). She is more likely to emit the warning when she is near her kittens, or adults from the same burrow, than when she is near other rabbits (Lockley, 1965). Lockley reports that a nursing mother rabbit will drive away large cats from her young (presumably when she could have avoided any personal risk by running away). These observations raise the question of whether a caregiving set goal of protection may have evolved before the proximity caregiving set goal. In the lack of direct evidence, I am inclined to offer a tentative speculation that protection without retrieval may have evolved separately in rabbits. This appears to have been a very narrow protection goal, restricted to immediate warning of a predator, but including neither teaching about such dangers ahead of time nor direct action against a threat.

Proximity caregiving motivation system. In rats and squirrels, with a somewhat larger neocortex and somewhat more differentiated limbic system than rabbits, caregiving behaviors include retrieval and licking. Breastfeeding is of course done by female rats, but other female and male rats form dyadic bonds with pups and nuzzle them and retrieve them (Panksepp, 1998; Rosenblatt, 1990). When rat pups wander from the nest, rat mothers respond to ultrasound squeaks from pups (produced when they are cold) by retrieving them to the nest. In rats, caregiving also includes protection of the nest. It is not clear whether protection of the nest is in fact caregiving for the pup or whether it is instead a geographical response (Vom Saal & Parmigiani, 1995). Retrieval behaviors also occur among squirrels (Gurnell, 1987). Adult squirrels make warning sounds at the sign of danger. It is not clear whether adult squirrels will retrieve baby squirrels under these conditions (probably not, since a freeze posture is a squirrel's usual response to danger and the warning will probably freeze babies as well).

Protection caregiving motivation system. Active protective caregiving behavior has been observed in the ungulates (hoofed mammals), from deer and elk to giraffes (Altmann, 1963; Masson & McCarthy, 1995). Protective caregiving behavior directed toward young is not only performed by mothers in these species but also by other adult herd members. An adult moose, for example, will attack and chase an intruder who approaches a moose calf. Such a system corresponds to the safety caregiving system proposed by Solomon and George (George & Solomon, 1999; 1996) and by Cassidy (1999) with a caregiving set goal of maintaining the safety of the partner. Ungulates also retrieve their young and keep them close.

Security caregiving motivation system. In felines and canines the caregiving system includes protection of the offspring from danger and adds some teaching of skills, such as teaching kittens and pups to find the nest and to hunt (Lopez, 1978; Schneirla, Rosenblatt, & Tobach, 1963). Teaching behaviors include play, modeling, and punishing (Rheingold, 1963). Cats do a lot of grooming (licking) of kittens (Schneirla, et al., 1963), as do dogs of puppies (Rheingold, 1963). Even after becoming mobile, kittens and puppies are in frequent interaction with their mothers using visual, auditory, and tactile contact. The goal of the dyadic caregiving motivation system in cats has expanded beyond proximity and the safety of the partner. This expansion in scope seems to correspond to the set goal of felt security in the Bowlbian caregiving system (Bartholomew, 1990; Heard & Lake, 1997; Sroufe & Fleeson, 1986; West & Sheldon-Keller, 1994).

Connection caregiving motivation system. In humans, caregiving adds a host of other behaviors to proximity, feeding, retrieval, protecting, teaching, and comforting. From teaching a wider variety of skills to meeting a wider variety of physical needs like clothing and transportation to maintaining the emotional security of the partner, the set goal of the human caregiving motivation system is to see that the needs of the partner are met (Bell & Richard, 2000a). For a caring parent, it is the full range of the child's needs that determines the parent's response (Blood, 1969; Erikson, 1963; LaRossa & LaRossa, 1981; Rapoport, et al., 1977; Ruddick, 1989). The caregiving evolutionary model proposed here shows the evolutionary continuity and development of the caring emotion.

THE CARING EMOTION

One may ask, what are the benefits of conceptualizing the caring emotion in this way, as an evolved motivation for caregiving? What can we explain using this concept of a caring emotion? The emotion of caring will be described in detail in Chapter 5. For now, I focus on two particularly important benefits of conceptualizing a dyadic caring emotion, called "dyadic" because it involves a motivation to be connected with another. First, the dyadic emotion, as it has evolved, has become increasingly responsive to social interactions. Second, over the course of its evolution, the emotion of caring has become associated with an increasingly wide attention to the other's needs.

The emergence of a caring emotion depended on the suppression of the stranger rejection system. The suppression of rejection was a completely general process, but the tolerance that emerged was a dyadic tolerance. That is, the tolerance and preference was directed toward one or more specific targets. The mammalian mother does not reject the infants who are around when her oxytocin and vasopressin levels are high. These are almost always her own offspring, but if another newborn is placed in her nest at this time, she will tolerate it as well (Panksepp, 1998). Thus the *mechanism* for the dyadic preference bond is not based on a genetic relationship with the object of the bond; however, the *consequences* of the bond will most often lead to proximity to an offspring who shares genes. From the point of view of the gene (as if genes had even metaphorical "views"), the establishment of a dyadic preference bond toward someone who is not an offspring is "misdirected, as it were by mistake" (Bowlby, 1969/1982, p. 132n; see also Clutton-Brock, 1991; Williams, 1966). Daly and Wilson (1983, p. 291) note that "the psychological mechanisms of parental love can be redirected to an unrelated child," although they are clearly uncomfortable with this conclusion. But from the point of view of the organism, such adoptions are a natural outcome of the neurophysiological process of dyadic preference formation.

The evolution of a smell-based preference had a critical effect on mammalian social organization. This smell-based preference is likely to develop in mammalian pairs who remain together for long periods and become accustomed to one another's smells (Filsinger & Fabes, 1985). Siblings, for example, are likely to develop preferences for one another over strangers. Extended family members who grow up in proximity are likely to develop preferences for one another. Mother-child pairs and extended family groups, preferring one another, are likely to develop a tendency to maintain proximity to one another. Proximity of an entire family group is likely to have positive natural selection effects. Because predators are more likely to take a solitary prey than a member of a group, the species members with a caring emotion who cluster in proximity will have an evolutionary advantage and the allele will spread as species members with a different version of the gene are disproportionately harvested by predators. Play behavior, although produced by a different motivation system from caregiving (Panksepp, 1998), is facilitated by the dyadic preference, and play may have "served originally to provide harmony in the nest, and then, later in life, affiliation among members of social groups" (MacLean, 1990, p. 397).

Caring develops over time as specific attributes of the dyadic partner become conditioned stimuli that deepen the relationship (LeDoux, 1996). The strength of the emotion generally develops with greater physical exposure. Proximity and strength of emotion are thus linked, so that a stronger caring emotion is likely to lead to more proximity and more proximity is likely to lead to a stronger directed emotion (Montagu, 1986). Second, in species with consciousness, this unconscious emotion gives rise to conscious feelings of preference toward the partner, feelings that the other's presence is pleasurable. Third, the dyadic emotion develops toward multiple partners. This multiple ability of the caring emotion is apparent in the dyadic relationships of parent to multiple offspring.

In the caregiving evolutionary model, the expansion of the caring emotion and the caregiving motivation system opened up multiple pathways for the development of a dyadic preference and caring emotion toward multiple partners. Exclusive, life-long heterosexual adult pair bonds are not common in most mammals (Carter, 1998a). However, multiple adult dyadic bonds are not unusual and are in fact pervasive among mammals. Attachment theorists, observing mother-dominated child rearing practices, have hypothesized a hierarchy of "attachment objects," with one person (usually the mother) unequivocally preferred when available (Bowlby, 1969/1982). The hierarchy metaphor has been useful when applied to attachment in children. It appears to be much less informative when applied to attachment in adults. Furthermore, the hierarchy metaphor seems even less appropriate when applied to caregiving. Most human parents appear able to experience approximately equal levels of emotional caring toward each of their children. Behavioral differences often appear because the caregiving motivation system focuses on the partner's need. Thus a younger and more dependent child will tend to be the object of parental nurturance more often than an older and more autonomous child.

If the caring emotion involved no energy expenditure, we would expect it to grow until an entire group felt maximum intensity of this dyadic emotion toward each other group member and the maximum operation of these caregiving motivation systems. However, to the extent that establishing and maintaining the caregiving system involves the expenditure of energy (such as from paying attention to, interacting with, or giving things to the partner), there will be upper limits on how far and how deeply these dyadic emotions spread (Dunbar, 1996). Thus, an organism is likely to have a small number of intensely motivated relationships reinforced by frequent contact and a larger number of relationships with moderate to low contact and moderate to low caring emotion.

Caregiving is not a sex-linked process, although some evolutionary scientists have explicitly or implicitly made this claim. "One can, in effect, treat the sexes as if they were different species" (Trivers, 1972, p. 153). A neurological structure for caring could, of course, appear on the X chromosome so that it could be genetically stronger in women. Since women have two X chromosomes and men have one, we would then have neatly solved the male-female differences that are in the back of our minds. Neurobiological evidence, however, reviewed in the next chapter, shows that male-female differences are quantitative rather than qualitative. That is, the caregiving system is initially strongest between mothers and newborns because of oxytocin secretion during birth and feeding experiences. However, although females usually have more caregiving neurons than males and these neurons are further increased by the action of gonadal hormones during childbirth, physical contact and social interactions lead to the growth of these neurons in both males and females.

As we will see in the next chapter, the density of neurons in caregiving circuits in the brain is related to gender. However, the neurobiological process by which these circuits are augmented and by which they operate appears to be pretty much the same in males as in females. The implicated subcortical brain areas where the unconscious caring emotion operates contain other emotions like fear that do not vary in a sex-linked way, and others like anger or aggression that are stronger in males. The dyadic caring emotion depends on contact as well as on gonadal hormones. Primary caregivers and children tend to develop the strongest emotional relationships because of their intimate physical contact and extensive interaction. The unconscious emotion, however, when activated, appears to operate identically in mother, father, child, and stranger, with differences in strength of emotion dependent on initial neuronal density and new neuronal growth related to amount of contact. Mothers and other female relatives tend to spend the most time with a child in contemporary cultures, so they are likely to consolidate more caregiving neurons than those who are less involved. The outcome of such a process is empirically sex-linked, but the mechanism itself is not.

Another effect of the dyadic caring emotion is what is often called "pair bonding" or monogamy. Once maternal caregiving and adult pair bonding have been established, the stage is set for biparental caregiving (Clutton-Brock, 1991). In humans, not only does the dyadic caring emotion protect children from predators, it also provides a basis for more intense parental involvement. Because human females during the period of evolutionary adaptedness probably averaged about three years between births while children required ten years or more of nurturance, the father's caring and nurturance would have had significant survival consequences (Mellen, 1981; Miller & Fishkin, 1997; Zeifman & Hazan, 1997). The development of a dyadic caring emotion, initially beneficial for its effect on survival of offspring, would probably soon have led to stronger pair bonding among parents and subsequently to more opportunities for cooperative caregiving by both parents. Neurobiological evidence suggests that an adult-adult bond is produced by the same system that produces the parent-offspring caring bond (Carter, 1998a). Furthermore, as I will describe in the next chapter, the caregiving system is, like the seeking system, associated with the dopamine happiness system, so that both oxytocin and dopamine act to solidify parent-child bonds. In some mammals, the oxytocin and dopamine systems are activated concurrently. In these species, adult pair bonding is monogamous; when the oxytocin and dopamine systems are uncoupled, monogamous pair bonding does not occur (Young & Wang, 2004).

True pair bonding, as for life, is quite rare among mammals, although somewhat more frequent among primates (Miller & Fishkin, 1997). The term "bond" itself is problematic, implying a kind of permanence and resistance against "breaking," but persistence is an assessment that can only be made in retrospect, so it is a weak criterion to use prospectively as an assessment of the strength or permanence of a bond. It is not clear what a bond is beyond a stronger than average preference. Adult dyadic caring is expected to reach a high level among consistent sexual partners as well as among those who cooperate in the nurture of children. The sexual experience, involving intense physical contact, and the feelings associated with the dyadic caring emotion, are mutually reinforcing neurochemically. It must be noted, however, that the dyadic caring emotion does not guarantee monogamy or fidelity. Group bonding has significant advantages over pair bonding from the point of view of protection from predators. Humans and prehumans, not being equipped with natural offensive weapons, rely on cooperation and coordination to effect a defense against large predators. An interaction-based emotional bond that enables group bonding leads to both monogamous pair bonding and to its threats. When the emotional gratifications of a caring bond deepen over time, monogamy can be sustained. However, because some of the direct gratifications of behaviors associated with the bond can decline with repetition, and because social organization brings members into contact with other potential partners, the way is opened for competing emotional bonds to develop.[4] The generality of the caring emotion can also be seen in inclination of humans to care for non-human animals (Archer, 1997).

Expanded domains

As the dyadic caring emotion evolved into more elaborate forms, its effects expanded beyond proximity and clustering. The increasing significance of the caring emotion was revealed when a predator stalked a peripheral member of the group cluster. The stalked member, say a youngster, may have raised a paw or hoof or hand or weapon in defense, but the rational predator, having targeted a member who was weak, would often have been successful. However, if another member of the group (a parent or other adult) had the allele for a stronger caring emotion, they would likely have been in proximity to the youngster, and the emotion may have led them to raise a paw or hoof or hand or weapon in support. The predator, now faced by *two* defenders, may have gone elsewhere for an easier meal. There is no reason to assume a strong or pronounced result the first time the stronger emotion appeared (Dawkins, 1987), and there may be many predators against whom a parent or other group member would not have overcome their own fear to help. But a slight statistical advantage in favor of the youngster and the rest of the group with the caring-motivated member could have been enough to give the group a slight competitive advantage over other groups.

One of the evolutionary changes that occurred subsequent to vivaparity was the growth of the neocortex in mammals. Warm-bloodedness probably was a beneficial co-occurrence along with vivaparity in order to supply the greater energy required in the new brain areas. Growth of the neocortex among successive species of mammals allowed for greater efficiency of the internal working model in memory and greater discrimination in the sensory cortex. The penalty for this improvement, however, was that the neocortex did not come with genetically predefined associations: the new cortex required learning. The neocortex was a place for new information: it was not filled up initially with good ideas for survival. The results of learning, recorded in the new neocortical areas, provided a greater capability and flexibility than instinct, but it took offspring longer to learn to use the new ability. Offspring who had to learn survival skills were more vulnerable than offspring who already knew survival skills. However, they could learn new survival skills in a lifetime rather than waiting for new instincts to evolve in evolutionary time. Parents did not "have to" provide protection and training to these vulnerable young. There was no mandate to parents to change genetically. And yet those parents who developed a mechanism for providing protection and training to their young would have slowly displaced the nonprotecting and nontraining parents as the unprotected and untrained young were disproportionately harvested by predators and accidents.

With the growth of the neocortex, parents were able to perceive a wider variety of needs in their offspring. In its evolution, the sensitivity of the caring emotion expanded from immediate needs of the child to longer term needs. Parents who were able to perceive that the child would eventually need certain knowledge and skills would have been motivated to provide appropriate training. Each expansion in parents' awareness of the child's needs, and action to meet these needs, would have provided an evolutionary advantage. In humans, parents became not just caretakers of the body but also teachers of the mind.

Caregiving in social context

Although we keep talking about genes, we need to keep in mind that nothing is "just" genes. As mammals evolved from the earliest forms about the size of a tree shrew to later mammalian forms, the brain increased in size along with the body. These size increases led to increases in capacity and also to changes in brain structure (Deacon, 1990). Brain structure within the developing fetus and infant changed as the brain grew and as external events activated different structures (Deacon, 1990). Thus the potential for caregiving and attachment structures were laid down in the fetal brain as the enlarging prefrontal cortex led to internal competition for neural connections. Then the infant's and child's experiences of caregiving led to the development of associational patterns that realized this potential (while another child who experienced little or no caregiving may have failed to form the associations necessary for later caregiving and attachment). Almost every egg and sperm has the genetic potential for caregiving and for attachment. Almost every properly nourished fetus will develop the physiological potential for attachment and caregiving. And almost every child who receives attentive and responsive caregiving will consolidate the appropriate neuronal structures for attachment and caregiving (Maestripieri, 1999).

Plotkin (1997) uses the metaphor of nested Russian dolls to describe these levels of evolutionary effect. This metaphor suggests a way to look at the conditions under which the caregiving motivation system is produced. The caregiving structure will emerge at full strength:

- If the genes first exist in the organism (true of all non-mutated humans).
- If the prenatal environment is congenial (an adequate nutritional and hormonal environment), so that genes are "turned on" at the appropriate time and underlying brain structures are laid down. If bad nutrition or excessive stress occurs during gestation because of poverty, drug use or other social factors, neurons in the caregiving and other systems may not be laid down in the developing brain (LeDoux, 1996; Panksepp, 1998).
- If appropriate social or other environmental stimulation occurs that leads the brain structures to consolidate and develop. Motivation circuits are highly plastic (Davidson, 1992). Their density and extent depend on appropriate social or other environmental stimulation that lead the brain structures to consolidate and develop. Physical contact contributes to the proliferation of caregiving neurons (Panksepp, 1998), which is why infants deprived of holding

often have trouble forming relationships (Hrdy, 1999; Montagu, 1986). For dogs (Scott, 1963) and monkeys (Mason & Sponholz, 1963), early social isolation leaves the animals unable to trust and form normal social relationships.

- If the child does not suffer the death or other disappearance of a parent (physical loss) or does not experience nonresponsive or rejecting parents (psychological loss). In the case of loss of an only caregiver, the caregiving circuit that was beginning to form with the parent may atrophy and be unavailable to later adult or parenthood relationships (Bowlby, 1980).

Once all biological prerequisites are in place, responsive caregiving will be expressed:

- If in parenthood an emotional caring bond develops between the parent and child. The child may be "unlovable" to a parent, say seriously deformed or otherwise nonresponsive (Egeland & Farber, 1984; Kagan, 1977). For example, parents of infants born blind often have difficulty forming a bond because the infants do not respond conventionally (they don't look in the parents' eyes). However, when these parents are trained to interpret hand movements as responsive, they are better able to care (Fraiberg, 1974; Stern, 1985).
- If cultural factors support caregiving. Culture may either enhance or inhibit motivation systems. In a culture where infants sleep in the same bed with a parent, parental nurturance can be delivered immediately before the infant becomes highly aroused (Doi, 1986; Montagu, 1986; Thevenin, 1987). On the other hand, where infants are routinely placed in separate rooms from parents for sleeping, the infant's attachment system may be regularly stressed as the infant experiences parental absence.
- If parental resources are available. Even if the caregiving neural system is fully formed and fully active, a parent's formal and informal educational background may make them unaware of appropriate or effective strategies to meet the child's needs, or the parent's economic or general social situation may make appropriate resources unavailable (Vaughn, Egeland, Sroufe, & Waters, 1979). Recognizing the needs of the child, developing strategies to meet the needs, and finding the resources to implement these strategies can be problematic in an adverse social environment. Other motivation systems may be activated along with the caregiving system that enhance its functioning (like play) or distort its

functioning (like compulsive fear and projection). An impoverished single parent may not have the money to pay for food or the energy to give adequate attention to the child.

- If, on top of the genetic, neural, cultural, and social factors that affect the *capability* of a person to perform caregiving, the person *chooses* to nurture. To a certain extent, parents may be conceptualized theoretically as objects of the caregiving motivation system that operates within them. But to a larger extent, parents are the subjects or authors of their actions (Crist, 1999), and the caregiving motivation system is one of the resources through which parents conduct their lives.

If these steps are not achieved successfully, then the internal caregiving motivation system will be reduced in strength and effectiveness, and external motivations like the threat of social sanctions may come more strongly into play.

What this analysis shows is that nothing is ever just genetic (see also Caporael, 1997). The complexity of the environment in which gene expression occurs means that there is always a substantial social and environmental component in development. Although I have talked extensively about evolution and genes, the organism carrying the genes may or may not survive, and if they survive they may or may not develop physically and psychologically in a species-normal way, and they may or may not be at any given moment in an environment that supports the expression of the genetic mechanisms. Genes and the neurobiological circuits they create are essential for the possibility of a person's caregiving. But the social and environmental history of the person are also a major part of this possibility for caregiving. Once the possibility is established by the laying down and activation of caregiving neural circuits, the expression of the caregiving motivation system is greatly influenced by the social, cultural, and interpersonal context of interaction.

With development of increased complexity in motivation systems, parents become designated teachers (children with a new, more complex motivation system do not have an evolutionary advantage unless they learn how to use it). As brain capacity and brain size grow, leading to developmentally earlier births and more helpless infants, the dyadic emotion motivates parents to nurture. A further benefit of the dyadic emotion relative to child survival is that it is compatible with adoption. A dyadic emotion can develop among unrelated persons and can develop at any time. In an environment of threats from predators where parents are at risk as well as children, the dyadic caring emotion allows for the continued protection of children even in the case of the loss of parents. To the extent that caring responds to need, then there will be a tendency toward adoption of unparented children, usually by close relatives or others who have formed some prior relationship with the children.

The benefit to children is not the only advantage of a caring emotion. In fact, the benefit of a parent-child caring relationship provides a rather small benefit in terms of protection from predators, so long as it is mainly the mother, with perhaps some help from the father, who protects each child. In the same way that the contact between mother and infant leads to the growth of the dyadic caring emotion between them and thus to greater closeness, a similar dynamic will grow up around other joint activities. In his only explicit example of protection from predators, Bowlby describes how, among pre-agricultural ground-living primates, "mature males, whether monkeys or men, combine to drive off the predator whilst the females and immatures retire" (Bowlby, 1969/1982, p. 62). In this example, it is the males who protect females and children from predators. Thus, a child who maintains close proximity to the mother is not protected against predators unless others—perhaps many others—with non-maternal dyadic bonds to that child maintain proximity and, further, cooperate. A simulation study by Macy and Skvoretz (1998) shows how increased interaction within a group facilitates the evolution of cooperation. The development of cooperation, supported by the dyadic caring emotion, has additional survival advantages beyond protection from predators. For instance, cooperation in hunting and gathering leads to benefits in terms of nutrition as well.

One advantage of an explanation focused on process and mechanism rather than function is that the mechanism can account for outcomes that are otherwise only interpretable as "mistakes" or "malfunctions" within a functional view. If we can give up the design metaphor with its value judgments of good (genetically efficient) and bad (inefficient), we are freed to look equally at the many (unjudged) outcomes of the dyadic caregiving motivation system. The motivation system supports parental nurturance of genetic offspring (usually, given an appropriate environment) and unrelated children (occasionally). It supports heterosexual parental bonds (usually) and philandering (often) and homosexual bonding (occasionally). It supports friendship and cooperation (usually) and deceit and manipulation (often) and passionate murder (occasionally).

Self interest seeking and caring

We see from this analysis how the caregiving motivation system has expanded exponentially in extent and effectiveness since the evolution of dyadic preference. From a simple preference, the caring emotion has broadened as a motivation to begin to compete with the self interest seeking motivation. Self interest seeking is often conceptualized in contemporary social science as a highly cognitive ("rational") process. However, the evolutionary origins of seeking in the earliest animals, animals without a cognitive neocortex, and its location in brain structures that are closely related to those of conventionally identified emotions, suggest that seeking is emotional in much the same way as fear, anger, lust, caregiving, and attachment. It is important to realize that both motivations have evolved. Self interest seeking has evolved from an initial search for food and exploration of the environment, eventually to include comfort, entertainment, and self-education within the enlarged seeking motivation. As the seeking motivation is manifest in many contexts and many forms such as exchange, power, social learning (Bell, 2008), so too is the caregiving motivation expressed in many different relationships, from parent-child to husband-wife to friendship, through many different behaviors.

Caring is not altruism

At this point it will be useful to consider what the proposed emotion of caring is not. It is not "altruism" as altruism is usually described in the evolutionary literature, as a general tendency to meet others' needs. Some evolutionary analysis has purported to show that altruism so conceived, such as protecting another from a dangerous predator, might never evolve (Boorman & Levitt, 1980; Wilson, 1975). In this evolutionary analysis, it is assumed that an altruist with an altruism allele may sacrifice for a non-altruist (with a different allele of the gene), who is unchanged by the altruism. This analysis has shown that organisms with such an altruism allele will disproportionately be selected out of the population because each has a lower rate of survival as a result of risking the organism's own life for other members of the species.[5]

In the caregiving evolutionary model presented here, however, the caring emotion allows for the creation of a relationship that can change the partner. Just as A's dyadic caring emotion for B grows over time that A spends in proximity to B and thus leads to A's intention to remain close to B, the very proximity that is the cause and consequence of A's dyadic preference for B is likely to lead to B's dyadic caring emotion for A. At the very beginning, when there are few organisms with the caring emotion, these organisms have a very small advantage because of their preferences leading to proximity. As their progeny survive, the initial one-way proximity seeking and protection (of a caring organism toward a non-caring one) will compete with two-way proximity seeking and protection (of caring organisms toward other caring organisms). Under these conditions those with the caring emotion will tend to cluster together and protect one another (each such relationship is sustained by *two* organisms' caring), with some caring organisms weakly attached by one-way bonds to non-caring partners, while the non-caring organisms will not cluster. The unpaired non-caring organisms will be most at risk. Within a caring-non-caring pair, the caring partner will initially be most at risk (because the non-caring partner will not undertake the risks of giving protection). However, for those non-caring organisms whose caring partners are harvested, their own subsequent status will be even more disadvantageous as they become unpaired. Under these conditions the non-caring organisms will have a serious selection disadvantage.

The concept of the caring emotion thus succeeds in explaining "altruistic" behaviors because it turns the usual analysis of altruism on its head. Instead of focusing on the non-caring organism's "deception" (e.g., Dawkins, 1976/1989), the analysis here focuses on the caring organism's motivation to help a partner who cannot be a stranger. Thus the only way for a non-caring organism to receive benefits is to remain in contact while the emotion builds strength—but this is just what the non-caring organism is unlikely to do. This model of the caring emotion does not invoke kin selection (Wilson, 1975), reciprocal altruism (Trivers, 1985), or group selection (Wilson, 1975) as *explanations* of caregiving. Instead it sees them as behavioral *consequences* of the caring emotion. Kin selection as an explanation presumes some sort of process that leads an organism to choose behaviors that benefit kin. The generic model of kin selection does not specify how such behaviors are motivated—only that such a motivation (if it were to arise) would produce positive benefits for offspring and their genes. Reciprocal altruism presumes some mechanism such as a social structure or psychological mechanism that enforces reciprocity, but like kin selection does not itself specify the mechanism. Group selection presumes the prior existence of groups who then compete, but does not specify the mechanism that produces groups, only the consequences of such a mechanism. Kin selection, reciprocal altruism, and group selection will occur as an outcome of the caring emotion and the caregiving motivation model presented here, but none of them is taken to be its cause.

The evolution of attachment

Within the mammalian line, after the evolution of caregiving, a second motivation system began to evolve as a complement to caregiving. It appears to have begun as a byproduct of the temperature regulation system (Panksepp, 1998). Early mammals were small and mammal babies smaller still. Because heat production depends on an animal's volume while heat loss depends on surface area, being smaller is disadvantageous. Some of the smaller mammals have a system (lacking in reptiles) apparently activated by oxygen imbalance of emitting high pitched sounds when cold. These ultrasonic cries are nonpurposive. The evolutionary model proposed here hypothesizes that at some evolutionary point after the emergence of dyadic preference and after the emergence of the primitive caregiving motivation system with a set goal of retrieval, some early mammalian mothers became capable of using these ultrasonic sounds to locate pups who had wandered from the nest and then to retrieve them. The cold-based ultrasonic sound system appears to be completely nonvoluntary and operates only until the pup can regulate its temperature unilaterally (Noirot, 1972; Smith & Sales, 1980). Rodent pups also have other systems, one activated by fear and one by loneliness, each with a different cry (MacLean, 1990). Each of these cries elicits the adult's caregiving motivation system and retrieval behaviors in contemporary rodent species. Mother rodents respond immediately to these cries and initiate retrieval behaviors (Smith & Sales, 1980); retrieval ceases when the young cease to give these ultrasonic cries.

The evolutionary model proposes that eventually, as adults began to offer more and more complex caregiving behaviors under the control of the caregiving system, the unconscious and nonvolitional crying behaviors were augmented by a more volitional (although still largely unconscious) attachment motivation system. Also built on and growing out of dyadic preference, the new attachment motivation system produced behaviors directed toward the adult caregiver that had the functional consequence of increased survival. As the early attachment motivation system probably had a set goal of proximity, so as the emerging attachment motivation system was developing from the dyadic preference, its early set goal was likely to be simple proximity. In these early species with limited cognitive resources, there was probably little calculation directed at achieving protection or support. It is likely that the volitional desire to achieve proximity was the beginning of a separate attachment motivation system. Thus, the desire to be close was occurring in adults at about the same (evolutionary) time that it was occurring in offspring.

Autonomous instinctive behaviors might emerge that, while not purposively directed toward a parent, might activate the adult's protection: behaviors like crying. There would be a comparative advantage toward behaviors that called forth protection from a caregiver, and we would call these behaviors "attachment behaviors." However, there would be no evolutionary advantage toward a mechanism that produced "attachment behaviors" until the caregiving motivation system was already in place and widespread within the gene pool of the species.

Early caregiving and attachment motivation systems were certainly weak. For example, each was likely to have been weaker than the fear (or defense) motivation system. In rabbits, rats, and hoofed mammals, the first response to danger is to freeze. As far as we know at this time, the caregiving motivation system does not under these conditions exert itself in rabbits or rats: they do not go to retrieve offspring in the face of a predator. In herd animals, on the other hand, adults will often jointly protect injured, ill, or young from predators (Masson & McCarthy, 1995). Thus the caregiving motivation system has become at least sometimes stronger than the fear system in herd animals. However, an attachment system, whereby a young animal in danger would run to the caregiving adult does not appear to occur in any of these species. Young in these species will cry when actually under attack (whether this cry is directed toward a specific caregiver is not yet known). By the time humans had evolved, the attachment motivation system had become allied with the fear system so that an afraid child will cry specifically for a caregiver. Human children will often cry for help when very young and run for help when somewhat older rather than freeze, even though freezing might often be more advantageous.

We turn now to look in some detail at the neurobiological substrates of caregiving and attachment.

Notes

* Portions of this chapter appear in Bell (2001).

1. See the discussion of activators on p. 25 above.

2. There are actually two motivation systems for thirst, one that reacts to intracellular salt concentration and another that reacts to blood volume (Panksepp, 1998).

3. Tomkins (1984), for example, lists 9 "affects": interest, enjoyment, surprise, distress, fear, shame, contempt, disgust, and anger. Ekman (1984) lists 6 emotions: happiness, disgust, surprise, anger, fear, and sadness. Plutchik (1984) lists 8 basic emotions: surprise, sadness, disgust, anger, an-

ticipation, joy, acceptance, and fear, and then derives more complex emotions by combining the basic emotions. Descartes, Kant, and William James, however, all include love in their lists (Masson & McCarthy, 1995). These emotion lists will be discussed in Chapter 4.

4. We will see in the next chapter that one of the special characteristics of the caring motivation is that neurochemically its effects do not decline from habituation.

5. Evolutionary logic suggests that in order for altruism to evolve successfully, altruists "must" have a reliable means to detect nonaltruists. Dawkins (1976/1989) considers the issue in terms of the "green beard problem" where a green beard (or other obvious mechanism) is the sign of an altruist. He points out that the sign is "vulnerable to a mutant arising," a green-bearded nonaltruist, who would again have an evolutionary advantage. Thus, over time, according to the usual evolutionary argument, risk-taking altruists will be more likely to die off than non-risky non-altruists. Authors like Dawkins who conceptualize the problem behaviorally consider it relatively easy for counterfeit behaviors to arise. On the other hand, it might be noted that when the problem is conceptualized emotionally, the evidence shows that emotions are extremely difficult to counterfeit. The muscles in the face under conscious control differ from those under emotional control, so fake smiles are demonstrably different from genuine smiles (Damasio, 1994). Thus, counterfeiting an emotion is very difficult to achieve.

Chapter 4. The Neurobiology of Caregiving and Attachment*

The neurobiology of nurturance is examined. Evidence from reptiles and mammals is examined to show how the fear system operating through the amygdala is responsible for the stranger rejection response. This response was altered in mammals by the evolution of a system (involving the neurotransmitter vasopressin) that suppressed the stranger rejection response and another system (involving the hypothalamus and the neurotransmitter oxytocin) that created a dyadic preference bond, at first between mother and child and later generalized to create bonds between others.

In order to proceed further to understand the nature of caregiving and attachment, we will look at the way the brain is organized, especially how motivation systems are embodied in brain structures. We will first review the literature on emotion to gain some perspective on how motivations might be conceived. Then we will look at the physiological evidence for motivation systems. Last, we will combine the two topics to consider how the emotional processes of caregiving and attachment appear to operate in the brain. Although evidence on caregiving and attachment in the brain is accumulating, there are still many unanswered questions. Nevertheless, a review of this literature will give us a set of concepts that we can use in the following chapters to propose some ways to enhance our understanding of caregiving and attachment.

APPROACHES TO EMOTION

What actually is emotion? The answer to this question turns out to be extremely elusive. In spite of over a hundred years of emotion research, there is as yet no consensus (e.g., Ekman, 1984; Harris & Saarni, 1989; LeDoux, 1996; Lewis & Haviland-Jones, 2000; Panksepp, 1998). The distinction between cognition and emotion is vague. Few authors attempt to define either, and, as we will see below, when they do make the attempt to define emotion, they are most likely to offer ostensive definitions (definition by example) or characterizations (what emotions are like) rather than nominal definitions (what emotions are).

Emotion is often described in a dualistic contrast with cognition. Cognition is conceived as clear and precise, and threatened by emotion. A number of authors see emotions as inhibiting factors that distort cognitive rationality (e.g., Coleman, 1990). Emotion is "a regrettable flaw in an otherwise perfect cognitive mechanism" (Scherer, 1984, p. 293). Others describe emotions as efficient automatic responses selected during evolution (Damasio, 1994). To begin to explore the nature of emotion, we turn now to the extensive, if fragmented, literature on emotion. This literature can be confusing; there are at least seven approaches to emotion that can be discerned.

1. Functional approach. Emotions are functional for the human species: emotions have consequences that help the human species to survive and thrive (Kemper, 1984; Plutchik, 1984). This is often taken to mean that emotions provide positive consequences for the individual as well as for the species. Early views of this type take emotions as biologically determined (e.g., McDougall, 1923; Watson, 1930). From this point of view, emotion is an adaptive response of the organism that has a consequence of contributing to the organism's survival and health. For example, we see a predator. The stimulus of seeing a predator leads us to be afraid (the emotional feeling). Being afraid, we run away (behavioral response). Because we run away, we survive. Unlike organisms who are not afraid and are thus eaten by the predator, we survive to produce and raise offspring who will be capable of the emotion of fear they inherited from us (natural selection). Fear is a reaction to danger and thus meets protection needs; lust is a reaction to a potential mate and thus meets reproduction needs (Ortony, Clore, & Collins, 1988; Plutchik, 1984).

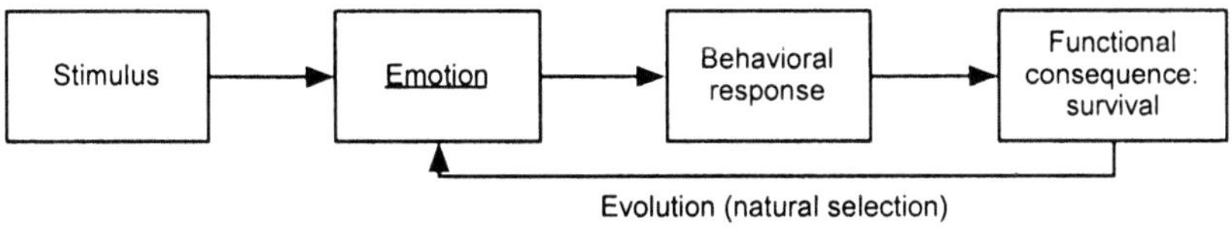

Figure 4.1. Functional Approach to Emotion

Functional definitions describe emotions in terms of survival consequences (the feedback arrow in Figure 4.1) or in terms of the survival or adaptive problems (functional consequences) that emotions solve. LeDoux (1996) raises the possibility that each emotion system may meet a different functional need and perhaps even do so with a neurobiological structure specific to that emotion. In the functional approach, as in most of the approaches we will examine, emotions are seen as reactive. A stimulus appears in the environment and the emotion is seen as a direct or indirect adaptive reaction to the stimulus. This is a standard stimulus-response process where emotion mediates between the stimulus and the response. "Emotions are total body reactions to the various survival-related problems created by the environment" (Plutchik, 1984, p. 214). Greenberg and Safran note that "emotion can be viewed as a biologically adaptive process that enables the individual to act in a potentially adaptive fashion" (1987, p. ix).

These definitions do not clearly differentiate emotions from cognitions. Most cognitions, like memory and planning, are also functional. Equally important, being a response to a stimulus is not a distinguishing characteristic of emotions. Memories are retrieved in response to stimuli, and plans are made in response to stimuli. But we must be careful not to conclude because cognitions and emotions are responses that they are *only* responses to stimuli or that they are always short term episodic phenomena. Some emotions are episodic, like the fear of seeing a snake or the disappointment when someone we look for is not there. And some cognitions are episodic, like a flash of memory about a previous experience with someone or a sudden decision to place a phone call. Other cognitions, however, endure over time. Plans can take a long time to formulate—and a longer time to carry out. Similarly, some emotions endure over long periods of time, like our love for a child, our passion for money, or our grief over the loss of a loved one.

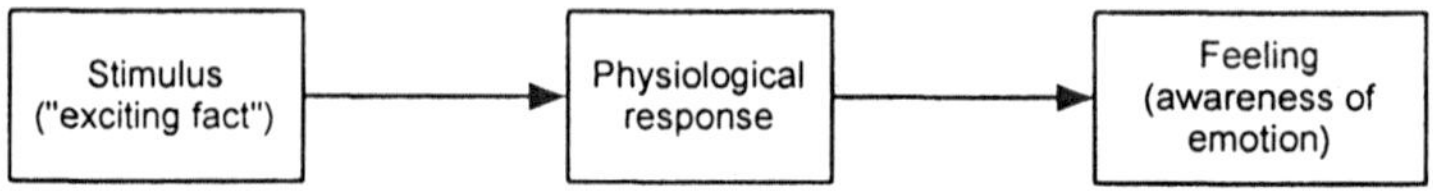

Figure 4.2. Physiological Perception Approach to Emotion

2. Physiological perception approach. Emotions can be seen as the conscious perception of a physiological state. In this view, emotions are feelings. James asserts that:

> bodily changes follow directly the PERCEPTION of the exciting fact, and that our feeling of the same changes as they occur IS the emotion (James, 1884, pp. 189-190, italics omitted).

In this view, our heart does not pound because we are scared, our face is not flushed because we are embarrassed: we are scared because our heart pounds, we are embarrassed because our faces are flushed. James believes that the person directly perceives internal and external states to construct a feeling. Cannon (1929) and Schachter and Singer (1962) agree with James that feelings are post-response constructions, but disagree that internal states are fast enough reacting or specific enough to contribute meaningfully. They emphasize the use of external cues in interpreting diffuse and imprecise internal experience. Nisbett and Wilson (1977) have pointed out, for cognitions as well as emotions, that people can be wildly mistaken in their interpretations. In a newer view, physiological sensations are seen as necessary for emotional feeling without being constitutive of emotion (Berscheid, 1983; Tomkins, 1984). Damasio (1994) argues that the healthy brain maintains a complex and continuously updated representation of the body's nervous, muscular, and hormonal state. The person's awareness of emotion (feelings) is built from this bodily representation. Thus facial configuration, autonomic nervous system arousal, skin sensor activation, and their mental analogues and associations provide information about emotional states.

> Emotion is a continuous read-out of consciousness, constantly integrating a large amount of information and forwarding it to us as feedback. [It] informs people of their response to situations (Greenberg & Safran, 1987, pp. 301; see also Burgess et al., 1971).

The importance of physical sensations is seen in our use of physical metaphors for emotions. Positive relationships are described as "feeling

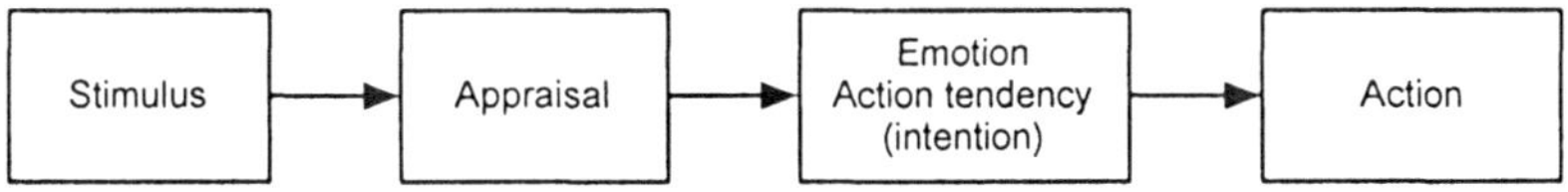

Figure 4.3. Intentional Approach to Emotion

warm" or "feeling close" to someone. Someone who is fearful is said to have "cold feet." "I feel hot" is a sensation metaphor for anger as well as lust. Many of our feelings seem to be more metaphorical associations with previous physical sensations than physical sensations themselves. Touch, for example, appears to be the sensation metaphor for caregiving.[1] When we connect, we "feel" close. For a number of authors, the awareness of an emotion is labeled a "feeling" (Damasio, 1994; LeDoux, 1996), and that terminology is used in Figure 4.2. When we find ourselves smiling, we realize that we are happy.

3. Intentional approach. For some authors, emotions are intentions; they are motivators. Emotions are not just "passions" that we passively experience, not just physical changes that we detect in our bodies. Emotions also motivate us to make changes, to take action (Leeper, 1970; Levy, 1984). That is, when we experience emotions, we want to do something: we intend to (want to) run away in the case of fear, we intend to (want to) share intimacy in the case of romantic love. For Arnold, the emotion is both the appraisal of something as good or bad and a stimulus for action:

> the emotion becomes a felt tendency toward anything appraised as good, and away from anything appraised as bad (Arnold, 1970, pp. 176, italics removed).

Appraisal is the central process in the intentional approach (although appraisal is also used in other approaches). A stimulus is appraised, either consciously or unconsciously, and an action tendency forms (Figure 4.3). This action tendency is the emotion in this view, and its evaluation in light of what is known about the situation produces conscious feelings. Some authors see the intention (the action tendency) as conscious and mutable (Arnold, 1970; Greenberg & Safran, 1987; Solomon, 1990). Other authors see the intention as a hard-wired automatic response to certain innate or conditioned stimuli (Bowlby, 1969/1982; Watson, 1930). Zajonc (1980) has shown that appraisal can occur without any conscious awareness of the stimulus.

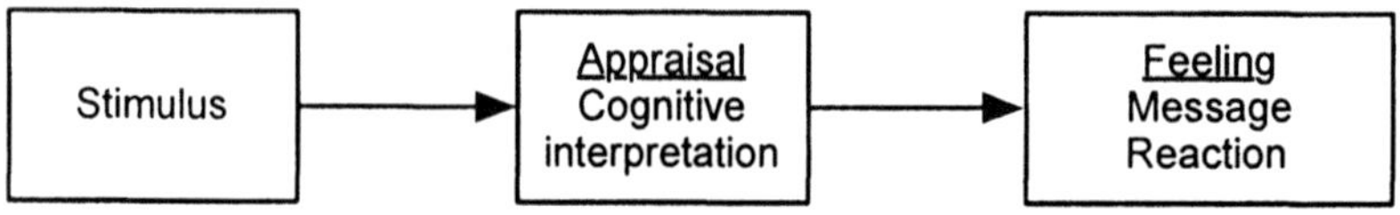

Figure 4.4. Cognitive Approach to Emotion

4. Cognitive approach. For some authors, emotion is information. We cannot feel anything unless we know what is happening. The emotion of fear, for example, is a message (information) that there is danger and that we need to act to protect ourselves. This approach is similar to James' physiological account, except that the cognitive approach emphasizes information about the stimulus rather than information about the body's response. Instead of relatively direct conversion of body changes into feelings, the cognitive approach emphasizes the cognitive processing of information about the stimulus.

This approach, like the physiological approach, focuses on conscious feelings as emotion. A stimulus leads to a cognitive appraisal of the stimulus (Figure 4.4). This cognitive appraisal then leads to a conscious feeling, a reaction to the stimulus, which serves as a message telling the person of the result of the cognitive appraisal (Berscheid, 1983; Lazarus, Coyne, & Folkman, 1984). For example, Ortony, Clore and Collins see emotions

> as valenced reactions to events, agents, or objects, with their particular nature being determined by the way in which the eliciting situation is construed (Ortony, et al., 1988, pp. 13, italics removed).

Sometimes the experience of emotion is stimulated by memory. We remember a prior experience in at least some of its complexity and clarity ("affective memory") and this memory shapes not only our interpretation of the situation but also our very emotional response to it (LeDoux, 1996; Leventhal, 1984). Cognitive information in memory thus contributes to the emotional experience. Even when we "feel," we do not always know *what* we feel (Schachter & Singer, 1962). Cognitive appraisal allows us to interpret our context and infer the meaning of our physiological reactions within that context.

5. Normative approach. Emotions are expected in certain social situations. Such socially situated emotions can be seen as norms, as socially organized and defined behavioral expectations:

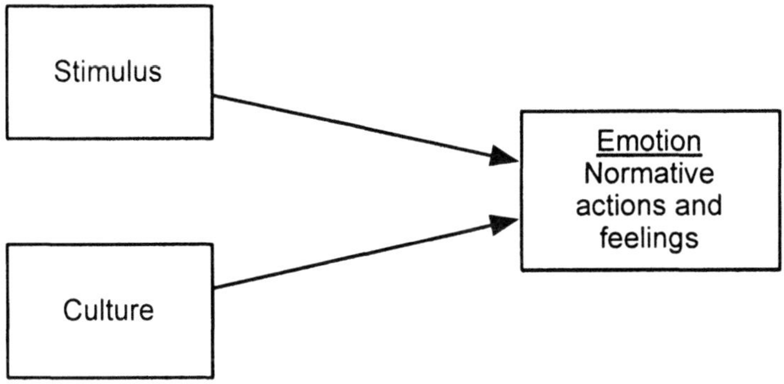

Figure 4.5. Normative Approach to Emotion

> emotions are *activities*. . . . We *do* them, and we *learn*, from our culture and our friends, from movies, books and, originally, from our parents, *how* to do them (Solomon, 1990, pp. 44, italics in original).

Social norms not only tell us how to behave when we experience an emotion; they also tell us when to feel the emotion and how it ought to feel (Hochschild, 1983). When a person is a parent, there are certain social expectations of caring and nurturance. These expectations define the parental role. Mothers and fathers are not only supposed to nurture their children; they are also supposed to feel an emotion of warmth, acceptance and love.

This view emphasizes how our feelings can be shaped by our culture and by our personal experience (Figure 4.5). There is a widespread assertion that the feelings and behaviors of the successful parent are determined by purported social norms of parenting, as discussed in Chapter 1. However, unlike many contemporary observers, I do not believe that parental love and nurture occurs primarily as a result of social norms (Bell, 2009a). I believe that in general parents love and nurture, and as a result society has come to expect caring and nurturance from parents. Norms are still very important: social norms—and accompanying social sanctions—may counteract the two a.m., cranky-infant, I-want-to-throw-you-against-the-wall feeling that may emerge in a parent. Nevertheless, norms have definite limits in explaining parental nurturance.

6. Intuitive approach. Emotions are intuitively apprehended. Emotions are an "intuitive appraisal" (Arnold, 1970; Greenberg & Safran,

1987; Leventhal, 1984). "Intuitive" in this context means "unexplained," and perhaps "unexplainable." A perhaps more coherent way of expressing this idea is to say that feelings may not be concrete enough to describe the underlying emotion. This view of emotion acknowledges ignorance, even enshrines ignorance. The acknowledgment of ignorance sometimes shades into mysticism. "Definitions" of emotion within this approach are usually characterizations. Emotions are characterized as "reactions" (Ortony, et al., 1988, p. 13; Plutchik, 1984, p. 214), a "readout of consciousness" (Greenberg & Safran, 1987, p. 301), a "transformation of energy" (Hillman, 1962, p. 287), or an "experience" (Leventhal, 1984, p. 271). We find this mystical approach in many characterizations of that most typical of emotions, love, (Singer, 1966/1984, 1984-1987, 1987). The "language of love," whether of love between persons or love of God, uses expressions that make little denotative sense. Brickman (1987, p. 81) refers to the "inarticulateness of love."

7. Neurobiological approach. A last approach to emotion has seen enormous advances in recent years. This approach to emotion has tried to identify the neurobiological structures of the brain that produce or carry out emotional process. For example, Panksepp (1998) has identified eight neurobiological emotions. In the previous chapter, six of them were discussed: seeking, fear, anger, sexual lust, caregiving, and attachment; the other two are pleasure and play. According to Panksepp, "emotions are the psychoneural processes that are especially influential in controlling the vigor and patterning of actions in the dynamic flow of intense behavioral interchanges between animals" (Panksepp, 1998, p. 48). Panksepp's approach has shown that many emotions are, at a fundamental level, social, in particular lust, caregiving, and attachment are almost always directed at a partner.

A conceptual map of emotion

Much of the apparent conflict in the many approaches to emotion is strictly terminological; they are primarily disputes over where to assign the label "emotion." Is the emotion the unconscious neurobiological process or the body's predictable physiological signals or the conscious feeling; is it the intention to do something or the consequence of it; is it the intuitive part behind the action or the social part? Each of these approaches identifies important parts of emotional processes.

In order to talk about motivation systems, I will need to use some relatively precise terminology. Figure 4.6 combines the seven approaches into a single conceptual map of emotion terms and concepts. The figure offers a map of the main concepts I will use and the terminology I will use to refer to them. For the purposes of this book, I will assign the term "emotion" to certain subneocortical neurobiological processes that serve as motivators of behavior. That is, certain circuits in the brain constitute emotional structures, and emotions, as I will use the term, are the operation of these circuits. To be precise, I am not claiming that the emotion *is* the circuit. The circuit exists even when the emotion is not experienced. Instead I am defining an emotion as the *operation* of the circuit.

Emotions are functional. Emotions, and the brain structures through which they operate, have been selected through natural selection because of the consequences of behavior produced by these emotional circuits (arrow 1). Vertebrates who were afraid of predators, and mammals who felt caring toward their children, for example, were more likely to pass on their genes. having been preserved through natural selection, emotions are conceptualized here as neurobiological processes operating in concrete brain circuits. These neurobiological systems receive information from the environment and channel it to cognitive resources that appraise the information (arrows 2). The result of appraisal affects (feeds the appraisal back to) the emotion system in turn (arrow 3). Neurobiologically situated emotions motivate actions by creating intentions (through plans formulated in the cognitive neocortex) which are enacted into behavior (arrow 4). Neural activation and body changes result in feelings that are cognitively and socially influenced (arrows 5, 6, and 7): how we feel toward someone depends on how our body responds to them and the social context of our relationship. At the same time, our emotion-based behaviors are influenced by social norms (arrow 8).

The figure suggests a scheme that conceptualizes social actions in terms of emotions, intentions, and behaviors. Behaviors have emotions as their motivators (more will be said about emotions as motivators below). If we follow authors like Zajonc (1980) and Berscheid (1983) who consider preferences to be emotions, then emotions can be seen as motivators for cognitive processes. Seeing emotions as motivators is not a new idea. Drive theory (e.g., Lindsley, 1951), popular in the first half of the twentieth century, often considered emotions to be drives that motivate behavior (Lazarus, et al., 1984).

In the model presented here, emotions can be consequences, as when the emotion of fear is caused by the sight of a snake—such emotions are reactions. Emotions can also be causes, such as the love of family that leads a parent to work two jobs. In this book, emotions will most frequently be investigated as the instigators of causal processes.

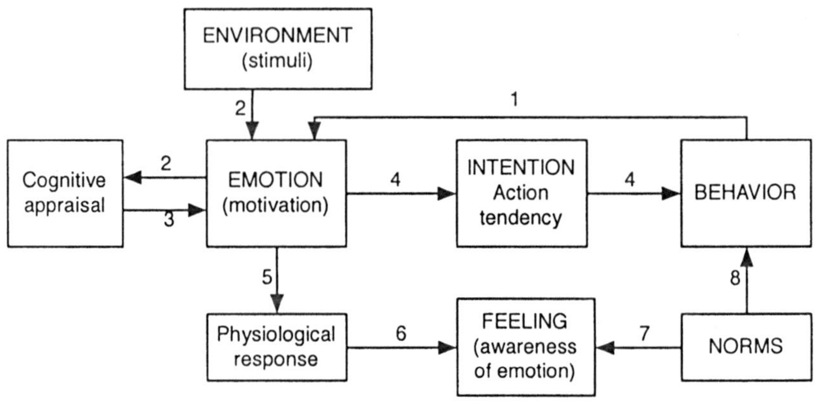

Figure 4.6. Emotion: A Conceptual Map

MOTIVATION SYSTEMS IN THE BRAIN

Functionalists and behaviorists, such as many ethologists and evolutionists, are often comfortable conceptualizing action in terms of "behavioral control systems," as Bowlby did. Focus on behaviors may be more comfortable than figuring out the largely unobserved processes operating in the minds of humans and other animals. However, when one is attempting to *explain* behavior rather than simply to *describe* its patterns, it is useful to focus on motivations. Thus we turn now to examine motivation systems in the brain. Some motivation systems are emotional, such as fear and caregiving. Other motivation systems are not, such as temperature control. The two types of system operate in similar ways, although I will emphasize systems that are emotional.

The conceptual map described in Figure 4.6 indicates how terminology will be used, but it does not map the concepts onto brain structures. As we turn to the brain, we will be most focused on the *emotion, appraisal,* and *intention* boxes, with some attention to feedback processes.

In the discussion of the evolution, neurobiology, and psychology of attachment and caregiving, I use the term "system," as Bowlby does, to refer to coordinated emotions, goals, and behaviors, and I use "circuit" to refer to the biological source of the system in the brain. Thus, in the terminology that I use, the "attachment circuit" refers to the brain's neurons

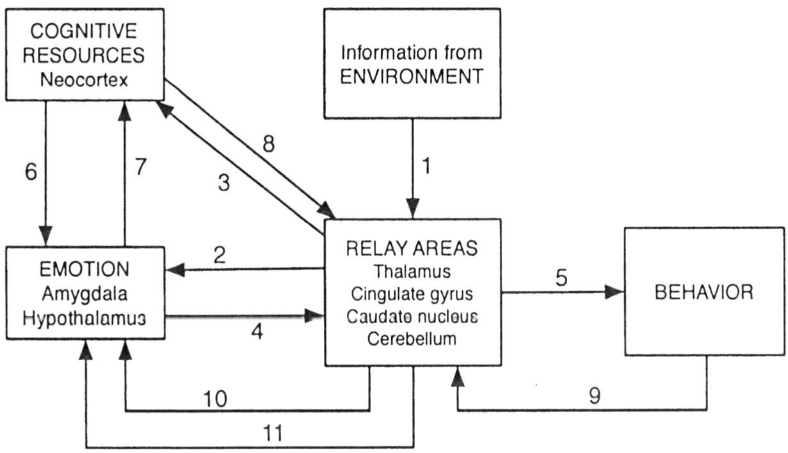

Figure 4.7. Simplified Functional Outline of a Motivation System

that are consolidated to produce the motivation to seek security and comfort from a particular partner.

We know a great deal about the physiology of learning, how associations between memories are formed and how memory structures are formed (Restak, 1995). Among emotions, the most is known about the physiology and biochemistry of fear (LeDoux, 1996). Less is known about the physiology of other emotions. However, research that has identified emotional circuits has suggested how these emotional circuits operate. Using LeDoux's (1996) excellent detailed analysis of the fear system as a prototype, but enlarged to include hypothalamic emotions, I present a simplified outline of the neurobiological locations of motivation systems (Figure 4.7).

There are six major parts of the central nervous system: (1) spinal cord, (2) medulla oblongata, (3) pons and cerebellum, (4) midbrain, (5) diencephalon, which contains the thalamus and hypothalamus, and (6) cerebral hemispheres, which consists of the cerebral cortex, the basal ganglia (including the caudate nuclei), the hippocampus, and the amygdala. For this discussion of emotional motivations, I will distinguish between emotion areas (generally the amygdala and hypothalamus), relay areas (thalamus, cerebellum, and other parts of the midbrain), and the cerebral neocortex.

Most information from the environment is received in the diencephalon via the thalamus as signals from the various senses (arrow 1). This is an operational activator. The amygdala and hypothalamus appear to be two of the locations in the brain where intentions to act are formulated. A signal is transmitted from the sensory neurons of the thalamus to the emotion center in the hypothalamus or amygdala (arrow 2) as well as to the sensory areas of the neocortex for more extensive interpretation (arrow 3) (LeDoux, 1996). Not all signals into the thalamus are sent to the neocortex. An animal might walk right past a water source and not even register it when the animal is not thirsty. Other times the sight of water may register and be interpreted by the neocortex but no action is taken because the animal is again not thirsty. Thus in the case of the thirst motivation system, action to drink may not be enacted unless the thirst drive is active, and thirst-relevant sensations may not even be interpreted if the thirst drive is inactive. When the emotion center determines that action is called for, motor activation is carried out by signals to the relay areas, specifically to the caudate nucleus for familiar actions, and thence to the cerebellum for habitual action components (arrow 4) (Jeannerod, 1997). These relay areas thus control bodily movements and other body responses to carry out the goals of the emotion (arrow 5).

On occasion, a lizard or mouse—or even human—while looking for water, may see a predator. Now the image of the predator will travel from the eye to the visual thalamus and thence to the visual cortex (arrow 3) where the predator will be identified and a message interpreting the situation as one of danger will be sent to the amygdala (arrow 6) to consult the internal working model for advice and thus to freeze or hide or run away. However, if this were all that happened, by the time the brain reached a decision, the lizard or mouse or human might be a meal.

When the sensory thalamus sends its message to the emotion center (arrow 2), the emotion center makes a "quick and dirty" evaluation of the sensory input and, if this preliminary evaluation suggests relevance, operates to actuate various body systems such as the endocrine system and the autonomic nervous system (arrow 4) (Damasio, 1994). In the case of the fear system, if the amygdala interprets the direct signal as a potential threat, the amygdala immediately activates the motor nervous system, tensing muscles (the "freeze" response), as well as the autonomic nervous system releasing adrenaline and raising the level of alertness.

Soon after the emotion center receives its raw sensory information, it receives a more textured interpretation from the sensory cortex (arrow 6). If the interpreted signal from the visual cortex, when it arrives, provides information that the image was not a threat (e.g., it was a curved stick instead of a snake or a bush instead of a bear), the amygdala turns off its arousal systems (LeDoux, 1996). However, if the image is interpreted as a threat, the initial direct response will have prepared the body to respond. The heart will already be beating faster to provide more oxygen to the muscles; sensory systems will be more alert. The body is ready to run, or to fight. Hormones and peptides are transmitted through the bloodstream to raise blood pressure and heighten awareness.

In beginning action, the emotion center accesses memory systems and planning systems in the neocortex (arrow 7). These include signals to direct attention to the stimuli that are of emotional interest (LeDoux, 1996). The emotion centers create what Damasio (1994) calls an "as if" loop, to stimulate those parts of the cortex that interpret bodily arousal so that they "feel" the emotion even in the absence of actual bodily arousal. Another part of this cortical stimulation is the activation of the internal working model, thus calling up memories that are useful for the current emotional process. Cognitive resources such as perception, memory, attitude formation, and planning are not just computing systems to store and process information. Their operation is affected by the emotional motivator that calls them, a process related to "affect infusion," whereby cognitive constructs such as beliefs are influenced by emotions (Forgas, 2000). In some cases, these cortical systems will report back to the emotion center for it to instigate appropriate action (arrow 6); in other cases they will directly send signals to the relay areas (arrow 8), for example, as plans formulated in the prefrontal cortex are downloaded to the caudate nucleus for implementation (Jeannerod, 1997). These intentions are then carried out as behaviors (arrow 5).

In the figure there is a clear distinction between an emotion and cognitive resources. The emotions occur as the activation of coherent circuits located in the lower forebrain and parts of the diencephalon, especially including the amygdala, hypothalamus, and nearby brain locations (Panksepp, 1998). Each of these identified emotional systems controls actions to achieve goals associated with the emotion.

Each motivation system can be seen to have an identifiable emotion at its center. The emotion of fear when the fear system is activated motivates behavior to achieve a goal of safety and security. The emotion of anger when the anger system is activated motivates behavior to achieve dominance or freedom. The emotion of caring when the caregiving system is activated motivates behavior to meet the partner's needs. The emotion of trust when the attachment system is activated motivates behavior to have one's needs met by the partner. The emotion of self interest when the seeking system is activated motivates behavior to achieve gratification of personal appetitive wants and needs. Note that these are emotional goals and not behavioral goals. Motivational goals are general and stable; behavior is specific and varying. A person may select a given behavior to achieve an emotional goal, but the person may switch to an alternate behavior if the original behavior is unsuccessful in achieving the goal (e.g., Bowlby, 1969/1982). Substitutability of behavior is one reason why many studies of parental caregiving that focus on specific behaviors have often found little consistency (Harris, 1998).

Motivation systems are goal-corrected feedback systems. That is, motivation systems are cybernetic systems that achieve a goal by correcting action when it deviates from the goal state (Bowlby, 1969/1982; Broderick, 1993; Buckley, 1967; Hill, 1971; Kantor & Lehr, 1975). For example, if running east does not achieve safety from a pursuing bear, maybe running south will help. If holding a crying infant does not stop the infant's crying, then maybe changing the diaper will meet the caregiver's goal of comforting the child. There are at least three feedback systems that have been identified in emotion systems.

Emotional feedback is depicted in arrows 9 and 10. Nerves in the thalamus and sensory cortex detect the success or failure of the current goal (arrow 9) (Eckman, 1984). Autonomic feedback involves both sympathetic and parasympathetic nerves (Porges, 1999). The brain also detects released chemicals in places like the area postrema, the nucleus basalis, and the subfornical organ, as well as in the hypothalamus (LeDoux, 1996). Neural and chemical pathways inform the emotion center of these results (arrow 10). One result of this feedback is to keep the emotion active even if the original stimulus is not present (LeDoux, 1996). One's awareness of the smile on one's face, once initiated, continues to sustain happiness. If you are being chased by a bear, you don't want to stop running just because you are faced away from the bear and thus are no longer receiving visual signals of the bear; you want your body systems to stay aroused and you want your motivation to escape to continue until you are sure of safety. Similarly, if you are preparing a meal for your child, you don't want to lose track of your goal just because the child is in the other room. This sustained emotional action contradicts the conception of emotion as simply reactive.

The dopamine reward system (arrow 11) also provides a unique kind of feedback. When a goal of some of the systems (seeking, caregiving, and probably attachment and lust) has been achieved, the nucleus accumbens is activated and dopamine is released, creating a feeling of pleasure. Some authors suggest that it is this pleasure feedback that makes some emotions "positive" (Berscheid, 1983; Bradley, 2000). At the same time, in ways that are not well understood, the reward system assists the neurons of the motivation system to become better organized. When the pleasure circuit is activated as a result of anticipating and/or achieving a goal, the neurons of the associated motivation circuit become more organized so that the motivation becomes more likely to produce the same behavior in the same circumstances again (Panksepp, 1998). Some contemporary theorists are beginning to incorporate these insights into social theories (Turner, 2002).

Feedback processes can be quite complex, with feedback occurring at many levels simultaneously. Consider, for example, a parent feeding baby food to his child (one could substitute a person feeding soup to an ill spouse or elder parent, or a person feeding grapes to a romantic partner). Under the direction of the caregiving emotional circuit, the executive system in the frontal neocortex selects a "feed the baby" plan, which is downloaded into the caudate nucleus (Jeannerod, 1997). The caudate nucleus sends a series of orders to the cerebellum: "pick up spoon," "load baby food onto spoon," and "insert spoon in baby's mouth." The cerebellum monitors muscular, tactile, and other nerve signals to move the arm and hand in well-practiced movements. Depending on observed results of these actions, the caudate nucleus may insert additional commands into the action stream (e.g., "pick up spilled baby food"). If the action plan is not working (e.g., the child keeps closing her mouth and refusing the spoon), then the prefrontal cortex may select a different plan or even devise a new plan that is expected to meet the emotional goal. For example, a "pretend the spoon is an airplane and then 'fly' the food to the child's mouth" plan may be downloaded. If this plan does not work, the executive system may signal that the goal of feeding the child cannot be met because the child is just not hungry now. In this case, the parent may switch from the frustrated caregiving plan to a different motivation system such as the play system.

The brain circuits depicted in the "emotion" box in Figure 4.7 lie in what is often called rather imprecisely the "limbic system" (MacLean, 1990). The main emotional centers in the limbic system include the amygdala and the hypothalamus. Important segments of the emotion circuits flow through areas that are not household words—the ventral tegmental area, the bed nucleus of the stria terminalis, the septum, and the nucleus accumbens, for instance. Emotional circuits provide the motivational "energy" for action (Levy, 1984; Panksepp, 1998; Salovey, Bedell, Detweiler, & Mayer, 2000). Sometimes emotional motivations are unconscious: they lead us to undertake some action without awareness of why we are undertaking it (Bargh & Barndollar, 1996). Other times we are aware of our emotion, in which case we refer to the conscious awareness of the emotion as a "feeling" (Damasio, 1994).

In the figure, "cognitive resources" refer to those neural circuits composed of neurons whose cell bodies are located largely in the neocortex. Some parts of the neocortex are specialized in processing sensory signals; other parts are specialized in motor processing. Plans are formed in the dorsolateral prefrontal neocortex, social planning and interpretation takes place in the ventromedial cortex, attention is focused in the anterior cingulate (Jeannerod, 1997). The neocortex is where most memory systems, language systems, and interpretation systems are located. I am using the term "cognition" to refer to those unconscious information transforming and manipulating processes in the brain that are not emotions.[2] It is reasonable to expect that some perception of the environment is probably cognitively mediated under the direction of an emotion, as when a fearful person searches the environment for danger, and that some cognitive resources are devoted to a particular motivation systems, such as an attachment internal working model in memory (Bowlby, 1969/1982).

In the presence of danger, a fear (or defense) system and an (unconscious) fear emotion are fully operational in the lizard. This fear emotion directly activates the autonomic system. The lizard also experiences fear-relevant cognitions as it interprets the danger and directs actions of self protection. Other parts of the mammalian system do not exist in lizards. The internal working model and the "as if" circuit have less neocortex to work with than in mammals, although these presumably exist at some level. Furthermore, the lizard does not (as far as we know) experience conscious *feelings* of fear. That is, the lizard does not reflect on its experience or have conscious thoughts about why it chose to freeze rather than run, or go to other lizards and tell them how scared it was.

We see in the above description how emotion circuits and other subcortical circuits interconnect and cooperate with neocortical cognitive circuits. In non-mammals, there is no neocortex, so the subcortical location of motivation is obvious. It is parsimonious to anticipate that subcortical circuits provide the motive force in humans and other mammals as well. Though humans clearly have much greater and more powerful neocortical resources (including expanded perception, evaluation, planning, and memory), and these cognitive resources clearly provide important information to subcortical motivation circuits, the subcortical emotional motivation of much behavior seems clear.

Some argue that subcortical structures like the amygdala are not sufficiently complex to handle the range of discrimination of which the human neocortex is capable (Matthews, Zeidner, & Roberts, 2002; Rolls, 1999). Like other claims of neocortical motivation (Turner, 2000; Wilson, 1975), this argument cannot be disproved. However, it seems implausible in the light of other evidence for the conservation of older neural systems. In less differentiated (more "primitive") brains like that of rats, the cortex makes a more finely detailed analysis than the amygdala alone is capable of, but in LeDoux's model, its result is then reported to the amygdala for action. Thus it seems plausible that the more highly discriminating neocortical structures in the human brain continue to perform these discriminations in service to the subcortical motivation systems, and that the subcortical systems are complex enough to make use of these discriminations. There are considerably more neural connections from the emotion systems to the neocortex than the reverse (Carter, 1998b; Panksepp, 1998). Furthermore, there is relatively clear behavioral evidence that feelings triggered by emotion often dominate behavior, overriding rational thought. Therapeutic and educational approaches, such as cognitive behavioral therapy along with the strengthening of mindfulness (Bell, 2009b; Hanh, 1999; Roemer & Orsillo, 2008; Segal, Williams, & Teasdale, 2002), seek to address this issue. Although hominids (*homo habilis*) with fully functioning emotional systems emerged some 2.5 million years ago, the modern prefrontal cortex where a cognitive motivation would be situated developed only 150,000 years ago, and the cultural forms that allowed the extensive use of rationality only began to emerge some 12,000 years ago (Massey, 2002). Most of the motivation systems discussed in this chapter predate the emergence of humans by hundreds of millions of years.

Emotions, intentions, and behavior. In a motivation system, then, emotion predominates over cognitive and behavioral subsystems (Aube & Senteni, 1996; Oatley, 2000; Salovey, et al., 2000). The emotion provides a goal as well as the psychological "energy" for action. Cognitive subsystems act in a mediating capacity to formulate plans and carry out the intentions of the emotion. In particular, the cognitive subsystems carry out informational intentions (interpreting environmental inputs) and strategy intentions (formulating and evaluating alternative courses of action). Then non-motivational limbic areas like the caudate nucleus and sub-limbic areas like the cerebellum monitor the carrying out of action. Depending on what motivation system is currently active (or "energized" by the corresponding emotion), the motivation system will employ various cognitive resources (perception, interpretation, memory, working models, executive functions to weigh alternatives) to carry out the intentions of the emotion (Oatley, 2000).

Within this model, emotions are self-regulating. Once an emotion is activated, feedback processes inform the motivational system about relative closeness to or distance from the goal, leading to increases in activation, decreases in activation, or modification of the goal. In these feedback processes, cognitive systems of perception, evaluation, and planning are necessary elements. These cognitive elements are instrumental in activating and deactivating the emotion. One must recognize the instrumental and supportive nature of these cognitive resources, however. One can of course claim that memory and evaluative systems cause subsequent action, but such "causation" may be like saying that a weather report "caused" me to carry an umbrella. One can equally claim that the environment, interpreted by the neocortex, "caused" the action, which is saying the potential rain "caused" me to take the umbrella. Yet, ultimately I carried the umbrella because I did not want to get wet, and knowing the weather report helped me achieve my goal. Thus, it is the motivation rather than the environment or the evaluation that I choose to emphasize as the cause of action.

WHAT ARE THE EMOTIONS?

I will make a short digression here to consider again what the emotions are. There have been two basic ways that distinctions among emotions have been formulated (Bradley, 2000). The one way is to distinguish emotions as discrete states, such as fear, anger, lust, and so on. This is the approach I have taken in this book. Support for this approach has been found in the discovery of identifiable and distinct structures in the brain corresponding to specific emotions. The second approach is to conceive of emotions more abstractly in terms of two independent parameters. This biphasic model conceptualizes emotions in terms of a direction parameter and an intensity parameter (Berscheid, 1983; Bradley, 2000). The two conceptualizations are not incompatible. They are in fact complementary (Bradley, 2000). Each has strengths, and each has weaknesses. As Izard (Izard & Ackerman, 2000) points out, one strength of broad dimensions (such as those in the biphasic model), is that these dimensions are easier to measure reliably than are specific emotions.

The biphasic model describes emotional intensity as the level of activation of an emotion. A picture of a snake may ordinarily not activate the fear emotion at all, unless the picture is presented unexpectedly and

Descartes	Kant	James	Tomkins	Ekman	Plutchik	Bowlby	Panksepp
(Masson & McCarthy, 1995)			(1984)	(1984)	(1984)	(1973)	(1998)
love	love	love				love	care
desire	hope		interest		anticipation		seeking
		fear	fear	fear	fear	anxiety	fear
sorrow	sorrow	grief		sadness	sadness	grief	sorrow
hate		rage	anger	anger	anger	anger	rage
joy	joy		enjoyment	happiness	joy		pleasure
astonishment			surprise	surprise	surprise		
			disgust	disgust	disgust		
	modesty		shame		acceptance		lust
			contempt				play
			distress				

Table 4.1. What are the Emotions?

dramatically. A real snake, especially if unanticipated, has the potential to activate the fear emotion at a very high level. Thinking about my child may not activate your caregiving system and the caring emotion at all, but thinking of your own child will do so.

This view of intensity is directly applicable to discrete emotions. The discrete emotion model suggests the importance of coherence in specific motivation systems. Most people are approximately equally capable of fear reactions, although lesions of the amygdala can produce the Kluver-Bucy syndrome, where the fear system becomes incapable of activation (Davis & Leinhardt, 1972). Persons who experience deprivation of parental caregiving in infancy may be unable or minimally able to form attachments to others (Hrdy, 1999; Main, 1999; Montagu, 1986; O'Connor, 2005; Zeanah, et al., 2005).

A problem with the discrete emotions model is identifying what the discrete emotions are. There are many lists, and few agree. Table 4.1 shows some early and contemporary lists of emotions. One of the differences in the lists is that, whereas some nineteenth century and early twentieth century philosophers (such as Descartes, Kant, and James) listed enduring emotions like love, hope, sorrow and grief, most contemporary emotion researchers (like Tompkins, Ekman and Plutchik) list only episodic short term emotions in their lists. These contemporary researchers have achieved a great deal by identifying neurobiological and psychological processes of some emotions. However, the fact that most of these researchers have so far excluded such critical emotions as love from their domain of study shows how far we have still to go. A major reason why such emotions have been excluded from contemporary emotion research may be that enduring emotions like love do not involve the clear start and stop points that can be relatively easily studied in the laboratory. This has led contemporary emotion researchers to focus almost exclusively on episodic short term emotional processes, those that can be stimulated by an experimenter. Two of the researchers who have studied enduring emotions are Panksepp and Bowlby. Of particular importance in this book will be the emotions of the caregiving, fear, self interest seeking, and attachment motivation systems as described by Panksepp.

The second phase of the biphasic model is direction. The direction parameter has been conceptualized in the biphasic model in terms of two qualities labeled "approach" and "withdraw" (Schneirla, 1959; Wundt, 1897), "protective" and "defensive" (Konarski, 1967), "attractive" and "aversive" (Dickinson & Dearing, 1979), "good" and "bad" (Arnold, 1960), and "appetitive" and "defensive" (Cacioppo & Berntson, 1994; Davidson, 1992; Lang, Bradley, & Cuthbert, 1990). In the earliest conception of the direction of an emotion, direction was seen as a single dimension with two poles (Konarski, 1967; Schneider & Younger, 1996; Wundt, 1897). More recent conceptualizations suggest that appetitive and defensive directions are separate and independent. The discrete emotional motivations of fear and anger are viewed as defensive or negative; the motivations of lust and self interest seeking are seen as appetitive or positive.

The distinction of defensive and appetitive motivations may have a neurophysiological reality as well as a conceptual one. Defensive and appetitive emotions may represent separate types of systems. The anger motivation system appears to have differentiated out of the fear system (Panksepp, 1998), so that even though the two systems now involve largely different circuits, perhaps they still represent a meaningful overarching system, both in terms of their origins and in terms of partially overlapping neural circuits. Similarly, lust and self interest seeking both produce dopamine, so there is a sense that they may have developed from a common origin and may now thus constitute a larger overarching system. On this ground, one might be inclined to include caregiving and attachment within this larger system because they produce dopamine too. On the other hand, one could argue that the emergence of oxytocin led to the creation of a separate motivation system.

THE NEUROBIOLOGY OF CAREGIVING AND ATTACHMENT

In the previous chapter, we considered the evolutionary evidence for three neurobiological processes that developed in reptiles, two of which enabled the emergence of mammals: a system of stranger rejection, a system to inhibit stranger rejection, and a system of dyadic preference (Bell, 2001).

The neurochemistry of stranger rejection. The stranger rejection response in reptiles is smell-based. Signals from the olfactory system carried by the peptide hormone vasotocin are processed directly in the amygdala and hypothalamus with less involvement of the neocortex than for other senses (Del Cerro, 1998; MacLean, 1990; Panksepp, 1998). In reptiles, vasotocin, operating through the amygdala where fear and anger are produced, induces agonistic aggression (competition for status) as well as sexual aggression (Panksepp, 1998). Vasotocin also controls sexual urges and stimulates pre-birth activities like nest building and during-birth activities like egg laying. In animals who depend on smell, the vasotocin system contributes to survival by activating the fear system in the presence of predators and creating emotional memories of dangerous locations and situations (LeDoux, 1996). This smell-based system, while contributing to the survival of both parents and offspring as each avoids predators, forces each individual from infancy to look to personal survival alone, for the "other" smell of a reptile infant would lead to its rejection and death at the teeth and claws of its parent or other adults.

Two hormones seem to have been involved in the evolution of mammalian caregiving: the peptide hormones vasopressin and oxytocin. Vasotocin, the sex, birth, and aggression hormone in reptiles, came to be differentiated into these two new peptides, each differing from vasotocin by a single amino acid (Carter, 1998a; Panksepp, 1998).

Neurochemically in mammals, vasopressin appears to have inherited the stranger rejection functions of vasotocin that lie behind attacks against the young. Vasopressin acts as a neurotransmitter from two olfactory systems (the main and vomeronasal systems) to the amygdala and hypothalamus (Del Cerro, 1998; Guillamon & Segovia, 1997). These neural circuits appear to be central to the anger motivation system. This system also evokes aggressive behavior in males, such as patrolling and combat as well as various forms of aggression (De Vries & Villalba, 1999; Numan & Sheehan, 1999). Vasopressin also increases blood pressure and affects heart function (Carter, 1998a), effects which support the aggressive aspects of vasopressin activity.

Male rats ordinarily have higher vasopressin levels and more vasopressin-sensitive neurons than females (Guillamon & Segovia, 1997) and are more likely to kill any new infants they meet (Del Cerro, 1998; Panksepp, 1998). Male rats have more neurons in the medial preoptic area (mPOA) of the hypothalamus (De Vries & Villalba, 1999), but nurturing rat fathers show a decline in mPOA neurons (Del Cerro, 1998). This is a particularly interesting result because it suggests that fathers have a natural caregiving motivation system that is initially suppressed by the mPOA and perhaps other systems. Thus fathers must overcome these inhibitions to become caregiving fathers.

Stranger rejection and its suppression have important sociological implications. Human fear and rejection of strangers has extremely deep evolutionary roots. Thus, ethnic and other distrust, competition and violence are biologically primed in humans, especially in human males. Such stranger rejection circuits probably account for the greater level of anger and status-based competition and aggression among men compared with women. However, unlike reptiles whose stranger rejection in uncontrolled, humans share with other mammals neurological processes that can counteract stranger rejection.

Inhibition of stranger rejection. There are several candidate mechanisms for inhibiting stranger rejection, but it is not as yet known for sure which effects are direct and which are indirect. One of the candidates for the inhibition of stranger rejection is oxytocin. As vasopressin evolved from vasotocin and carried out its stranger rejection functions, oxytocin also evolved from vasotocin. Vasopressin and oxytocin are chemically similar and each can activate the other's receptor sites at reduced efficiency (Carter, 1998a; Panksepp, 1998). Oxytocin appears to reduce stranger rejection by operating on the mPOA through the amygdala and the bed nucleus of the stria terminalis (BNST) (Kendrick, et al., 1997; Wellman, et al., 1997). Projections from the mPOA to the ventromedial nucleus (VMN) and the septum inhibit aggressive behaviors (Numan & Sheehan, 1999). One mechanism within the inhibition process may involve chemically preventing messages of strange odors from reaching the amygdala. Infusions of oxytocin into the olfactory bulb of sheep reduce rejection behaviors (Kendrick, et al., 1997). Injection of oxytocin into virgin wild mice suppresses infanticide. For both mice and voles, in those species where both males and females nurture the young, the size of the mPOA is about the same size in males and females, while in species where only mothers nurture, the mPOA of males is larger (De Vries & Villalba, 1999; Gubernick & Kurz, 1993). It has been speculated that oxytocin produced during sex may explain why male mice are least likely to attack young around three weeks after mating, which coincides with the expected time of birth of the infant (Panksepp, 1998).

In addition to oxytocin, there may be several other neurotransmitters which have a role in inhibiting stranger rejection. Part of the complexity comes because at the same time the parent's rejection of the offspring is inhibited, the parent's defensive rejection of other adults (who might threaten the offspring or the nest), and even of the infants of other mothers, is heightened (Vom Saal & Parmigiani, 1995). Other potential candidates for inhibition of stranger rejection are norepinephrine (Nelson & Panksepp, 1998) and serotonin (Insel & Winslow, 1998). Inhibiting stranger rejection is critical before caregiving behaviors can be initiated. This is not only logically true, but has been empirically demonstrated. Procedures in rodents that increase infanticide toward strange pups (that is, procedures that either increase stranger rejection or decrease its inhibition) tend to reduce parental caregiving behaviors (Panksepp, 1998).

The inhibition of stranger rejection is thus produced by one or more of the above systemic neuropeptides. Blood from a female rat who has just given birth transfused into a virgin female leads to maternal behaviors in the virgin rat (Panksepp, 1998). The suppression of the stranger rejection response appears to have a lasting effect in mother rats (Del Cerro, 1998). First-time (primiparous) rat mothers apparently take longer to inhibit stranger rejection before they can bond to their pups; multiparous rat mothers bond much more quickly.

Dyadic preference. As discussed in the previous chapter, it was not enough for the emergence of mammals that reptilian mothers stop killing their young—they needed to come to prefer them. This preference took the form of an unconscious emotional dyadic preference in the parent toward the child, a preference whose predictable result was to keep the child near. There is consensus that the neurotransmitter associated with this preference is oxytocin (Keverne, et al., 1999; Maestripieri, 1999; Panksepp, 1998) acting as a transmitter from the main olfactory bulb to the paraventricular nucleus of the hypothalamus (PVN). Oxytocin is synthesized in two areas in the hypothalamus (Carter, 2005; Insel, et al., 1999; Panksepp, 1998; Uvnäs Moberg, 2003). In many mammalian species, the emotional bond is associated with a preference for the smell of the offspring (Kendrick, 2000). There are more oxytocin receptors in the brains of the social prairie vole compared to the solitary mountain vole

(Nelson & Panksepp, 1998), and female mammals tend to have more oxytocin-producing neurons than males (Del Cerro, 1998; Nelson & Panksepp, 1998). In the days before and just after giving birth, the mother's brain creates more oxytocin receptors and more hypothalamic neurons to create oxytocin. In addition, the oxytocin-producing cells begin to work together. Oxytocin is released in women during birth and nursing and in all humans with close personal contact and interaction (Carter, 1998a; Hrdy, 1999, 2005; Insel, et al., 1999; Panksepp, 1998). Mothers who deliver vaginally have higher levels of oxytocin than mothers who deliver by C-section (Nissen, et al., 1996). Mothers who have skin-to-skin contact with their infants immediately after birth bond with them more strongly (Klaus, et al., 1972). Furthermore, oxytocin is provided to the infant in the mother's milk and is further produced in the infant as a result of being held. Oxytocin in this way promotes development of a close relationship. Greater mother-child physical contact increases the production of oxytocin over the child's life course, which is associated with more rapid formation of pair bonds (Carter, 2003). Oxytocin thus initiates bonding, the active dyadic preference for a known partner in rats, prairie voles, sheep, and humans (Carter, 1998a; Insel, et al., 1999; Nelson & Panksepp, 1998; Panksepp, 1998; Young & Wang, 2004).

Oxytocin reduces anxiety levels in general, at least partly by causing the release of endogenous opioids. In human mothers, oxytocin levels are associated with decreased anxiety, an increased desire to please, and increased social interaction (Uvnäs-Moberg, 1998, 1999). Formation of a dyadic emotional bond reduces stress and improves one's sense of well-being (Maestripieri, 1999; Sachser, Dürslag, & Hirzel, 1998). Mitani and Watts (1997) note that among primates, older siblings who remain in their natal groups tend to care for their younger siblings. One consequence of this "allocaretaking" is that mothers feed infants better under these arrangements (probably because they experience less stress). The quality of maternal nurturance in humans appears to be reduced by the level of fatigue and increased by spousal and other social support (Fleming & Anderson, 1987).

Although mammalian females are closely associated with parental caregiving, oxytocin is not produced just in females. Sexual experiences in male rats increase oxytocin levels, reduce aggression, and make them more nurturant (Carter, 1998a; Panksepp, 1998; Uvnäs-Moberg, 1998). The bonding process takes longer in nonmothers than in mothers: several days longer for mice (Del Cerro, 1998), several weeks longer for primates (Mason & Mendoza, 1998), and several months longer for humans

(Maestripieri, 1999). The bonding of a biological mother to her child can occur almost immediately or can take several weeks (Fleming & Anderson, 1987; Robson & Kumar, 1980).

Both oxytocin and vasopressin are involved in live births (as vasotocin induces egg laying in reptiles, so do oxytocin and vasopressin promote uterine contraction in mammals). Oxytocin, already part of the muscle contraction and pain management systems involved in egg laying and then live births, also was adapted to the mammary system. Oxytocin, stimulated by the infant's sucking at the nipple, is known to regulate the milk letdown response (Panksepp, 1998). This association of oxytocin with the nipple eventually generalized to other touching and even non-touching social interaction. Touching is associated with the release of oxytocin in humans and other mammals (Carter, 1998a; Uvnäs-Moberg, 1998) and with feelings of sociality in human mothers (Carter, 1998a; Montagu, 1986). Without continued physical and social stimulation from the infant, the caregiving bond declines (Fleming & Anderson, 1987).

The caregiving motivation system

As we saw in the previous chapter, dyadic preference, while important for maintaining the proximity of parent and child, is not enough to produce protection, support, or teaching. A caregiving motivation system, growing out of the dyadic emotional preference, produces these behaviors. Furthermore, as it has developed, the caregiving system has become at least partially independent of the original dyadic preference. While oxytocin is the central neurotransmitter in the creation of a dyadic preference, oxytocin is not required in the same way for the operation of the caregiving system. When an oxytocin antagonist is given to a rat mother (Russell & Leng, 1998) or sheep mother (Carter, 1998a) at birth, no dyadic preference forms. If the oxytocin antagonist is given after a dyadic preference has formed in a rat, caregiving behaviors are still performed (Kendrick, et al., 1997). Once an oxytocin-based emotional bond has formed between mother and child, the removal of oxytocin-producing neurons does not eliminate parenting behaviors (De Vries & Villalba, 1999; Panksepp, 1998; Russell & Leng, 1998).

Even if oxytocin is not required for caregiving, it still seems to play a large part in the normal operation of the caregiving system. Oxytocin produced by the supraoptic nucleus (SON) and PVN of the hypothalamus is projected throughout the subcortical brain, especially the ventral tegmental area (VTA) and nucleus accumbens, resulting in the release of the opiate dopamine (Carter, 1998a; Gingrich, Liu, Cascio, Wang, & Insel,

2000; Keverne, et al., 1999; Uvnäs-Moberg, 1998; Vernotica & Morrell, 1999; Young, Wang, & Insel, 1998). An opiate antagonist reduces grooming, nurturing and protecting of infant rhesus monkeys. The opiate antagonist does not, however, reduce nursing, which appears to be under separate endocrinological control. One of the effects of dopamine appears to be that it operates to reinforce and consolidate memories of the partner (Carter, 1998a). Chemical disruption of the dopamine system in the nucleus accumbens apparently interferes with the storage of memories of caregiving behaviors (Lee, Li, Watchus, & Fleming, 1999). The dopamine effect is the same effect that is tapped by most addictive drugs. However, although a person may receive some of the same "high" that cocaine or heroin provide, caregiving does not become "addictive." This is because the oxytocin has another very useful function. Oxytocin inhibits tolerance to opioids (Kovács, Sarnyai, & Szabó, 1998; Panksepp, 1998). This means that, unlike cocaine and heroin that produce a high by producing or releasing dopamine but that then prevent the reuptake of dopamine (so that more and more of the drug is required to give the same effect), oxytocin prevents the blockage of dopamine reuptake and thus allows the "high" of caregiving to continue over time without habituation.

In evolution, the beginning of the caregiving motivation system probably involved oxytocin release from the PVN (initiated by nursing) that activated the dopamine system associated with the dyadic bond (Panksepp, 1998). By reinforcement, the enjoyment to the mother from nursing assured that nursing would continue (Hrdy, 1999). In early mammals, that was probably it. However, as the neocortex grew, the dopamine release associated with nursing became a secondary reinforcement of helping the child. Specific attributes of the dyadic partner become conditioned stimuli that will deepen the relationship (LeDoux, 1996). The strength of the emotion (and its associated feeling) is likely to increase with greater physical exposure. Proximity and strength of emotion are thus linked, so that more of the feeling is likely to lead to more proximity and more proximity is likely to lead to more feeling (Montagu, 1986). Later other subcortical processes probably developed to support the caregiving motivation system.

The growth of the caregiving motivation system occurs with the laying down of emotion neurons (LeDoux, 1996; Panksepp, 1998). For example, the oxytocin transmitted to the hippocampus stimulates the creation of social memories (Carter, 1998b; Nelson & Panksepp, 1998; Panksepp, 1998). These memories become a part of the caregiving internal working model. In species with consciousness, the unconscious emotion of caring gives rise to conscious feelings of preference toward the child, feelings that the other's presence is pleasurable. These feelings are probably formulated in the ventromedial sectors of the prefrontal cortex (Panksepp, 1998).

The primary addition of this hypothetical model of a caregiving motivation system over previous work on caregiving in the attachment tradition is its ability to identify an emotional motivator for caregiving. In addition, this hypothetical model locates the emotional motivator in the hypothalamus. As Izard (1993) points out, either emotions (like joy, sadness, anger, or fear) or drives (like hunger, thirst, fatigue, or sex) can serve as motivators for action. A particular advantage of conceptualizing an emotion motivator for a motivation system is that identifying the emotion or the drive helps to identify the set goal. For example, if the drive is thirst, then the set goal is to achieve adequate water. If the emotion is fear, the set goal is safety. The nature of the caring emotion can also be used to identify the caregiving set goal of meeting the needs of the partner (see Chapter 5).

The attachment motivation system

The fear process is particularly relevant to Bowlby's model of attachment, because Bowlby's prototypical attachment metaphor is the child confronted by a predator (Bowlby, 1969/1982). An adult confronted by a fox or other small to medium sized predator will experience an immediate fear response from the sight of the predator and will immediately look for a weapon and/or run or back away carefully. A child will do something different. Instead of looking for a weapon, the child will look for a caregiver. The child may run to mother or call for father. At first glance, this attachment behavior appears to be parallel to the adult's search for a weapon. The child could be choosing an adult as the analog of a weapon. The child, however, does not choose the most competent adult. The child does not "evaluate" the situation, select a competent adult, and act. Instead the child calls immediately and automatically for Mom or Dad or whoever has cared for the child. The child's emotional fear response is directed toward a specific person who has provided nurturance in the past.

The neurobiology of distress attachment

A simplified depiction of the attachment motivation system emerging from neurobiological research is given in Figure 4.8.[3] The fear system

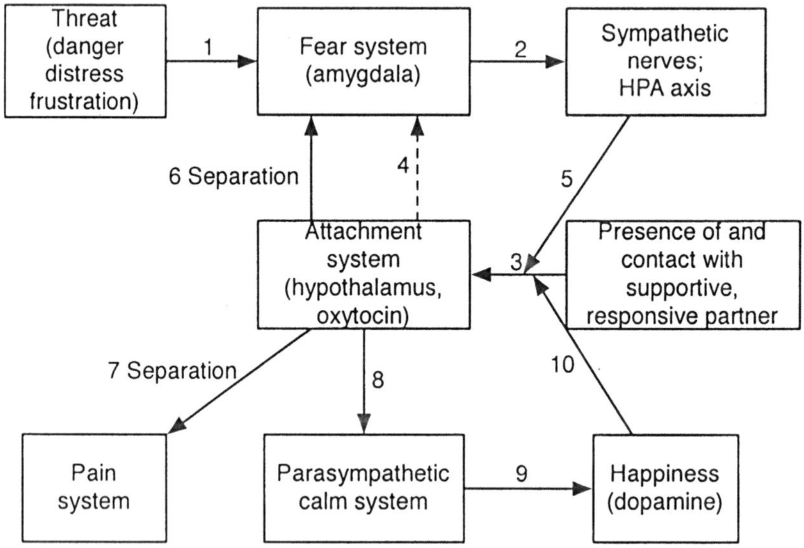

Figure 4.8. Neurobiological Map of the Attachment Motivation System

continuously assesses environmental threat (arrow 1). Safety has always been an issue for mammals, including humans. The earliest mammals were small animals surrounded by large, and in fact enormous, predators. The fear system is centered on the central nucleus of the amygdala (Carter, 1998a; Damasio, 1994; LeDoux, 1996). With the detection of actual or potential threat, the fear system activates two related systems (arrow 2).

First, the fear system activates the fast-acting sympathetic nerves (Porges, 2005): adrenaline is released, the heart rate increases, muscles tense, and respiration, scanning, and vigilance increase. Second, the amygdala activates the longer-lasting hypothalamic-pituitary-adrenal stress system (the HPA axis) which controls reactions to stress and regulates the immune system and moods (Panksepp, 1998). Thus, the body is prepared for a fight-or-flight response. The fight-or-flight response may be enhanced in interaction with androgen and thus is more easily activated in males (Taylor, 2006).

It has been shown that, in a variety of species, the presence of a bonded partner (arrow 3: an attachment figure in the human literature) inhibits the fear process (arrow 4, shown as a dashed arrow because of its inhibiting effect), at least under moderate levels of fear and uncertainty (Carter, 2005; Sachser, 2005; Sachser, et al., 1998). These are not just immediate effects. Infant monkeys raised without a mother to down-regulate their fear system show a lifetime increase in fear and depression (Harlow & Harlow, 1965). Fear reduction is achieved by oxytocin, which inhibits the fear system in the amygdala and thus down-regulates the HPA axis to relieve stress (Carter, 1998a; Uvnäs-Moberg, 1998) as well as the sympathetic nervous system to reduce adrenalin and other fight-or-flight responses. In general, fear-induced fight-or-flight defense systems are inhibited when a person feels safe (Porges, 2005). Hazan and colleagues (2006, p. 55) refer to this effect as "the attenuation of arousal responses to threats and stressors."

Contrary to some assertions of Bowlbian attachment theory, which imply that only bonded partners moderate the fear system, non-bonded familiar partners also show effects on the fear system. Familiar partners who are not bonded (that is, who do not generate separation distress) also reduce fear, although the reduction is not as immediate as it is with bonded partners (Uvnäs Moberg, 2003). In guinea pigs (Hennessy, 1999; Sachser, et al., 1998) and squirrel monkeys (Hennessy & Kaplan, 1982), surrogate mothers act like familiar partners, but not like bonded partners. Gump and colleagues (2001) found that female college students had higher stress responses (higher blood pressure) when they experienced a stressor with a stranger than with a romantic partner. Such a differential response did not occur, however, when the stranger was supportive (Carpenter & Kirkpatrick, 1996). Bonded partners may be preferred, but persons under stress are likely to turn even to relative strangers (Shaver & Klinnert, 1982). Fontana and colleagues (1999) found supportive strangers to be as effective as friends in reducing the stress response.

The cardinal assumption of Bowlby's attachment model, that the fear system activates the attachment system (arrow 5), has been verified by extensive research (Carter, 1998a; Insel, 1997; Panksepp, 1998). Taylor and colleagues (2006) found that adult women with lower levels of contact with their social network (and thus presumably higher separation distress) had higher levels of oxytocin. This is what Taylor (2002) refers to as the "tend and befriend" response to distress. Simpson, Rholes & Nelligan (1992) found that for female undergraduates who expected a stressful experience, level of anxiety was associated with the level of seeking comfort from their male romantic partners. Note, however, that the fear system only activates an existing attachment system by this route—it does not create attachment neurons.

We have seen that the attachment system reduces the fear response (arrow 4). Other evidence suggests that fear, in turn, can promote attachment bonding through the stress system (arrow 5). Adrenal steroids associated with fear and other stressful experiences appear to facilitate the formation of a bond (Carter, 2005; Montagu, 1986). These findings suggest that persons who are under stress are more susceptible to developing new relationships. This may be the process observed in the Stockholm syndrome, where prisoners develop bonds to their captors, as well as in other forms of abuse (Crittenden, 1995; DeLosier, 1982).

One of the defining characteristics of attachment is that separation from an attachment partner is distressful. Panksepp's (1998) review of the neurobiology evidence shows that separation distress has two components. First, separation increases fear (arrow 6). Brain scans show that the amygdala and related areas are highly active when people experience social exclusion, a form of social separation (Eisenberger, Gable, & Lieberman, 2007). This effect of separation is described in the attachment literature in terms of insecurity. Once an attachment bond has formed to a partner, separation not only activates the fear system (arrow 6); it also reduces the inhibition of the fear system (arrow 4) (Panksepp, 1998).

However, separation does not always activate the fear system. In squirrel monkeys, separated juvenile and adult female squirrel monkeys showed elevated levels of vocalization, indicating an activation of the attachment system. However, no activation of the fear system occurred as indicated by a lack of excess production of cortisol, a marker for fear and anxiety (Mendoza & Mason, 1999). In guinea pigs, if the pup is in a familiar or safe environment, maternal separation does not induce a fear-stress response (Hennessy, Hornschuh, Kaiser, & Sachser, 2006).

The second effect of separation from an attachment partner comes largely from non-fear circuits (Panksepp, 1998). Separation leads to activation of parts of the attachment circuit in the periaqueductal gray, in an area where physical pain processing occurs (arrow 7) (Eisenberger, et al., 2007; Eisenberger, Lieberman, & Williams, 2003; Panksepp, 2003). Thus the painful feelings of grief that Bowlby (1980) described in persons who lost an attachment partner are more than just metaphorical pain (Panksepp, 1998).

The neurobiology of nondistress attachment

As Panksepp (1998) points out in his summary of research on the neurobiology of emotions, social comforting is the positive side of the same coin for which separation distress is the negative side. Bowlby also noted that the attachment motivational system is a bifurcated system: attachment behavior is "activated by fatigue or illness as well as by a situation that causes fear" (Bowlby, 1973, p. 90). In this view of the attachment system, the caregiver can be both "comforter and protector" (Bowlby, 1973, p. 201). In addition to high intensity attachment characterized by clinging, rapid locomotion, and crying, Bowlby also identified a "low intensity" version of attachment characterized by "smiling, relaxed locomotion, watching, and touching" (1969/1982, p. 250). Low intensity attachment is soothing and comforting (Mikulincer, 2006); there is a focus on "being understood and accepted" (Rothbaum & Kakinuma, 2004, p. 36). This operation of the attachment system leads a child to respond to caregiving behaviors such as rocking and being talked to with contentment (Bowlby, 1969/1982, p. 294) or comfort (Bowlby, 1973, p. 180). Low intensity attachment produces emotions of joy, love, happiness, and pleasure. In adulthood, this form of attachment leads one "to collaborate with [another] person in such a way that a mutually rewarding relationship is initiated" (Bowlby, 1979, p. 104).

In addition to "high intensity" stress reactions that act to reduce fear by involvement with a caregiving partner, neurobiological research has verified a parallel "low intensity" attachment process that is not a reaction to fear and distress. The attachment system also operates on the parasympathetic nervous system (arrow 8) (Uvnäs-Moberg, 1997). Independent of its effects on the fear system, neurons using oxytocin as a neurotransmitter extend from the attachment system in the medial hypothalamus to the parasympathetic system and produce calming effects (Porges, 1998; Uvnäs-Moberg, 1998).

Activation of the parasympathetic system results in a drop in blood pressure, a slowing of the heart rate, and in general produces calm (Porges, 2005). Levels of oxytocin are associated with lowered blood pressure in humans, as well as with self reported number of hugs in a monogamous couple, although only for women (Grewen, Girdler, Amico, & Light, 2005; Light, Grewen, & Amico, 2005). As we have seen, breastfeeding women produce oxytocin at high rates: such women are calmer and show increased levels of social interaction compared to bottle-feeding women (Uvnäs-Moberg, 1998). In a study of cohabiting and married couples, blood pressure monitors were worn for a week (Gump, et al., 2001). The researchers found that, compared to interacting with a person who was not a significant other, interacting with a spouse or other significant other was associated with lower blood pressure, less arousal as well as greater intimacy and emotional support (Gump, et al., 2001). Significant partner and non-significant partner interactions were seen as equally negative, positive, instrumentally supportive, and with equal strain, so it does not appear that the non-significant partner interactions were more stressful than significant partner interactions.

These findings show how the oxytocin of the attachment system produces calm independently of fear and distress. The nondistress attachment system creates short term and long term calm, contentment, relaxation, and dyadic trust and love (Uvnäs-Moberg, Arn, & Magnusson, 2005). While the activation of the HPA axis of the sympathetic nervous system can facilitate an attachment bond (arrow 5), parasympathetic activation also facilitates an attachment bond. Panksepp (1998, p. 223) uses reinforcement terminology to describe how the attachment system provides "satisfying feelings of social gratification" in the presence of the partner (arrow 9). In this way, "comfort seeking" reinforces the attachment bond, creating "a conditioned association between the mother and feelings of security" (Hazan, et al., 2006, p. 55). Hazan and colleagues suggest that this association conditions a person to prefer a calming partner (see also Carter, 1998a). Thus, the rewarding experience of the attachment-driven calming system acts to maintain and strengthen attachment relationships (arrow 10).

As well as occurring separately, nondistress attachment can also occur alongside security attachment. A number of attachment researchers have noted that the reduction of fear has a soothing effect (Mikulincer & Shaver, 2007).

Boundaries of caregiving and attachment

There is a good bit of confusion in the attachment literature about nondistress attachment. On the one hand, a number of authoritative accounts have claimed that attachment terminology should be restricted to the joint fear-attachment system (Ainsworth, 1989; Berman & Sperling, 1994; Cassidy, 1999; Mikulincer & Shaver, 2007; Simpson & Rholes, 2000). Bowlby himself drew a boundary around the protection/safety function of fear-attachment and explicitly excluded behaviors and motivations with other functions, such as feeding, play, and companionship (Bowlby, 1969/1982). Within the traditional conceptualization of attachment as associated with fear and distress, when the child is hungry, she is seen to go to the parent for food under the control of her hunger system. When thirsty, she is seen to go to the parent for a drink under the control of her thirst system. When she wants a toy to play with, she is seen to go to the parent under the control of her play system. When she wants to explore, she looks to the parent as "secure base," but the exploration is motivated by the exploration system.

On the other hand, we have seen above that Bowlby also described a form of attachment that is not activated by fear. Of the emotions Bowlby lists that accompany attachment, anxiety, sorrow, anger, and security can be linked to fear-attachment. Other stimuli that lead to attachment behaviors, hunger, cold, fatigue, illness, and unhappiness (Bowlby, 1969/1982, pp. 203, 258) are not generally related to fear. They are most likely to reflect discomfort rather than distress. Nondistress attachment is consistent with love and joy (Bowlby, 1969/1982, p. 209) as well as intense pleasure (Bowlby, 1969/1982, p. 242), emotions that are not easily linked to fear. When the child smiles and babbles and the parent strokes, pats, and hugs the child, both partners are expressing joy (Bowlby, 1969/1982, p. 246).

Bowlby also described many of the cognitive components in the attachment process. He identified the internal working model in the person that contains a cognitive representation of the partner and the relationship. Children and adults tell us of their *feelings* of safety and trust with a caregiver. What has been missing, however, both physiologically and functionally, has been a description of the *emotion*, largely unconscious, that accesses the attachment internal working model and produces attachment behaviors and feelings. Equally missing has been an account of the largely unconscious emotional processes of caregiving. Work I have summarized in this chapter provide the beginnings of an understanding of the physiological mechanisms that underlie caregiving and attachment. There is clear evidence for specialized caregiving and attachment neural pathways and processes in the brain.

In the next chapters, theoretical descriptions of caregiving, attachment, and related processes will be developed.

Notes

* Portions of this chapter appear in Bell and Richard (2000a), Bell (2001), and Bell, Brown and Montoya (2004).

1. There are other potential metaphors of human contact. However, I clearly do not mean the metaphor of hitting, control and dominance.

2. One could of course use "cognitive" for all information processing in the brain, but then "cognitive" would be simply a synonym for "brain." All emotions require information processing (for example, you have to identify that thing as a snake—or at least a potential snake—before you are afraid of it: e.g., Damasio, 1994). The sole purpose of the emotion-cognition distinction I make here is to be able to distinguish the "emotional" desire to avoid the snake from the "cognitive" decision of where to run. There has been a debate for some time among psychological action theorists about the relative primacy of motivation and cognition (Gollwitzer & Bargh, 1996). Much of the dispute in this debate, it seems to me, stems from linguistic questions about how to use words rather than psychological questions about processes in the body and brain. The definitions used here are not necessarily better than other definitions, but they help us get on with the goal of creating theory. My advice to readers who do not like my use of "emotion" is to substitute the term "motivation."

3. A more detailed discussion of this biological model is given in Bell (2009a).

Chapter 5. Caregiving

The focus in this chapter and the next is on dyadic relationships. This chapter describes the caregiving theoretical orientation. This chapter builds on the evolutionary and neurobiological evidence of the previous chapters to develop a psychological model of the caregiving motivation system. Extending Bowlby's concept of a caregiving system, this chapter reviews evidence showing how the dyadic emotion of caring produces empathy (the intention to know the partner, called "sensitivity" in Bowlby's scheme), and responsibility (the intention to meet the partner's needs, called "responsiveness"). These proactive intentions in turn explain parental and other dyadic nurturance.

Let's imagine a human parent who hears a cry from an infant offspring; it is the startled cry when the infant encounters a snake. The incident of the child and the snake is exactly the kind of incident that Bowlby means as the prototype of survival-related caregiving and retrieval. When the parent hears that cry, the parent experiences the classic signs of fear, including an adrenaline rush and heightened attention. However, the parent does not generally move away from the snake like a lizard would. Instead the parent moves to the child even though this may mean moving toward the snake at the same time. The parent is not exclusively or even predominantly motivated by a self-focused fear emotion here. Of course, if the snake is big enough and the parent's fear of the snake is great enough, the parent may be overwhelmed by this fear and may be unable to approach the child. But in the case where the parent's fear of the snake is small to moderate, and thus manageable, the parent may even attract the attention of the snake toward the parent and away from the child. The system that is activated in the parent when the child is threatened is fear for the child rather than the parent's self-fear.

It is clear, of course, that something is occurring alongside of fear in the example of the child and the snake that motivates the parent to protect the child. Consider other examples of parental nurturance in which the fear system is not activated. For example, a young child comes to the parent and holds both hands up. The parent responds by picking up and holding the child. Or the child shows signs of sadness, such as crying, and the parent responds by holding and comforting the child. Or the child says, "come see," and the parent goes to see. In each of these cases the parent and child have increased their proximity. But there are other cases. The cranky child says, "go away," and the parent leaves the child out of respect for the child's feelings. Or the child may indicate hunger by asking verbally, by sucking her thumb, or by whimpering or crying, and the parent responds by leaving the room to go prepare a meal.

In Chapter 1, I examined many of the self interest theoretical orientations and some social bond theoretical orientations that have been used to construct theories of parental nurturance. I do not consider any of the self interest explanations to account adequately for caregiving, neither reciprocity nor social norms nor any of the others. As indicated above, these explanations are logically unpersuasive. In addition, they violate the subjective experience of the caregiver. Instead of viewing caregiving as self interest in disguise, the view presented here looks to an emotional motivator that produces caregiving. Chapter 2 examined in detail how John Bowlby applied a functional logic to derive a theory of the evolution of attachment and a cybernetic theory of the child's relationship to the parent. We saw, in fact, that there are a number of cybernetic theories of attachment. The examination showed how, in spite of its success in accounting for the child's attachment behavior, the attachment approach has not provided an adequate theoretical account of the parental (caregiving) side of the parent-child relationship. Chapter 3 showed how a caregiving motivation system had to have evolved in mammals before attachment and how stages in the evolution of the caregiving system correspond to the different versions of caregiving logic. Chapter 4 explored the neurobiological basis for parental nurturance and showed how the human caregiving motivation system is built on top of an earlier premammalian system for dyadic preference.

It is not enough to identify neurobiological structures and processes to explain behavior such as parental nurturance. If one remains at this level of explanation, then the behavior of humans as well as other animals is taken as "caused" rather than "authored." Humans and other animals are taken as objects rather than purposive subjects of their own lives.

> [A] technical-causal language of behavior extinguishes authorship from the animal world, or alternatively translocates it onto causes that are theoretically identified—for example, neurophysiological mechanisms, environmental stimuli, or genetic programs. An experiential outlook upon the world is swept aside, for its existence has no role to play in the production of action. Animals become portrayed as vessels steered by forces they neither control nor comprehend, and as a consequence, behaviors emerge as events that happen to animals, rather than as active achievements (Crist, 1999, p. 203).

This loss of authorship can also occur in theory about human behavior if explanation remains at the genetic or neurobiological levels. In this chapter, I am going to explore the human psychological dynamics of the brain circuit associated with caregiving in all mammals.

CAREGIVING AS AN ACTION SYSTEM

The volitional nature of motivation is of critical importance in systems such as those that create parental nurturance. The concept of volition involves two issues of importance here. First, volition involves a recognition that an actor is the author of action. That is, actors make choices. While it might be convenient to say at the neurobiological level that one motivation system "inhibits" another (as attachment was said to inhibit fear in the previous chapter), in fact in most cases actors make choices (I'm angry, but I'm still going to be polite; I love my child, but I'm not going to give her candy for dessert; I'm afraid, but I'm still going to protect my child). The second aspect of volition is that it presupposes motivations as variable. Parents often choose to lower the activation level of their own self interest seeking motivation system and increase the strength of their caregiving system because a child has needs that the parent decides must be met. Thus individuals make continual choices, whether to nurture the partner at all or to protect the self, whether to nurture a child or a spouse, how much to nurture, whether to nurture overtly or covertly, whether to say "yes" to gratify a child's desire for candy or to say "no" to meet the child's need for healthy nutrition, and so on.

In the connection theoretical system, caregiving and attachment are considered to be action systems. Action is a more inclusive concept than behavior. In general, social scientists give behavior a common-sense meaning: it is any human movement that we can see. Action, however is a more complex concept. Action, like behavior, is something that people do. But not all behaviors count as actions and not all actions are behaviors. For some philosophers, only those behaviors that result from thoughtful deliberation directed toward a purpose count as action (e.g., Aune, 1977); for other philosophers, action is what "an agent does, as opposed to what happens to an agent (or what happens inside an agent's head)" (Blackburn, 1994, p. 5). For some sociologists, only those behaviors count as action that are directed toward a social goal (e.g., Alexander, 1988; Parsons, 1937) or behavior that is rationally motivated (Borgatta & Borgatta, 1992). Action, moreover, is not just observable physical behavior. Sometimes action includes unobservable things like thoughts. For some authors, thoughts seem to be outside of action (e.g., Aune, 1977). For other authors, some thoughts are included within action, especially thoughts that embody social norms and cultural values (e.g., Parsons, 1937, 1951).

For my purposes, I will consider action to include motivations and intentions as well as behaviors (see Bell, 2008 for a more extensive discussion of action and action systems). In this usage, action involves caused behavior. Action thus includes both behavior and the causes of behavior (e.g., Habermas, 1981). Thus behaviors and other things that are not observable behaviors, like thoughts and emotions, become actions when we conceive of them causally in relation to behaviors (Giddens, 1979). An action system, as I will use the concept, consists of motivation, intention, and behavior.

Motivation. The most important question in an action system is one of motivation. As described in the previous chapters, the motivations of interest here are emotions.[1] Motivations are conceptualized as basic "movers" and fundamental causes of behavior. They are what "move" the agent, who causes the action (Linton, 1945; Taylor, 1966). Motivation conceptually turns "behavior" into "action." Motivation provides the emotional energy for action. Motivations vary over time for a given actor. At one time we look after our own interests (self interest motivation is high), at another time we care for another (caregiving motivation is high). Furthermore, motivations vary across actors. Some people are more self-interested than others; some people are more active caregivers than others. The formulation of an action system considered here makes explicit the importance of emotion (and thus motivation) as a variable concept.[2]

Intention. The causal mediator between emotional motivation and behavior is found in intention. A given motivation leads the actor to formulate intentions. Intentions are taken as variable concepts that refer to conscious or unconscious processes that help to implement the goals of the motivation. Intentions may be conscious (within the actor's awareness, often called "volition" or "will"), unconscious (generally outside the actor's awareness, like strategies that repress painful memories), or nonconscious (without the actor's awareness, including some pain instincts and some processes of calculating the values of rewards).

Behavior. Behaviors are the end-points of action. In the action systems I describe, behaviors are seen as variables. I am interested in explaining a parent's amount of nurturance, the frequency with which a husband supports his wife, the level of encouragement from one friend to another.

The caregiving theoretical orientation, as we will see, provides a conception of caregiving that is more phenomenologically grounded than Bowlby's cybernetic model. As a behaviorist, Bowlby focused his cybernetic models of caregiving and attachment on behavioral outcomes rather than internal psychological processes. Internally, he only described appraisal and cognitive comparison processes. Bowlby's cybernetic view of caregiving thus treated the caregiving motivation system as a cognitive process with no explicit internal emotion (Bowlby, 1969/1982). First, according to Bowlby, the caregiver completes an appraisal of the stimulus, "appraising the baby as something to be comforted. . . . as something to be ignored or even as something to be shouted at" (1969/1982, pp. 116-117). Appraising the baby as "something to be comforted" activates the security caregiving behavioral control system in the caregiver to comfort the baby. In this process of appraisal, information is the major determinant of behavior (Sroufe & Waters, 1977). There is no explicit description of an emotion or other motivation within the caregiver that motivates the caregiving behavior. There is no particular reason to believe that Bowlby intended the caregiving process to be seen as purely cognitive. However, he didn't specify any emotions internal to the "black box" of the caregiving system. The only emotions he explicitly described were *outcomes* of the caregiving process, not *components* of it (see Chapter 2).

Bretherton's (1980) and Hinde's (1982) characterization of behavioral control systems as computer programs extends this purely cognitive view of caregiving. As far as the published cybernetic model of the attachment system is concerned, attachment and caregiving behavioral control systems operate as a result of biological and environmental stimuli without explicit volitional control (Bell & Richard, 2000b). Bowlby is aware in his clinical descriptions that the determinants of attachment and caregiving behavior are complex, and he shows that parents can be and are proactive in nurturing their children, but he does not bring any explicit concept of voluntary motivation into his cybernetic model, where action is mechanistically governed by a discrepancy between the current state and the set goal.

Within the model of caregiving proposed here, ego's emotional motivation takes center stage. There can be at any time an inherent conflict between ego's emotional motivation to meet alter's needs and ego's motivation of seeking self interest. To clarify this conflict, we must conceptualize how caregiving behavior arises from an autonomous motivation that can successfully compete with self interest seeking.

THE CAREGIVING THEORETICAL ORIENTATION

Turner (1991) has shown the importance of considering motivation in the explanation of any social interaction. One way motivation has been conceptualized is as need. If a person has a need, then the person's behavior can be explained by the need. Turner shows how a large part of social science theory imports (and often smuggles) concepts of need, from need for survival, to need for freedom and for cooperation, to need for a sense of reality or need for human contact, to need for sex and for sustenance. Emotion theorists have long claimed that emotions are responses to needs (Greenberg & Safran, 1987; Maslow, 1971; Ortony, et al., 1988; Plutchik, 1984). Maslow says that basic needs are

> objectively and subjectively perceivable demands or wishes [that must] be gratified or else illness (or diminution of humanness, i.e., loss of some of the characteristics that define humanness) would result (Maslow, 1971, p. 365).

Many attachment authors have given needs an important place. Griffin and Bartholomew (1994, p. 430), following Bowlby, describe the "universal human need to form close affectional bonds" (see also Bardwick, 1974; Bowlby, 1977; Van IJzendoorn & Tavecchio, 1987). Fairbairn "highlights the longing, the hunger for contact and connection, that propels human relationships. . . . The child does not *seek* caring connections with others; rather, the very structure of his needs for satisfactions and his responsiveness to anxiety in others pulls him into those connections" (Mitchell, 1988, pp. 28, italics in original). Solomon and George (1996, p. 186) invoke a "need to protect and nurture the child." Shaver and Hazan (1988, p. 479) describe "wanting best for other, wanting to give to other" as "reactions" to feelings of love for the partner. For

Miller, it is wanting to preserve and be in the relationship that is the motivation (Miller, 1991).

However, moving beyond these conceptualizations in terms of actors' own needs, we can see actors in terms of their motivations towards the needs of others. For parents, we see that the parent has a *motivation to meet the needs of the child.*

> Parents want the world for their children. They want their children to be healthy, happy, and independent, to be curious about life, to be loving and responsive, to develop healthy relationships, to feel secure and good about themselves, and to weather difficult life situations (Klaus, et al., 1995, p. xvii).

When we emotionally care for someone, we want them to be happy, to be complete, to be fulfilled, to be successful; we want their needs to be met.

This conceptualization of caregiving as grounded in a motivation to meet the needs of the partner emerges both from the observation of the evolutionary expansion of the caregiving goal from the earliest mammals through humans (Chapter 3), and from the phenomenological experience of parenting and partnering. In addition, although a number of attachment theorists have suggested a more restricted meaning for caregiving (e.g., safety by Heard and Lake, and security by Solomon and George), parents do not just meet the child's safety and security needs. Parents also meet the child's needs for satisfying their self interests, for entertainment, for stimulation and novelty, for learning. The parent meets the child's felt need for distance as well as the felt need for proximity; the child's needs for exploration as well as for protection and holding; for independence as well as for warmth. One might, and some attachment authors do, assert that the term "caregiving" should only be used to describe the parent's behaviors that meet the child's proximity, safety, or security needs, and that other terminology should be used when parents meet other needs. However, the preponderance of the biological evidence suggests that the parent's motivation to protect the child comes from the same brain system as the parent's motivation to feed, clothe, house, teach, and soothe the child.

Within the connection theoretical system, the motivation of the caregiving system is conceptualized as the unconscious emotion of caring. There are three related concepts that should be distinguished: the caregiving bond, the caring emotion, and the feeling of caring.

The caregiving bond

Bowlby and other attachment theorists have had relatively little to say about caregiving and thus little to say about the nature of the affectional bond that governs caregiving. In developing a psychological understanding of the caregiving bond, I want to start at the biological level. Biologically, it is clear that the "bonds" we are speaking of are internal to the individual—not some conceptual entity that exists in the space between two people. The child's attachment bond with her mother is neurologically the number of attachment neurons associated with her mother. The caregiving bond is a similar set of organized neurons in the mother's brain. Thus, the caregiving system exists in the brain of a single person, but this caregiving system is dyadically oriented toward a specific target.

From oxytocin release during the birth process, to oxytocin release as the mother nurses the infant, to oxytocin release as the parent holds the infant, to oxytocin release as the parent looks meaningfully into the infant's eyes and sees a gleam of response—in each of these incidents, neurons in the brain of the parent are created and become organized and consolidated into a dyadic caregiving circuit devoted to this relationship with this child. In this neurobiological view, the caregiving bond can vary from zero, when no caregiving neurons have been organized for a given relationship, to strong. The bond can increase by small or large increments as caregiving neurons are consolidated, or decrease over time as relatively unused neurons atrophy or are consolidated to support a different motivation system. Thus, at a given moment, ego has a certain level of caregiving bond to alter that depends on the density and organization of caregiving neurons devoted to the ego-alter relationship. In most cases, the caregiving bond, both neurological and subjective, remains relatively constant over time periods of weeks, months and even years. In this view, the caregiving bond *is* the caregiving circuit. That is, to have a caregiving bond is to have a caregiving circuit.

> **Definition (biological definition).** Ego's caregiving bond to alter is the level of consolidation of the caregiving neurons in ego's brain related to alter. It may be seen simplistically as the number of caregiving neurons in ego's caregiving neural circuit related to alter.

This definition is not a practical guide for measuring the caregiving bond. For one thing, we do not yet know where all the caregiving neurons are to be found. For another, we certainly have no way of distinguishing between a caregiving neuron for alter, another caregiving neuron related to a different alter, or a third neuron shared by two alters. And it is certainly overly simplistic to assume that the caregiving circuit is undifferentiated and that a count of neurons, if it could be carried out, would necessarily be the correct metric. I am using number of neurons as a conceptual metric to emphasize that a caregiving or other bond, and a caregiving or other motivation system, should be seen as concepts that vary from a theoretical minimum of zero to some biologically maximum amount. Nevertheless, this definition gives a concrete meaning to the caregiving bond, and it allows one to begin thinking about the values that such a bond might take. Furthermore, it should be also be clear in the above definition that a child is not the only person who can be an alter toward whom a bond is formed. Lovers, spouses, siblings, parents, and good friends as well as children can be the "alter" in a caregiving bond. I choose to assume that all relationships have some value of a caregiving bond. For many relationships, the value will be so close to zero as to be undetectable, and for many others the value will be very low. This approach will encourage us to give considerable attention to what is happening in a given relationship as the level of the bond grows until it crosses whatever imaginary line distinguishes a non-bond from an affectional bond.

The emotion of caring

In juxtaposition to the neurological caregiving bond, which refers to the number and consolidation of caregiving neurons, is the caring emotion, which refers to the level of activation of the caregiving circuits. Since the caregiving bond is biologically seen as the number of caregiving neurons, caring is seen as the number of *activated* caregiving neurons. Obviously, if the level of the caregiving bond (related to the number of neurons in the caregiving circuit) is low, the maximum potential activation of the caregiving circuit is low. The level of the caring emotion varies much more rapidly than the caregiving bond, often on a minute-to-minute basis.

> **Definition (biological definition).** Ego's emotion of caring for alter is the level of activation of ego's caregiving neural circuits related to alter.

Caring according to this definition is no more susceptible to direct measurement than is the caregiving bond. This definition encourages the theorist and researcher to think about levels of caring in a given relationship in a given context at a given moment.

A mother may have a very strong (consolidated) caregiving bond to her one-month-old infant, call its level 100 on some arbitrary scale of caring. Yet in a particular moment, for example, while the infant is asleep and Mother is relaxing and being held by her partner, her caring emotion for the infant is low, say 10, simply monitoring (while her attachment system to her partner is activated at a high level). If at the next moment Mother hears what appears to be a cry from Baby; her caring emotion shoots to 100, and she rushes to Baby. If the baby is just hungry, Mother holds and feeds him, and her caring emotion settles in at an unstressed 75. Baby falls asleep nursing and Mother holds him a moment longer, then puts him down. As Mother leaves Baby to sleep, she thinks she ought to shop for a new blanket for him and, her caring emotion at say 40, she goes to write it on her to-do list. Having made this note, her caring emotion reduces again to 10, monitoring for signs from Baby, and she goes about attending to other tasks and other relationships.

We might compare this mother with another mother who also has a one-month-old infant. This mother had a lonely and perhaps painful childhood and in adulthood has few caregiving neurons, say 20 on our imaginary caring scale. Perhaps her caring emotion monitoring her infant is at 2, so she doesn't notice his cries as soon or respond as quickly as the first mother. After identifying her baby's cries, her caring emotion rises to 20, the most she is capable of. Perhaps she is somewhat uncomfortable touching her baby, so she bottle-feeds him, maybe propping up his bottle with a pillow so that she does not have to hold him. As soon as her baby seems satisfied with the bottle, this mother leaves, her caring emotion returning to 2, and she goes about her other activities. In most cases in this book, I will be focusing on the caring emotion, on the level of the emotion, rather than on the caregiving bond, the number of neurons in the caregiving circuit, which define the potential maximum level of the caring emotion.

Caring is, as some authors note, a natural response (Noddings, 1984), a human response (Doi, 1981). I offer this psychological definition of caring.

> **Definition (psychological definition).** Caring is an unconscious emotional preference by an actor (ego) that orients ego toward meeting the needs of the partner (alter). Ego cherishes alter.

Caring is both dyadic and situational. I care about all of my children's needs even though they are now old enough to meet most of them themselves. I care about my students to the extent that they want to learn about sociology and sociological methods; I cherish them in their exploration and self improvement, but I do not feed them or help them pay the rent. Across the many relationships in our lives, both long term and short term, the amount of our caring, and the domains to which our caring applies, vary from one relationship partner to another.

By basing the psychology of caregiving on a variable caregiving bond and its (variable) momentary expression as the emotion of caring, the caregiving theoretical orientation is able to capture and describe the entire development of the caregiving side of a connection relationship from an initial inactive state where the caregiving bond can vary from weak (few neurons) to strong (many neurons). And at any point on that trajectory, we can describe the level of activation of the caregiving system neurons. It may react in an instant to a stimulus, but may also be sustained actively over extended periods of time.

Caring, like all the conceptual variables of the connection processes, is conceived as an unobservable nonnegative ratio concept. That is, caring, as a variable concept, is assumed to have order (more and less), to have equal intervals, and to have a meaningful zero point.[3] Caring thus varies from zero to some high positive value. When ego's caring for alter is at a level of zero, then ego is emotionally nonresponsive to alter, ego is not oriented toward meeting the needs of alter. Ego does not cherish alter. At a high level of caring, ego is emotionally very responsive and open to alter; ego likes alter a lot, perhaps loves alter, and has a lot of warm feelings for alter. While there is a conceptual zero point, there is no conceptual ceiling value. There is presumably some limit on the number of neurons that could embody the caregiving bond to a given alter, but it is not clear how one could ever determine such a number, or to represent "perfect" caring.[4] The concept of caring developed here is not consistent with "negative" caring. As defined, caring cannot take on negative values. I explicitly reject such conceptions as hatred or loathing as the "opposite" or "negative" of caring (Bengtson, Olander, & Haddad, 1976; Lowenthal & Chiriboga, 1975). Concepts such as hatred or dislike are assumed here to be different concepts from caring. They operate by a different logic from caring (probably involving the emotion of anger) and thus are not usefully seen as existing on the same continuum as caring. Also conceptually distinct from caring is the feeling of overprotective control (based on a touching metaphor of grasping rather than caressing, and derived from fear), which may be (falsely) interpreted as caring.

The conscious feeling of caring

Although the emotion of caring is unconscious, awareness of it and of the caregiving bond are embodied in the conscious feeling of caring. Thus, much of the *evidence* for the human emotion of caring and its consequences will involve descriptions of the feeling of caring.

Caring as a conscious feeling can be described metaphorically as contact. Caring involves the feeling of emotional "contact with the soul of another person" (Hillman, 1962, p. 279). "Feeling is not *all* that is involved in caring, but it is essentially involved" (Noddings, 1984, pp. 32, italics in original). Caring involves an emotional sense that we are reaching out (metaphorically) to a special other.[5] Caring produces an emotional feeling of warm, tender contact with the other.

The contact experienced in emotionally caring for another has sometimes been described as a "merging" (Freud, 1961; Singer, 1966/1984; Viorst, 1986). If we start from an assumption of fundamental self interest, such merger is necessary to give meaning to caring. A selfish actor cares only about the self, so to encompass caring, the other has to be seen as merged into the self so that the actor can have "interest" in the merged other. Within the self interest view, "otherness" is always suspect, is always dangerous because the other is by assumption fundamentally self-interested as well. A self interest logic of caring may support the metaphor of merging to the extent that it is seen as erasing the other's "otherness" by erasing the boundary between self and other. This conception leads to an intrinsic logical confusion of self and other. Jordan (1991, p. 70), using such a model, asserts the dangers "as distinctions between self and other blur experientially" so that "one could become lost in the other's experience." But within the caregiving theoretical orientation, caring explicitly recognizes the other's uniqueness, the other's specialness. Caring involves contact with another who remains "other."

Authors have been writing about the related concept of love for over two millennia and have reached little agreement. Caring is conceived as a more focused concept than the usual diffuse concept of love. Most conceptions of love consider it a conscious feeling rather than an unconscious emotion. Maslow (1987, pp. 182-183) defines love as a "feeling of tenderness and affection with great enjoyment, happiness, satisfaction, elation and even ecstasy." Similar comparisons occur with other definitions of love. Cancian's (1987) four-component definition of love includes behavior (expressing affection and giving care) and intention (maintaining affection for a long time and giving the loved person priority) within its conceptual umbrella (see also Kelsey, 1981). While concepts reflecting intention and behavior are included within the caregiving process, I see them as logically separate from caring (an emotional motivation). Nevertheless, for want of a better term, I will sometime use the verb "to love" to describe the caring process as a verb (in preference to "to care for," which can be confused with a behavior, or "to care about," which has overly cognitive overtones). In the noun and adjective forms, I will refer to the motivation as "caring." Another reason I refer to the motivation of the proactive connection process as "caring" rather than "love" is that the term "love" in American society is frequently taken to mean romantic, sexualized feelings.

We turn now to the processes that intervene between the emotion of caring and achieving the goal of meeting the partner's needs. A distinction will be made between the strategic planning aspects of the caregiving process and the perceptual aspects. These two aspects will be identified as *responsibility* and *empathy*.

RESPONSIBILITY

Caring is an emotion that is focused on a specific, special other person. In the psychological analysis of caregiving, the emotional motivation of caring toward a special other becomes manifest in two emotional intentions. The one of these intentions is a commitment to the fulfillment of the other's needs. The other, discussed in the next section, is a commitment to learning the other's needs.

A particular advantage of conceptualizing a motivation for a system such as caregiving is that the motivation helps to identify the set goal. For example, if the motivation is thirst, then it is easy to see that the set goal is to consume adequate water. If the motivation is fear for one's life, it follows that the set goal is safety. From ego's emotion of caring we infer the caregiving motivation system's set goal of meeting the needs of alter. In a parent-child relationship, the goal of the parent's caregiving motivation system is to meet the needs of the child.

The caregiving set goal of meeting the other's needs, within the caregiving theoretical orientation, goes beyond limited goals such as proximity or safety. While the assumption of a set goal limited to proximity, safety, and security is a natural result of Bowlby's functional analysis of attachment, it is challenged by both the evolutionary account of Chapter 3 and the neurobiological account of Chapter 4. In the caregiving theoretical orientation I present here, the caring emotion generates a set goal of meeting alter's needs. These needs may include food and shelter, safety and security, growth and achievement.

The proposed set goal of meeting alter's needs is general enough to serve for most parenting activities. Furthermore, meeting alter's needs is an appropriate goal for adult caregiving as well. Two points must be made about meeting needs as a set goal. First, needs are developmentally variable (Bowlby, 1969/1982; Erikson, 1963). The needs of an infant, a one-year-old, a five-year-old, and an adult are different, so the behavior associated with meeting the set goal will be different as well. Second, needs are subjectively perceived, so ego, alter, and an observer may all differ in the needs they identify (Pierce, Sarason, Sarason, Joseph, & Henderson, 1996). But since ego's set goal derives from ego's caring, the set goal for ego will be to meet alter's needs as interpreted by ego. These issues are discussed further below.

Responsibility is ego's emotional intention to meet alter's needs. Responsibility is what Peck uses in his conception of love as "the will to extend one's self for the purpose of nurturing one's own or another's spiritual growth" (Peck, 1978, p. 81). Peck limits his concept of love and responsibility to spiritual needs. In my model, however, as emotional caring is focused on alter's needs as a whole, responsibility also focuses on all of alter's needs. In Davis' notion of sympathy (Davis, Kirkpatrick, Levy, & O'Hearn, 1994), "the observer's emotional response to the distress of another leads the observer to feel desire to take action to alleviate the other person's suffering" (see also Baron-Cohen & Wheelwright, 2004).

Responsibility, as I use the term, is ego's goal-directed intention and commitment to finding ways of meeting alter's needs. The concept of responsibility within the caregiving theoretical orientation includes accessing a caregiving internal working model: a record of prior caregiving experiences, a model of ego as a caregiver, and a model of alter as a recipient of nurturance. Between a parent and child, because the child's needs are multiplex and because they change developmentally (on a yearly, monthly, and even daily basis), a parent is continually challenged to go beyond previously successful behaviors and previously met needs recorded in the working model to nurture the child. As Bowlby pointed out, because the child's needs change developmentally, attempts to measure parental caregiving with specific behavioral measures will be unsuccessful because specific parenting behaviors change with the development of the child (Bowlby, 1969/1982).

Responsibility involves emotion, cognition, and behavior. A parent commits to meeting his child's needs. The parent's responsibility is expressed behaviorally by reading manuals on child care, learning songs the child enjoys, and observing other parents. Cognitively he considers his child's needs and how they might be met. Cognitive comparisons lead to choices between alternate behaviors he might enact in order to meet his child's needs. When the child cries at two a.m., he cognitively plans the route from bed to the infant, he chooses between rocking or walking, and perhaps chooses a song to sing.

The intention of caregiving responsibility is also deeply emotional. One may "intend to read *War and Peace*" with an intellectual force that means "if nothing else comes up." But a parent "intends to protect this child" with an emotional force that means "no matter what."[6]

Responsibility expresses ego's subjective awareness of the importance of the relationship with alter. To satisfy the emotion of caring, ego makes a commitment to the satisfaction of alter's needs. Thus responsibility is both a feeling, an awareness of an emotional contact with alter, and a foundation for the nurturance of alter (Befu, 1986). "Caring requires me to respond to the initial impulse with an act of commitment: I commit myself either to overt action on behalf of the cared-for (I pick up my crying infant) or I commit myself to thinking about what I might do" (Noddings, 1984, p. 81). Ruddick is another author who sees a relationship between caring and responsibility.

> For many women, mothering begins in a fiercely passionate love that is not destroyed by the ambivalence and anger it includes. Many mothers develop early a sense of maternal competence—a sense that they can and will care for their children (Ruddick, 1989, p. 29).

Within the self interest seeking motivation system, commitment is a constraint: commitment is "the degree to which the individual has committed himself to the particular contents of this role-identity, has gambled his regard for himself on living up to certain imaginations of self" (see also Levinger & Rausch, 1977; McCall & Simmons, 1978, p. 75). Marriage, in this view, is a commitment to the extent that ego has internally and externally agreed to give up the freedom and potential rewards of choosing other partners. Self interest commitment is a loss of potential gratifications given with the hope of greater countervailing gains. Responsibility within caregiving, however, includes commitment and is defined by addition, not subtraction. It is an intention to do more, not to get more. And the "more" that is done is for the other, not for the self. It is not based on a fear of what generalized others will think or even what the self will think: it is based on the emotion of caring, the cherishing of the other person, and a resulting commitment to the other's needs.

We often use emotional terms to describe responsibility. We say that metaphorically we have a "feeling" of responsibility or a "sense" of responsibility. Sometimes we use negative metaphors, as when excessive responsibility takes on the metaphor of a heavy weight, a burden, to emphasize the self-interested motivations that are not satisfied because of the responsibility for another. These negative metaphors may represent a cultural sense in the United States that responsibility is a response to social norms, that it is something imposed on us. But other metaphors are positive. For example, there is the description of children as a joy, a blessing, an adventure.

Responsibility is similar to "responsiveness," one of the two characteristics of good caregivers noted by attachment researchers (Ainsworth, et al., 1978; Belsky & Isabella, 1988; Berman & Sperling, 1994; Bowlby, 1988; Feeney & Noller, 1996; Solomon & George, 1996; Sroufe, 1988). However, the term "responsiveness" is less consistent with the proactive emphasis of the model here. "Responsibility" better captures the proactive emotional intention.

Responsibility is a conceptual variable that can vary from zero to some high value. If ego has a responsibility of zero toward alter, ego's actions will be directed toward goals other than alter's needs. If ego's caregiving bond (the number and density of neurons in the caregiving system) is at a low or moderate level then the maximum level of ego's responsibility will be low or moderate. When ego has a high level of responsibility toward alter in the moment, ego is highly attuned in the moment to the needs of alter. A large part of ego's attention will be given to considering how to meet alter's needs; ego gives a great deal of attention to developing plans to meet alter's needs. There is no assumption of a fixed overall amount of available attention, so attention given to alter's needs does not necessarily mean a decrease in attention given to ego's needs and wants, although this can happen. It is possible, but not certain, that ego can increase attention to both alter's needs and to ego's wants and needs. In the strongest relationships, such as many family and some friendship relationships, responsibility is high and unconditional. In such relationships, the partner's need is a primary consideration. And if that need is great—as in the case of a life-threatening illness or other crisis—then responsibility can be commensurably great. In some cases, responsibility can impel the risk of ego's life. However, not all responsibility is effectively directed. Responsibility can be misdirected, especially when needs are misunderstood. Or it can be ineffective when ego chooses an inappropriate strategy for meeting alter's need.

Responsibility does not mean selflessness. Responsibility is directed at the other's needs. If alter's needs are great, then when responsibility is at a high level, the sheer magnitude of effort needed to meet alter's need may preclude the satisfaction of some of ego's needs, and ego is likely to sacrifice ego's own comfort and convenience to meet alter's needs. But when alter's needs are less or when ego's needs are more or when ego's responsibility is low, it is likely to be ego's needs that take precedence. When we speak of parent and child, the needs of the child are usually greater than those of the parent. American culture and social science have mythologized this tendency in the social norm of the all-sacrificing parent, invariably a mother (Chodorow, 1978; Epstein, 1988).

We often describe responsibility with terms like "ought to" and "have to." These are terms that can also be used to describe external forms of compulsion and morality. These terms go with expressions such as "I had to do it or I would have been punished" or "You ought to do it because it is right." When associated with compulsion and morality, "ought to" and "have to" indicate an external constraint. In the final chapter, I will look at the probable origin of these emergent moral norms. But within the caregiving theoretical orientation, responsibility is a voluntary, self-selected intention. It is metaphorically a "force" coming from within the person.

> **Caregiving assertion 1**. The greater ego's caring for alter, the greater ego's responsibility toward alter, because ego's cherishing of alter makes alter's happiness (fulfillment of needs) important to ego. To encourage and support alter's happiness, ego directs attention to the fulfillment of alter's needs.

The causal relationship between caring and responsibility is shown in Figure 5.1. Caring motivates the actor to take responsibility. Because ego loves alter, ego responds emotionally to alter's needs. When ego comes to be committed to providing for alter's needs, ego has taken responsibility. In order to carry out ego's responsibility for alter, ego needs to make judgments based on ego's capabilities (is ego able to perform the behaviors that will meet alter's needs?) and on alter's capabilities (can alter meet those needs without help?). These judgments are based on an inter-

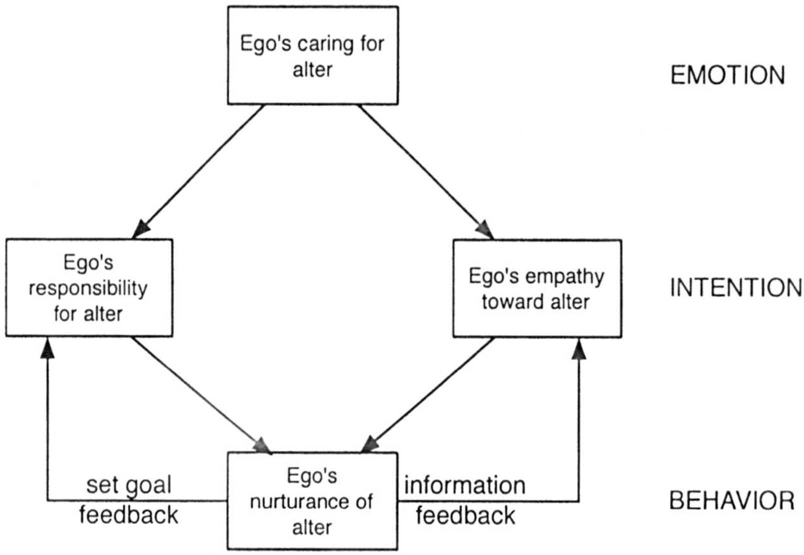

Figure 5.1. The Caregiving Process

nal working model that encodes ego's knowledge of self, of alter, and the history of their relationship, and of its potential future.

The effect of ego's caring on ego's responsibility is such that an actor who has a high level of caring for another will come to take a high level of responsibility for the other. The potential maximum level of responsibility is limited by the level of the caregiving bond (biologically, the number of caregiving neurons); its momentary value is determined by the momentary value of the caring emotion, the level of activation of the caregiving system (biologically, the number of activated caregiving neurons). Correspondingly, an actor with a very low level of caring will take little responsibility for meeting the other's needs. When the first glimmerings of emotional contact begin to be established in a newly-forming relationship, when caring is still tentative, responsibility is also tenuous. As caring grows within the relationship, responsibility increases as well. Like all assertions, this one has an implicit *ceteris paribus* ("all things being equal") restriction. Caring is only one causal antecedent of responsibility. For example, an actor who has a low level of caring for a specific dependent but who also has a high level of moral commitment may take a high level of responsibility for alter as an expression of some abstract and general moral principle. In Chapter 7, we will consider some other processes that create exceptions and additions to the effect of caring on responsibility.

Even thirty years ago, it would have been virtually impossible to contemplate how a complex process like responsibility could be tied to specific neuronal circuits or localized in the brain. We still know relatively little, but some of the neural pathways are beginning to be tentatively identified. As we saw earlier, the caring emotion appears to be centered in the paraventricular nucleus (PVN) of the hypothalamus. The hypothalamus appears to access the caregiving internal working model. It is not clear exactly where memories of past nurturing are stored, but their storage appears to involve the hippocampus and the temporal lobes (LeDoux, 1996). On the basis of information from memory, the hypothalamus seems to instruct the prefrontal cortex to formulate an action plan (like loading a computer program through the hippocampus), which is then transmitted to the anterior cingulate which focuses attention and selects information, and then apparently notifies the caudate nucleus which copies and implements the plan (like executing a computer program) by sending signals to appropriate effector body systems (Bretherton, 1980; Hinde, 1982; Jeannerod, 1997). I would hypothesize that it is in the hypothalamus that the behavioral outcome is evaluated in some way in terms of the discrepancy with the complex caregiving set goal, and the process continues until termination, usually by achievement of the set goal or a change in motivation systems.

EMPATHY

Within the model proposed here, we have seen that the first effect of caring is responsibility. The second effect of emotional caring about a partner is that we want to know them. This process leads to empathy. For the purposes of the caregiving theoretical orientation, I define *empathy as the emotional intention to know the other*.

Innumerable definitions of empathy have been proposed in the literature (Batson, 2009). For orientation, I offer here a brief description of those meanings I do *not* intend. I do not mean "cognitive empathy" (Preston & de Waal, 2002), the ability to perceive alter's emotions, or "empathic accuracy," the accuracy of that perception (Ickes, 1993). I do not mean feeling the same emotion as alter: "emotional contagion" (Hatfield, Cacioppo, & Rapson, 1994) or "affective empathy" (Zahn-Waxler, Robinson, & Emde, 1992). I also do not mean "empathic distress," one's distress upon recognizing alter's suffering (Batson, 1991; Hoffman, 1981) or "sympathy," feeling for alter when alter is in need

(Darwall, 1998; Sober & Wilson, 1998; Wispé, 1986). I will discuss some of these concepts below.

Empathy in the caregiving theoretical orientation means emotionally attending to the other for the purpose of knowing the other's needs. It involves being emotionally receptive to the other's reality (Noddings, 1984). The empathy that I am talking about is the intention to know. It is emotional because, like responsibility, it is derived from the emotion of caring. Thus, there is an emotional immediacy and energy that gives force to empathy. Sympathy for another's unmet need helps to activate empathy. Empathy is cognitive; it involves processing, storage, and retrieval of perceptions. Knowing about alter is a puzzle: verbal and nonverbal cues must be perceived and interpreted. Empathy thus produces a focused attention on the other and the other's needs. This focus includes the senses of sight, smell and touch as well as listening, all channels through which we can learn about the other. Empathy is also behavioral. It involves behaviors of listening and observing. Effective empathy involves responsiveness and feedback, what we sometimes call "active listening." Empathy thus involves not only passive receptiveness to alter's actions, but also more active attempts to elicit information and to respond to what is learned. To understand alter and alter's needs, ego attends actively to alter, perhaps directly questions alter and arranges to have access to information about alter, perhaps public information, perhaps personal. Empathy, like responsibility, can generate a goal-directed feeling, a conscious awareness that ego wants to know alter.

> **Caregiving assertion 2**. The greater ego's caring for alter, the greater ego's empathy toward alter, because ego's cherishing of alter makes alter's happiness (fulfillment of needs) important to ego. To encourage and support alter's happiness, ego directs attention to learning alter's needs.

The Japanese word for empathy is *omoiyari*, which literally means "giving thought." But in Japanese, the character for "thought" is 思い (*omoi*). This kanji contains the character, 心 (*kokoro*), which means both "mind" and at base "heart." Thus "giving thought" in Japanese involves thinking from the heart. It is this meaning that is intended here. Ruddick describes a similar concept as "attention" or "attentive love." "Attention is at once an act of knowing and an act of love. . . . Attentive love, or loving attention, makes truth serve lovingly the person known" (Ruddick, 1989, p. 120).

Anglo-American cultural traditions emphasize both verbal expression and independence. In American culture there is a cultural bias toward verbal (oral) communication. If you want to communicate with someone you must put it in words. Thus we sometimes think of empathy as "mind reading" because it goes beyond verbal communication. But other cultures, such as Japanese, emphasize nonverbal expression. In contrast to the American reliance on words, Japanese culture tends to mistrust verbal communication.

> The Japanese glorify silent communication, *ishin denshin* ("heart-to-heart communication"), and mutual "vibrations," implying the possibility of semitelepathic communication. Words are paltry against the significance of reading subtle signs and signals and the intuitive grasp of each other's feelings (Lebra, 1976, p. 115; see also Bell, 1989).

The phenomenal ability of the Japanese to "read" facial and body language speaks to the importance of gathering knowledge of the partner in a connection-based culture (Lebra, 1976). The Japanese even have a common term, "*aizuchi*" for the aural but nonverbal "ers" and "mms" of spoken language. These nonverbal components of conversation convey important information about social relationships. By listening and attending, one can understand the other's needs, one can *sassuru* (infer the other's needs, primarily by nonverbal means). In Japan, empathy is a central cultural value. This cultural tradition emphasizes parental caregiving as intuitive and proactive (Doi, 1981, 1989).

Because of the relative homogeneity of Japanese culture, the relatively greater extent of shared values, the nurturing person may be more easily able to empathize than tends to be the case in the more heterogeneous American culture. Japanese children are taught to pay attention to the face, to read nonverbal cues and to listen well. In American society, we put less attention to sensitivity and perceiving subtle cues than we do on expressing oneself clearly. The concept of empathy as attentiveness, as used here, draws on both traditions and emphasizes ego's proactive efforts to learn the child's needs by attending to covert as well as overt signals. Even though most Anglo-American parents are not trained from infancy to read nonverbal and covert signals (like most Japanese parents), most Anglo-American parents still learn to recognize many nonverbal cues from their infants. These parents are motivated to learn to read nonverbal signals because of the way they feel about their infants. Empathy as conceived here is concerned with the gamut of the child's needs, the ability to read overt and covert signals of those needs, as well as the parents' proactive attention to needs not signaled by the child.

Empathy is a conceptual variable that varies from zero to some high value. At a level of zero, ego has no concern to know about alter and in fact is indifferent to information about alter. At a high level of empathy, ego is highly committed to knowing about alter. Empathy is defined in terms of intention rather than outcome. Thus empathy as conceptualized here does not mean accuracy of knowledge. "Intending to know" does not necessarily successfully lead to knowing. Sometimes for all of our best efforts, we are unable to read the other's signals accurately. But the attention given to alter will often pay off: we can anticipate a generally high consistency between empathy and accuracy. Thus, although empathy is not *defined* here in terms of accurately knowing another's feelings, one's empathy will very frequently include knowledge of the partner's feelings.

In the caregiving theoretical orientation, the emotion of caring motivates ego toward empathy. It supports a desire to know alter in order to meet alter's needs. When the level of caring is low, the system produces a low level of empathy. A person who has a low level of caring has little emotional commitment to seek information about the other. When the level of caring is high, there is a high emotional commitment to knowing alter. Loving alter orients ego to alter's needs and emotions, and this makes ego open to those needs and emotions. The ability to understand alter's state (Preston & de Waal, 2002) or to perceive alter's emotion ("empathic accuracy") partially depends on ego's desire to know, but also depends on ego's prior training and other experience, in which one develops the "capacity to think and feel oneself into the inner life of another person" (Kohut, 1984, p. 82). Because ego's desire to know alter's needs is energized by ego's caring, to the extent that ego perceives alter's needs, ego will respond positively in regard to these needs; this emotional response is called "sympathy" by Baron-Cohen and Wheelwright (2004) "compassion" by Berscheid (2006) and simply "empathy" by Batson (2002). In the view I describe here, there is no assumption that ego's desire to know alter's emotion will lead ego to share alter's emotion. I can perceive that my child is angry without becoming angry in return.

In the caregiving process, responsibility and empathy tend to be at the same level because both are caused by ego's caring. Ego's wanting to help meet alter's needs (responsibility) activates ego's desire to know what the other needs (empathy). but in addition to being a result of ego's responsibility, empathy can itself activate responsibility. Batson has found this effect. Batson's approach to empathy is somewhat different from mine because he has studied empathy primarily among strangers in laboratory settings where knowledge of alter's needs and how to meet them have been manipulated by the investigators (Batson, et al., 1989; Batson, et al., 1988). I suspect that the caregiving process is very much like Batson's model, but that our concepts have slightly different boundaries because of his focus on altruism between strangers. There is no prior relationship between ego and alter in the situations in which he is interested, so for Batson caring is not aroused until ego learns of alter's distress: the emotional response of caring and the emotional intention to know occur at the same time and thus appear to be combined in Batson's concept of empathy.

If ego cares about alter and perceives that alter is afraid, ego is likely to attempt to comfort alter. Ego does not want alter to be afraid, and alter also does not want to be afraid, so ego's comforting is consensually directed at meeting alter's need for safety and security. It is possible that ego will be afraid also, but it is clear that ego will comfort alter even when ego is not afraid. Similarly, if ego cares about alter and perceives that alter is angry, ego is again likely to attempt to comfort alter. It would be unusual in such a situation that ego would feel the same anger felt by alter (and in fact, alter's anger may be directed at ego). Ego will want to reduce alter's anger because ego perceives that alter needs calm, and not because ego has become angry in turn. Thus, the definition that I gave above emphasizes that it is ego's perception of alter's needs (not necessarily perception of alter's emotions, and not necessarily alter's perception of own needs) that will affect ego's response. When I fail to give my daughter what she needs, it may be painful to me. However, I do not feel her pain. Although I may perceive her pain, it is my own pain of failed responsibility and guilt that I feel. Caring rather unconditionally produces empathy, the intention to know alter. The successful knowing of alter, of course, depends additionally on skills of perception, of imagination, as well as similarity of experiences.

The connection concept of empathy is related to, but is differently nuanced than the more cognitive concept of "role taking." Role taking is a "cognitive process [that] involves taking the perspective of another into account when acting" (Stets, 1992, p. 166). Empathy involves taking the *person* into account emotionally as well as cognitively. Furthermore, empathy as used here means a positive focus on the other. When we feel caring, we focus on how we can help.

The information relevant to empathic intention can arise externally, as from hearing the child cry (reaction to partner stimulus) or from seeing a predator (reaction to environmental stimulus), or internally, as when the parent decides to build a fence when no predator has been seen (proactive responsibility). One of the ways that empathy works is to create and update an internal working model. One of Bowlby's important contributions was to note that an actor has multiple internal working models, a working model for caregiving and giving nurturance, for example, and a working model attachment and asking for nurturance (1969/1982). *Ego's caregiving working model*, as identified by Bowlby and by Solomon & George (1996, 1999), encodes an image of the self as a nurturer, alter as an object of nurturance, and the history of ego's nurturing relationship with alter. There is also *alter's caregiving working model* that encodes alter's experiences of alter as nurturer, ego as recipient of nurturance, and alter's nurturing relationship with ego. As we will discuss in the next chapter, in association with ego's caregiving working model, there is *alter's attachment working model* that encodes information about alter as a recipient of ego's nurturance, ego as a giver of nurturance, and alter's history of experience of receiving ego's nurturance.

In addition to a caregiving internal working model and an attachment internal working model, individuals have other working models, including an internal working model that encodes experiences of individuation. Although some of Bowlby's language seems to imply that the various internal working models are completely separate, other language seems to imply that one internal working model has access to information from other models. Other authors write as if an actor has a single internal working model containing models of self and other in various relationships (Bretherton & Munholland, 1999; Stern, 1985; Winnicott, 1965b). Conceptually, it makes sense to distinguish the various internal working models, but practically we must acknowledge that sharing of information is probably widespread within the brain.

Very little of the neurobiological structure of empathy has been investigated, except for memory. Relationship episodes seem to be recorded initially in the hippocampus, where they are consolidated and from which they are stored into long term memory in the neocortex (Carter, 1998b). Storage of some memories relevant to caregiving appears to occur through the nucleus accumbens (Lee, et al., 1999). Many social memories, especially those that involve inferring someone else's state of mind appear to be stored in the left medial prefrontal cortex (Carter, 1998b; Panksepp, 1998). Other social memories may be stored in the piriform cortex and the orbitofrontal cortex (Kendrick, et al., 1997; MacLean, 1990).

It is important not to idealize the empathic process. Most parents probably know their child's needs fairly well, albeit with some error. And most parents are aware that needs change developmentally. Infants need constant nurturance, children need comfort and encouragement, adolescents need trust and autonomy within the relationship. Culture, education, experience, and self interest affect these perceptions of need. Parents have folk theories, some of which are culturally transmitted and preexist the child, but many of which the parent learns directly from the child (Bowlby, 1988).

The parent's perception of the child's needs may differ substantially from the child's understanding. Thus a child may cry for a deeply desired military toy observed in a television commercial while the parent attributes to the child a need for nonviolent playthings. Both parent and child may engage in direct or subtle attempts to modify the other's perceptions. Furthermore, the parent's and child's perceptions may differ from an observer's perception. In addition to simple errors of perception, there are also more serious distortions that can sidetrack the intention of empathy and reduce the accuracy of empathic perception. The parent's own interpersonal history may create obstacles to effective expression of the parent's empathy, for instance by leading to the projection of the parent's needs onto the child (Bell, Bell, & Nakata, 2001; Brazelton & Cramer, 1990; deMause, 1974). If accurate perception of need were easy, the caregiving process would be simpler.

In its emphasis on emotion, the concept of empathy in the caregiving theoretical orientation goes somewhat beyond the concept of "attentiveness" or "sensitivity," identified by attachment researchers as characteristic of good parental caregivers (Ainsworth, et al., 1978; Berman & Sperling, 1994; Bowlby, 1969/1982, 1988; Feeney & Noller, 1996; Heard & Lake, 1997; Solomon & George, 1996). The emotional term "empathy" is preferred for the proposed model of connection caregiving because it emphasizes the active intention to know, while "sensitivity" seems to imply a generally passive awareness of the partner.

The perception of children's needs varies with culture and social class. Constantine (1986) highlights how different family structures are adaptive in different social contexts. A parent in the United States, especially a middle class parent, may infer that the child needs to develop independence and self reliance skills in order to succeed in life, where a parent in Japan may infer that the child needs to develop interdependence skills to be successful within the culture. A parent raising a child to survive in a violent society may infer that the child needs to be aggressive and insensitive to succeed within that world.

A major threat to empathy is fear. Ego may sometimes repress knowledge of a loved one's weaknesses if acknowledging those weaknesses would activate ego's insecurities; or being afraid, ego may project ego's feared thoughts, feelings, or needs onto alter and thus misperceive alter's actual thoughts, feelings, and needs. Furthermore, because empathy successively carried out involves awareness of the other's feelings and needs, it can be affected by our own feelings and intuitions about the other as much as by our perceptions of them. But it is also the emotion behind empathy that can support accurate knowing. It is our caring for the other that encourages us to watch them over time and thus come to know them better.

Although empathy has a direct association with caring, it has a curvilinear association with information-seeking behaviors. New relationships that involve little emotional contact show little empathy. Information seeking is low. There may be much talk, but with low empathy, there is little emotional commitment to the information, so mostly passive attention is given to the information content of the talk. If some emotional contact develops or if the initial interaction raises awareness of a potentially significant relationship, the emotional intention to know the other will grow. This increase in empathy produces greater attention and thus greater effort to seek information. In the developing stages of a relationship, when empathy is at a moderate level, ego seeks a broad range of information to help understand the kind of person alter is (Murstein, 1970). As the relationship develops (if it does), ego comes to seek more narrow and specific information as ego explores the depths of alter's character. In even later relationship stages, for these partners who have continued to build caring, information gathering becomes more casual, aimed at reassurance and confirmation rather than toward the gathering of new information. Much of the intention to know has been satisfied by earlier learning.

The curvilinear association between empathy and information-seeking helps us make sense of the often observed pattern of inattention in close relationships. When a close relationship is stable, empathy is high, but the search for new information about alter's needs may be low (however out-of-date the previous learning may have become). Each assumes (rightly or wrongly) that they know each other well, and both seem to be getting what they need.

> People are hardly aware of needs currently being well served, but they tend to be keenly aware of needs not being well satisfied (Glenn, 1991, pp. 268-269).

If either partner were to enter a crisis, the other's responsibility would be activated to meet the need. But without a crisis, there is often no apparent unmet need. It is in such a stable relationship where needs are less salient that one partner may feel "taken for granted." Needs must be uncovered through an active process of attention. But, as the connection grows, as we learn more and more, we eventually become satisfied that we know enough. We've heard the other's history and stories, and we begin to experience diminishing returns from careful attention. This growing disinterest (or rather, fully satisfied interest) may be seen—at least on the cognitive side—as the central fact of taking the other for granted. Taking one another for granted is seen as a healthy sign in Japanese family relationships (Lebra, 1984). It means we already know. Of course, if the partner does not really love and feel responsibility, then "taking for granted" is a sign of disinterest or power (Berscheid, 1983).

This discussion emphasizes the importance of taking in information in the caregiving process. Learning about the other is a consequence of caring. The easiest way (from the point of view of an American emphasis on verbal communication) for ego to learn about alter's needs is to wait for alter to express those needs in a demand for ego's action. If this sort of demand were common, then empathy would be achieved by a very simple process of verbal listening. However, the stating of demands is only one method of communication, and even this method is effective only to the extent that the listener is paying attention. Empathy includes not only an openness to the other's explicit and intended expressions of need, but also to subtle and often unintended expressions.

The opacity of the judgment process is an important aspect of caregiving. There is no currency for converting ego's need and alter's need to the same denomination. Ego feels and thus knows ego's own needs. But ego also knows ego's wants, and there is always some ambiguity. A self-interested caregiver is fully aware of both own wants and own needs and strives to satisfy both as a primary goal. When connection is salient, when ego is oriented to alter's needs and wants, ego may devalue own needs and wants. Thus, relative to an unconnected actor, a connected ego tends to undervalue own needs. Stating this as a moral principle, Aristotle notes in the Nicomachean Ethics that "the virtuous man tends to take less than his share" (Aristotle, 1952, p. 384). On the other hand, when ego considers alter's needs, ego's information is more limited. Because of ego's orientation toward nurturance, ego may have a bias toward seeing alter's behavior as expressions of need. Furthermore, when there is no explicit statement, ego must try to imagine what alter's needs might be. This may lead to a tendency to nurture the other to a higher degree than oneself. When we are oriented toward self interest, we generally feel that we have not received enough; when we are oriented toward caregiving, we generally feel that we have not given enough.

NURTURANCE

Behaviorally, raising children is a matter of nurturance, of not just caring emotionally but of giving care behaviorally. Nurturance is the behavior of providing for the other's needs. Nurturance, within caregiving logic, is strictly voluntary. When the child asks for a favor or expresses a need, she will not be nurtured unless the parent chooses to nurture her. Nurturance within the caregiving theoretical orientation is always conceptualized within a specific relationship.

Nurturance is defined specifically as a behavior. Both responsibility and empathy involve behavior as well, but of a different sort. The goal of empathy is knowing the other and thus involves behaviors of watching, active and passive listening, asking questions and other forms of attention. It is through these processes of active and passive empathy that ego detects alter's needs. If ego perceives (and/or feels) alter's unmet needs, ego takes responsibility to meet those needs. The process of responsibility involves planning for meeting alter's needs and thus involves the behavior of information gathering about the constraints and opportunities in the social context. Accessing memories encoded in the caregiving internal working model, ego selects previously successful behaviors as well as formulating new behaviors to enact that are expected to achieve the set goal of meeting alter's needs. Both knowing and planning often involve asking questions and seeking advice. The feelings and behaviors of responsibility and empathy provide the ability to meet alter's needs, but they do not themselves meet those needs.

Of course, this situation is not unambiguous. Alter's perception that ego is listening and that ego is taking responsibility may itself be interpreted as meeting some of alter's needs. If ego is listening with the purpose of showing alter that ego cares—knowing that alter "needs" to feel cared for—then I would be comfortable classifying the listening behavior as nurturance (and if ego is really listening, the listening expresses empathy as well). But in the ordinary course of listening as an outcome of ego's emotional caring toward alter, then I would consider listening behaviors to be part of empathy. Fortunately, we are concerned here with the unobservable imaginary realm of explanation so that the ambiguities of multicausal observable reality and the design of measurement instruments do not concern us.

Ego's nurturance of alter is the behavior of ego that is directed toward meeting alter's needs. By this definition, nurturance need not be successful. It is the goal of the behavior rather than its effect that defines it as nurturance. This definition differs from that of Noddings (1984), who limits nurturance to successfully meeting the other's needs. I prefer to leave the outcome out of the concept. Emotional caring leads one to *try* to meet the partner's needs. Many other factors can influence the success of the attempt. The effect of ego's nurturance on alter will be considered later as a separate conceptual variable, alter's *acceptance*. Nurturance is a conceptual variable that can vary from zero, when ego undertakes no action directed toward meeting alter's needs, to a high positive value, when many of ego's actions are directed toward meeting alter's needs.

The ultimate indirect outcome of the emotion of caring finds expression in the behavior of nurturance. Giving behavioral nurturance is the result of emotional caring, as the caring is given direction through the intentions of responsibility and empathy.

> **Caregiving assertion 3**. In the face of alter's need as perceived by ego, the greater ego's responsibility to alter, the greater ego's nurturance of alter, because nurturance is the behavior by which ego carries out the intention of responsibility.

> **Caregiving assertion 4**. In the face of alter's need as perceived by ego, the greater ego's empathy toward alter, the greater ego's nurturance of alter, because ego can perform behaviors to meet alter's needs only through knowledge of alter's needs.

Ego takes responsibility for meeting alter's needs. Responsibility in turn expresses itself in nurturance. Ruddick describes this association as: "Mothering is an activity governed by a commitment" (Ruddick, 1989, p. 70). This causal relationship was shown above in Figure 5.1. When ego assumes responsibility for alter and for the relationship with alter, ego effects responsibility by giving nurturance, by nurturing those needs for which ego has taken responsibility. The maximum level of nurturance depends on both very high responsibility by ego and very high need in alter as perceived by ego. Even at the highest level of responsibility, the amount of nurturance will be near zero if alter has no current known needs.

There is not only a direct effect of responsibility on nurturance. In addition, there is a feedback effect from nurturance to responsibility. Ego's intention to meet alter's need can be modified by the results that ego perceives from the nurturance. To the extent that the nurturance is not achieving the intended goal of meeting alter's need, ego can then modify the nurturance strategy to identify other behaviors to better meet alter's needs.

Ego cannot expect to give alter what alter needs unless ego knows what alter needs. When ego assumes a responsibility toward alter, ego can only nurture alter to the extent that ego understands alter well enough to know what alter needs. Thus ego's preparedness to listen and be empathic is a major component in successful nurturance.

The effect of empathy on nurturance interacts in complex ways with alter's needs. First of all, if there are no needs for ego to perceive through empathy, low nurturance will result from high empathy. Second, even if alter has high needs, if ego's empathic skill is unable to detect the needs or if some other factor like fear prevents ego's empathy from operating effectively, then alter's *perceived* needs will be minimal and nurturance will be low. Even when alter's needs are accurately perceived, ego may lack the resources to meet those needs—or may be unable due to other concerns or obligations. Finally, some other factor like ego's insecurity may lead ego to *misperceive* alter's needs, and ego's nurturance may be both highly active and ineffective, or even harmful.

The possibility of inaccurate empathy creates the basis for harmful nurturance. The parent who sees her own fearful weakness in the child may perceive a need in the child to eradicate the weakness, may take responsibility for eradicating the weakness, and may as a result perpetrate child abuse in attempting to nurture the child. A heterosexual man who loves a dating partner may, because of his own need to be loved, inaccurately perceive that she loves him as much as he believes he loves her, may be perplexed by her reluctance to have sex with him, and may rape her in an attempt to express the love he feels she needs. These and other ways that caregiving processes can lead to abuse and other negative consequences are discussed in Chapter 7.

In addition to a direct effect of empathy on nurturance, there is an information feedback effect from nurturance to both empathy and responsibility. As behavioral nurturance occurs, ego observes the effects of the nurturance on alter and is thus able to modify ego's expectations and intentions. If nurturance is having the intended effect, no modification is needed, but if the effects of nurturance are not those intended, ego may need to increase empathic efforts in order to clarify needs. In addition, ego may need to refocus responsibility, enact additional strategies, and modify nurturance behaviors accordingly.

The caregiving theoretical orientation explains the source of nurturance not only in the desire for knowledge about the other (empathy out of caring), but also in the emotional intention to meet those needs (responsibility, also out of caring). Nurturance is seen as arising out of a special emotional relationship between the caregiver and the nurtured. Furthermore, the caregiving process provides an account for nurturance in relationships outside of the purview of social norms.

In the caregiving view, it is the causal link from ego's responsibility that provides the impetus for the nurturance. It is the causal link from empathy that provides for accuracy of knowledge of alter's needs and thus for successful nurturance. These two causal links have more than an additive effect. If this were an additive association, empathy and responsibility would be substitutable: more empathy could be substituted for less responsibility to achieve the same final effect. It is more reasonable to hypothesize that empathy and responsibility have a multiplicative effect. In a multiplicative effect, a zero level of empathy even coupled with a high level of responsibility would produce near zero nurturance because ego would have no notion of how to direct the attempted nurturance. This is not only a question of accuracy of knowledge of alter's needs. At zero empathy, accuracy is not an issue: ego is not even trying to understand alter. Furthermore, a zero level of responsibility even coupled with a high level of empathy would produce near zero nurturance because for all of ego's awareness of alter's needs, ego would have no emotional commitment to taking action.

By identifying the caregiving affectional bond with the consolidation of caregiving neural circuits and identifying the emotion of caring with the level of activation of this bond, we have accomplished three important goals: (1) we have identified a motivation system that does not depend on Freudian drives, a major goal of Bowlby's analysis (Bowlby, 1969/1982); (2) we have identified a volitional motivation for caregiving; and (3) we have identified a dyadic motivation that varies in strength.

From Theoretical Orientation to Theory

The caregiving theoretical orientation is an abstract explanatory construction. As with any theoretical orientation, its purpose is to construct theories in empirical domains where the logic operates. A caregiving theory of parenting, like Bowlby's attachment theory, emphasizes the parent's empathy and responsibility that leads to the nurturance of the many needs of children. The caregiving theoretical orientation also provides the basis for a caregiving theory of child nurturance to explain the nurturance that children provide to parents, siblings, and peers. When children love and an adult has needs, the child can become the caregiver to the adult. The child's behavioral repertoire may be limited, but within these limits, the child can nurture a teacher, parent, or grandparent. The emotional dynamics of the nurturing parent, the nurturing child, the nurturing friend, and the stranger who is "touched" by another's needs—all are explained by the same logic of caregiving, by the same emotional dynamics of the relationship.

When caregiving is viewed through the lens of caring, it can be seen that there is no theoretical inconsistency between caring for a child and caring for a spouse or caring for an acquaintance in need. Adult partners exercise empathy toward one another at a level consistent with their caring and similarly take responsibility for the partner's need. For example, I believe that the caregiving system and the affiliation (or sociability) system described by some authors (Bowlby, 1969/1982; Cassidy, 1999) are at base the same system. This conception of caregiving is not based on preponderance of resources (Bowlby, 1988), or on being "stronger and wiser" (Bretherton & Munholland, 1999; Cassidy, 1999; Shaver, et al., 1988). A caregiving system resides in even young children who are neither stronger nor wiser than their parents and yet are motivated by caring to nurture their parents. Nurturing behavior in a caring relationship is based on the availability of resources and on a perceived need toward which resources are directed.

It is easy to describe the logic of the caregiving process as a smooth sequence in which caring is followed by an equal level of responsibility, empathy, and nurturance. But in daily interaction, the process does not necessarily operate smoothly. As actors move out of sight of one another, as each becomes more or less engrossed in one or another of life's activities, the sense of emotional contact varies. And, as we have seen, misperception can lead to harmful rather than helpful nurturance. As demands for attention from multiple relationships ebb and flow according to changing contexts, responsibility changes even when caring remains constant. Furthermore, the multiplicity of alter's needs means that even with perfect responsibility and perfect empathy, the attempt to provide nurturance for one need will often entail a failure to meet a conflicting need.

Chapter 8 will develop a connection theory of adult relationships that will apply the logics of the caregiving and attachment theoretical orientations to the initiation, development, and dissolution of adult romantic relationships.

Notes

1. Self interest seeking is often conceptualized in contemporary social science as a highly cognitive ("rational") process. In this usage, rationality is considered a synonym for self interest. By this definition, a parent cannot be "rational" in nurturing a child if nurturing is not a self-interested act. However, the evolutionary origins of self interest seeking in the earliest animals, animals without a cognitive neocortex, and its location in brain structures that are closely related to those of conventionally identified emotions, suggest that self interest seeking is emotional in much the same way as fear, anger, lust, caregiving, and attachment (Damasio, 1994).

2. Many theoretical orientations, especially among those emphasizing the motivation of self interest, treat the motivation of self interest as a constant. This assumption is most likely to be made when the theorist believes that the self interest motivation is the only motivation for all actors and all contexts.

3. This way of specifying the properties of these conceptual variables is quite simple, since all the variables are rational constructions of the theorist and thus imaginary. We can conceive of them as we will. Of course, to measure them is a different problem.

4. However, of course, that an unobservable concept has an undefined limit does not imply the existence of unlimited values of a corresponding observable variable.

5. I will later discuss altruism as a generalized emotional response that reaches out to many others without a personal relationship, but I regard altruism as strictly derivative of the dyadic caring for a specific special other. Caring in this view is very definitely *not* a subcategory of altruism directed toward a specific partner; instead altruism is seen as an expansion (and partially dilution) of emotional caring directed toward one or more nonspecial others.

6. Caring is the starting point—and engine—of the connection caregiving process, but it was the last concept to be added to my personal understanding of the process. In an early version of formulating the caregiving process, before I was able to acknowledge and understand the fundamental importance of emotion, I had placed "commitment" at the root of proactive caregiving. Commitment was cognitive, calculating, separate, safe. However, I could never find a persuasive cognitive process by which commitment could be produced and grow within a connection relationship. I had to realize—to feel—that the growth of commitment is based on emotion, not cognition. Study of the neurobiology of parental nurturance gave me a physiological basis for emotional caring.

My initial goal was to understand *amae* behaviors (proactive dependency: Doi, 1981): the temper tantrum, the sulk, and the taken-for-granted request (next chapter). It became clear that amae depended on giving, on voluntary nurturance. This led to my awareness of trust as a critical intervening concept. But whence the origin of nurturance? Nurturance, it appeared, had to depend on commitment. For about a year I went about filling my theoretical model with empathy and responsibility, maturity and security. But the effort felt sterile until I became aware that I was describing the process of parent-child nurturance with no notion of love. I had earlier started with love (especially, Singer, 1984-1987). but had moved away from it because all the conceptions seemed to treat love as a commodity, something to be given for profit. But then I began to see the emotion behind commitment, what the Japanese call *ninjo*, a "human feeling." I was able to see caring as a human emotional response rather than as a cognitive calculation. This led me to see an emotional basis of trust as well.

Chapter 6. Attachment

This chapter describes the attachment process of the connection theoretical system. Corresponding in several ways to Bowlby's concept of secure attachment, this model of attachment describes emotional processes operating in an actor who seeks and accepts warmth, comfort, protection, and other nurturance. In this model, attachment is motivated by trust, evolved like caring from dyadic preference. Trust in attachment is complementary to caring in caregiving. Similarities and differences with Bowlby's model are discussed.

Most theories of human intention must deal with the problem of double contingency (Parsons, 1951). That is, ego's interaction with alter must take into consideration alter's response to ego's actions. At the same time, alter's actions are affected by alter's anticipation of ego's response to alter's response. In Chapter 1, we reviewed a number of theoretical orientations that describe the logic of relationships where ego and alter are both motivated by self interest seeking. The various exchange theoretical orientations for example, describe the logic by which two self-interested actors mutually adjust the values they give and receive when they are relatively equal in the resources they control. Each actor in an exchange relationship makes an exchange offer while taking into consideration the partner's anticipated willingness to agree. The power theoretical orientations, in turn, describe the logic by which a self-interested high-resource ego will be aware of a self-interested low-resource alter's ability to resist in attempting to exert power.

Double contingency is also characteristic of relationships involving caregiving. Ego, a caregiver, constructs actions that meet alter's needs or that help alter meet alter's needs. Ego's actions are contingent on alter's communication of needs, as well as on ego's anticipation of how alter will accept this help. At the same time, alter's actions to get needs met are contingent on ego's willingness to take responsibility and offer nurturance. In this chapter I will explore the ways that alter adapts to ego's caregiving. In this telling, I will reverse the approach of most attachment explanations. Most Bowlbian attachment descriptions of the parent-child relationship focus on the child, whose attachment behaviors are seen to elicit caregiving behaviors from the parent (in this approach, the parent is seen mainly in the background and is thus seen as passive until "activated" by the child). Instead, I will examine how alter's attachment actions emerge as a response to ego's largely proactive caregiving, and how alter's expectations of ego's caregiving affects alter's pursuit of attachment goals. The nature of the double contingency is particularly salient when examining what is known as attachment "styles." Attachment styles are usually described in terms of alter's response to ego's response to alter's needs. The issue of attachment styles will be discussed near the end of the chapter.

What we have just examined in the previous chapter was the proactive, giving side of the connection relationship of giving and receiving. Our focus was on ego, the caregiver. We saw alter only through the eyes of ego. Ego's proactive caregiving process may have occurred at a high level: ego's great caring for alter led to high empathy and high responsibility and thus yielded a high level of nurturance of alter. Or the process may have occurred at a lower level: ego's minimal level of caring for alter led to only a small amount of empathy and responsibility and yielded a minimal amount of nurturance. Or in spite of ego's high or medium level of caring, some barrier may have interfered with the expression of the caring, reducing or eliminating nurturance by ego's ignorance or inexperience (inability to "read" alter's expression of need or ignorance of how to meet the need), by a physical or mental ailment or by some other barrier. Now let us turn to the receptive side, the receiving side. For the sake of simplicity and clarity, I will continue to refer to the caregiver as "ego" and to the care-receiver as "alter."

THE ATTACHMENT GOAL

As discussed in previous chapters, I conceive of the goal of ego's caregiving as to meet the needs of a special alter. I conceive of the caregiving system as providing for alter's hunger, thirst, temperature control, modesty, comfort, safety, companionship, play, and self interest seeking needs. Neurobiological evidence now supports the proposition that multiple functions are served by the same caregiving process. For example, the strongest evidence that the caregiving system is associated with feeding in addition to security is the association of oxytocin release with breast feeding (see Chapter 4). Thus, within the caregiving theoretical orientation, ego's caregiving goal is to meet any of alter's needs, as perceived by ego. This is the proactive side of connection relationship. Ego's caregiving system may respond to alter's need for comfort when alter is angry. This is a need not necessarily felt by alter; alter may not perceive a need for comfort when angry. Alter may perceive a need for revenge, retribution or another form of attack. But it is ego who perceives that alter needs to be comforted. When alter is hungry, ego will provide nourishment for alter's hunger need, and will provide comfort in the meantime if food is not yet available. Caregiving is often claimed by attachment researchers to be subsidiary to attachment in that a caregiver is said to respond to attachment behaviors (Ainsworth, et al., 1978; Cassidy, 1999; Feeney & Noller, 1996). However, as we saw in the previous chapter, a great deal of proactive caregiving behavior occurs in the absence of attachment behaviors. At the motivation level, ego's caregiving motivation can be active when alter's attachment motivation is quiescent. The reverse can also be true.

Now we turn to the receptive side of a connection relationship, where alter is primed to take advantage of ego's emotion of caring. The evolutionary development of attachment followed a similar path to that of caregiving by continually expanding the domain of the system. In rats, the attachment squeak appears to be an involuntary reaction to cold. In hoofed mammals, there appears to be volitional seeking of proximity and vocalization to elicit proximity and perhaps also to elicit protection. Cats and dogs seek proximity and comforting. In humans, the attachment system as described by the connection theoretical system has an expanded set goal that includes, in addition to a desire to relieve distress, the desire to be understood, to be supported, to be cherished.

We saw earlier that Bowlby and many other attachment researchers have insisted on a relatively narrow set of goals for attachment: proximity, safety, and felt security. A lack of proximity, safety or felt security is experienced as distress, in each case caused by high level fear or low level distress—fear of separation, fear of danger, fear of loss (Bowlby, 1969/1982). However, Bowlby implicitly acknowledged a broader scope for attachment by identifying a "low intensity" version of attachment, discussed in Chapter 4. Low intensity attachment soothes and comforts, understands and accepts. Low intensity attachment is characterized by joy, love, happiness, and pleasure. Note that this process of low intensity attachment is not stimulated by fear and not goal directed at reducing distress (Bell, 2009a).

In Bowlby's theoretical system, while the attachment system is characterized by a single function, felt security, the caregiving system is characterized by two functions, what Bowlby called the "secure base" and the "safe haven" (Bowlby, 1969/1982, 1988). As Bowlby made clear, the function of a *safe haven* is to further security—that is, to reduce (regulate) fear and distress—and thus is clearly related to the Bowlbian attachment system. Using the caregiver as a safe haven often involves attachment behaviors—looking at the caregiver to feel safe, asking for a hug to relieve distress, imagining the caregiver's availability. Thus, the attachment system acts in many situations to activate the caregiver's safe haven behaviors to reduce fear and distress.

However, the caregiving system also has the second function of a *secure base* to foster exploration (Bowlby, 1969/1982). Exploration is possible because "As long as the child experiences 'felt security' . . . the attachment system is quiescent" (Hazan & Shaver, 1994). When alter is secure and the attachment system is quiescent, then alter activates the exploration/seeking system and treats the caregiver as a secure base (Bowlby, 1969/1982). As toddlers begin to be capable of independent action, parents usually begin to refocus their caregiving actions toward the child's needs for autonomy and effectiveness (Brazelton & Cramer, 1990; Mahler & Bergman, 1975). The child's self effectiveness needs (conceptualized here as deriving from the self interest seeking motivation) are promoted by the parent's acknowledgment of the child's individuality and independence, and may involve the parent's "letting go" of protection-focused caregiving in certain areas (Bowen, 1978; Clark & Ladd, 2000; Grossmann & Zimmermann, 1999; Kerr & Bowen, 1988; Main, 1999).

Other adult attachment researchers have suggested expanding the boundaries of attachment. Goldberg and colleagues (1999) have suggested that felt security should be considered to include general well-being. Rholes and Simpson have suggested that the goal of attachment behavior is to achieve "physical or psychological contact" and to experience "comfort and emotional support" (Rholes & Simpson, 2004a, pp. 3-4). It is important to note that, in the connection theoretical system, an actor with whom one satisfies attachment needs need not be, even temporarily, "stronger and wiser," need not exhibit a fundamental inequality in strength and wisdom. This approach diverges from much attachment literature (Bretherton & Munholland, 1999; Cassidy, 1999; Main, 1999; Shaver, et al., 1988).

My view of attachment, conceptualized as a receptive process within the connection theoretical system, does not focus on goals because it takes goals as derivative. As I will describe below, the emotional motivation of the system is trust, trust in the partner's emotion of caring. When we see attachment as energized by trust in the caregiver, we see how the goals to which attachment intentions and behaviors are directed may be as broad as the caregiver's dependability. Rather than assuming a priori that attachment is directed only to a particular set of needs, I will initially open the concept of attachment fully and will depend on subsequent research to identify needs that are never met by depending on a partner. I will take as the goal of the human attachment motivation system to have one's needs met by another. If we are willing to expand the meaning of "distress" so that it encompasses many unmet needs in addition to a need to relieve fear, then we can agree with Bowlby that the attachment set goal is to relieve distress. It is important to recognize that the attachment system operates in the context of other motivation systems, in particular the self interest seeking system by which one attempts to meet one's needs by one's own actions. But some of one's needs cannot be met by autonomous action. The attachment system is alter's mechanism for having needs met by ego.

THE CONNECTION THEORETICAL SYSTEM

I have suggested that ego's caregiving system can respond to all of alter's needs and desires. That is, ego's caregiving motivation responds to just about any of alter's needs where ego can provide support. If we follow Bowlby and see ego's caregiving and alter's attachment as a matched pair of motivations, then alter's attachment motivation must be seen to be matched with these same needs, not just with fear. Instead of saying that the attachment system determines alter's partnering with ego only to meet safety, security, and comforting goals (the view of Bowlbian attachment theory), the connection theoretical system suggests instead that it is alter's attachment system that chooses ego to provide for any of alter's needs. Alter's trust in ego is not just trust in ego's protection and comforting—it is alter's trust in ego as a nurturing partner. Thus, alter's attachment system chooses ego to support and help control alter's fear system (what is usually called "safe haven attachment"); but alter's attachment system also chooses ego to support alter's exploration motivation ("secure base attachment"), chooses ego to support alter's hunger motivation ("hunger attachment"), affiliation desires ("affiliation attachment"), sexual desires (lust or "sexual attachment"), and desire for companionship and intimacy (intimacy or "love attachment").

When we use the connection theoretical system to view the interaction of the caregiving and attachment psychological systems, we see a view like Figure 6.1. Figure 6.1 views a connection relationship from the viewpoint of the caregiving system. The caregiving system in ego is directed toward meeting alter's needs: exploration needs (on the left), needs for relief from fear (in the center), as well as alter's other needs (summarized on the right).

A number of attachment researchers have referred to attachment as an affect regulation system (Bartholomew, 1990; Feeney & Noller, 1996; Mikulincer & Shaver, 2007; Sroufe & Waters, 1977; West & Sheldon-Keller, 1994). In the light of our preceding discussion, this is a slightly misleading characterization. Actually ego's caregiving system is the one that regulates alter's emotions: reducing alter's fears (ego is a safe haven), supporting alter's exploration (ego is a secure base), increasing alter's comfort and happiness (ego's nurturance supports alter's low intensity attachment). One could say in this case that alter's attachment is an *emotion-regulation-elicitation* system. We can say that alter's attachment system regulates alter's emotions on those occasions where alter's attachment actions activate ego's caregiving. But this formulation obscures all of ego's proactive nurturance to regulate alter's emotion.

We see here that the attachment system can act in a service function facilitating the regulation of multiple emotional needs: attachment serves to facilitate the reduction of fear and it serves to facilitate seeking/exploration. Thus, the attachment system functions as a mechanism to select an appropriate partner and to elicit that partner's cooperation to meet one or another of the actor's needs.

THE ATTACHMENT BOND

Parallel to the definition of the caregiving bond in the previous chapter, I define the attachment bond in terms of the density and consolidation of attachment neurons in the brain (biological definition). As before, this is not a practical definition; there is no known way to count the number of attachment neurons. Furthermore, attachment is a dyadic phenomenon. There is not only no known way to distinguish the neurons associated

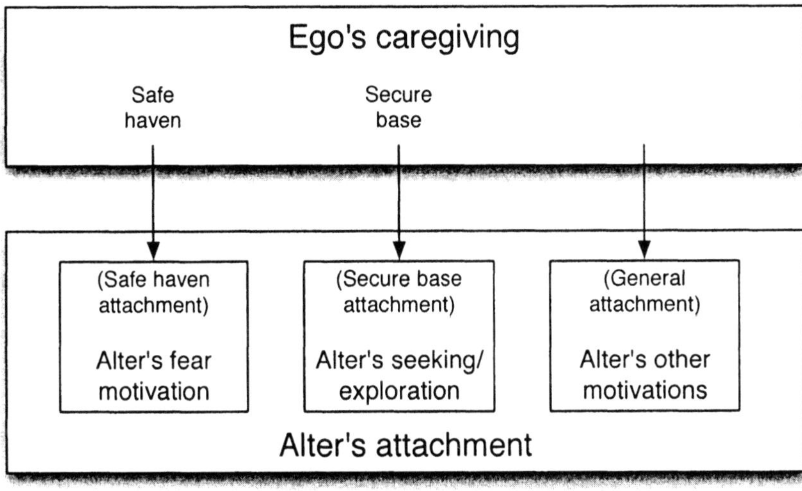

Figure 6.1. The Connection Theoretical System

with the attachment to one person from the attachment to another, but also there is certainly such an overlap and multi-tasking of these neurons that such a measurement is effectively impossible. Of course, scientists regularly find ways to measure unobservable phenomenon. Nevertheless, this definition emphasizes that the attachment bond is being conceived in terms of the capacity that an actor has to engage in attachment relationships with a given partner, a capacity that depends on a neurobiological substrate. The attachment bond in this conceptualization represents the maximum level of attachment that an actor can exhibit toward a given partner. This definition also implies that levels of the attachment bond are not fixed. New neurons can be created in resonance with new or old relationships, or they can atrophy. It is important to recognize that this conceptualization recognizes that all relationships start from an attachment bond strength of zero. Furthermore, it is important to remember that the attachment bond is an intrapersonal construct. The attachment bond is a psychological description of neuronal patterns in alter's brain which represents alter's trust of ego and motivates alter to depend on ego.

In the attachment literature, an attachment relationship is defined by the existence of an attachment bond. That is, a relationship with an attachment bond is an attachment relationship, while a relationship without an attachment bond is not. There is a range of conceptualizations of the attachment bond among attachment researchers. One set of attachment researchers conceives of an attachment bond as a dichotomy: one has a full-blown attachment bond or one has no attachment bond at all (Ainsworth, 1972, 1989; Bowlby, 1969/1982; Main, 1999; Simpson & Rholes, 2000; Sroufe & Waters, 1977; Weiss, 1982). In these views, there is no such thing as strength of a bond or level of attachment—the bond either is or it is not. Other theorists conceptualize an attachment bond that can vary in strength (Berman & Sperling, 1994; Kahn & Antonucci, 1980; Levitt, et al., 1994; Troll & Smith, 1976).

In the model that I present here, two people can differ in the strengths of their attachment bonds: each has their own number and consolidation of attachment neurons. These neurons also can be activated at different levels in the moment, from zero to an individual maximum determined by the strength of the bond. We can now turn to an examination of what it is that is being activated.

TRUST

Caring is the emotion that I see as driving the proactive process of caregiving. Trust is the emotion that drives the receptive process of attachment. Unlike caring, no neurobiological locations or neurotransmitters have yet been identified that specifically produce trust. At this point trust will have to remain a purely hypothetical construct which accounts for the attachment motivation. The trust that I wish to talk about is better known through its conscious feelings than as an unconscious emotion. The conscious feeling of trust, like the conscious feeling of caring and love, is based on a metaphor of physical contact; trust involves the feeling of being held, protected, and supported, with feelings of warmth and contact. Cognitively, the feeling of trust involves a belief in the other's caring, in the other's ability and willingness to provide protection, comfort, and support. But while caring derives its warmth and meaning from reaching out emotionally to the other, trust derives its warmth and meaning from the other's metaphorical warm and gentle touch. While the metaphorical prototype of caregiving is the mythological all-giving mother, the metaphorical prototype of attachment is the held child.

We saw in Chapters 3 and 4 that a dyadic preference develops in mammals (based on oxytocin) between mothers and children. In many mammalian species, it also develops in fathers and other adults toward the child and in the child toward the parent or adult. It is this neurobiological dyadic preference, emerging through natural selection, that forms the basis for the emotion of caring that lies at the center of caregiving. I believe that the dyadic preference also serves as the neurobiological foundation on which the dyadic emotion of trust is built. It is this emotion that provides the primary motivation in the process of attachment. The similarities of warmth and calm, and a desire for physical and social contact indicate a common basis for caring and trust. In my model, trust grows in response to caring, by physical contact and other direct social interaction. The emotion of trust is the brain's response (a) to the partner's continued contact and interaction and (b) to the partner's manifest caring. In this way, trust can be seen as an emotional awareness that one is cherished by the other.

In the earliest (and since relatively unchanged) evolved mammals like rabbits and rats, the emotion of trust is hardly distinguishable from dyadic preference. Young rabbits and rats show comfort in the physical presence of their mothers when they are infants, but aside from nuzzling to find the nipple and movement to find the warmer spot in a pile of siblings, they show little proactive behavior toward the caregiver. In rats, a high frequency squeal is a reaction to cold and to the lack of familiar scent and tactile feel. Experiments with rats have shown that the physical loss of the caregiver leads to emotional arousal and distress (Hofer, 1994), as indicated by ultrasonic calling. This squeak is used by the mother to retrieve a lost pup, but in the pup, the squeak is not a goal-corrected intentional signal. The squeak has the evolutionary consequence of survival because the mother is motivated by her caregiving motivation system to retrieve the pup. Neither rabbits nor rats, as far as the ethological evidence indicates, use the mother as a secure base for exploration. In hoofed mammals, the young do not run in the presence of a predator unless their mothers run. In herds, the young move to the center of the herd. This behavior represents a rudimentary level of trust, with limited cognitive components. Higher levels of trust can be observed in domesticated dogs and cats, who can often communicate rather clearly their expectation of food, and then wait for food to be provided. Anyone who has taken a dog or cat to the vet (after the pet's first negative experience) can see the animal's trust warring with fearful memories.

Trust is a conceptual variable that varies from zero to a high positive value. At a level of zero, alter has no awareness of or belief in ego's emotional presence: alter does not feel cherished. This is our experience with strangers and some acquaintances. At a high value of trust, there is a strong awareness of and belief in emotional contact and support, belief that the other is fully committed to helping one meet one's needs. At lower levels of trust (greater then zero) alter may feel ego's presence and support only intermittently, or only in alter's most basic needs of survival and physical health. As the level of trust increases, alter feels supported as well in more personal (e.g., psychological and social) needs.

> **Attachment assertion 1**. The greater the positive social and physical interaction with ego, the greater alter's trust in ego, because social and physical interaction increases the dyadic preference in alter that is the basis for trust.

As we explored in Chapter 4, oxytocin is released both through physical touching and through social interaction. Thus, the level of both physical contact and social interaction contribute to oxytocin production, which in turn creates and consolidates the neurons that make up the dyadic caring circuit. I suspect, but do not have evidence for, a direct effect of alter's experience of ego's caring on alter's trust, probably also supported by oxytocin release.

> **Attachment assertion 2**. The greater the caring that alter perceives from ego, the greater alter's trust in ego, because ego's caring means to alter that ego will be emotionally present and that ego will take responsibility to help meet alter's needs.

The cognitive aspect of trust, alter's perception of ego's caring, is not built on a direct experience of ego's emotion of caring. I do not believe this is a process of direct experience of the other's feelings. Instead, I believe that alter's perception of ego's caring is an experience, a feeling, and an inference that is built out of ego's observed actions. The actions that serve as indicators of caring are ego's direct expression of caring, and alter's experience of ego's empathy, responsibility, and nurturance. These components of the inference of caring are shown in Figure 6.2.

To the extent that alter intuits and experiences ego's emotional contact, alter feels the warmth and comfort, the protection and encouragement of ego's emotional presence. Alter's trust is thus logically derivative of—enabled and elicited by—ego's caring as it is felt, perceived, and experienced by alter. The causal effects involve both the (unconscious) emotional and the (conscious or unconscious) perceptual bases of trust.

> **Attachment assertion 3**. Alter's perception of ego's caring is an inference based on ego's verbal and nonverbal expressions of caring, and on alter's experience of ego's empathy, responsibil-

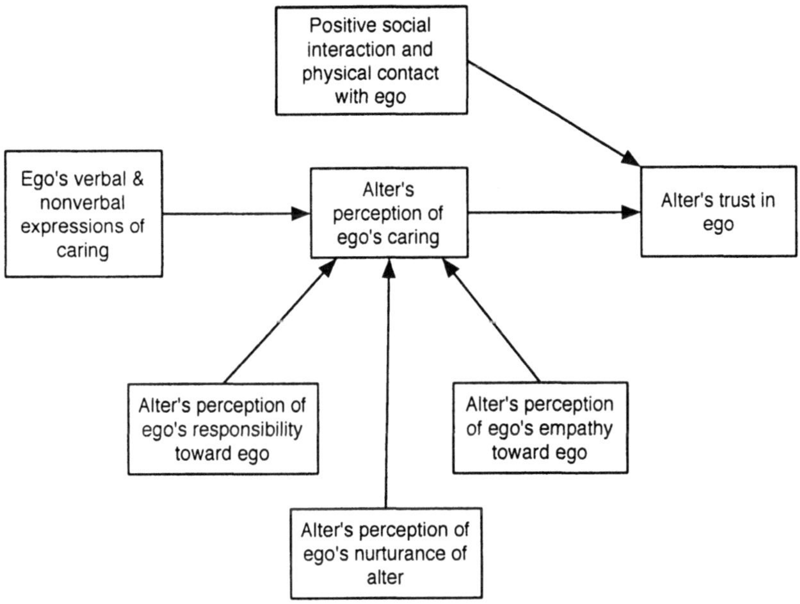

Figure 6.2. Causes of trust

ity, and nurturance, because unobservable caring must be deduced from observable action.

In principle, the highly cognitive American cultural predisposition suggests that the best way to know if someone cares for us is to ask them. We may actually do this, especially when they have done something to hurt us, when we ask for an explanatory account (Orbuch, 1997; Scott & Lyman, 1968). In practice, however, asking is an unreliable method for learning about the other's caring. Of greater value, although harder to detect, are nonverbal cues, especially those that are not under conscious control. Thus we look for eye contact and open posture; we listen to tone of voice. Caring is also deduced from overt behavior. If the other nurtures us regularly, and when we are most in need, we feel most safe in trusting.

Inference from empathy. Empathy is not entirely a matter of observation, a passive taking in of information. Empathy also involves active communication. In order to understand the other, we mirror: we reflect their communications back for confirmation. "Did you mean. . . ?" helps to verify our understanding. It also communicates our acceptance of the partner and the partner's views. As an expression of caring, empathy thus gives information as well as receiving it. Empathy validates the other, it tells the other that they are important, that they are cherished. "To the extent that the other is in tune with one's inner world, . . . then the person will experience her individuality as being confirmed. . ." (Roland, 1988, p. 189). Validation does not necessarily mean agreement. Because we cherish someone, we want to know about them. But caring does not mean that we have to be the same. Caring about the other means that we cherish who the other is and what the other thinks and feels. In many cases disagreeing with someone shows that we respect them and their ideas. This expression of respect shows our empathy.

Inference from responsibility. Responsibility is an internal emotional intention, but it often has an outward manifestation. We see evidence of the other's planning in their anticipation of our needs, as well as in verbal declarations of their commitment. We also see a sign of their responsibility in their sacrifices, as we become aware of the price the other has paid to support us. And we see a sign of their responsibility in their guilt and regret when they have failed us.

Inference from nurturance. When the other offers us something in an exchange relationship we must calculate how much we are willing to pay to consummate the transaction. But if instead they give us something without reservation, we have no contractual obligation. Gifts are unique. They not only have the objective value of a good or service; they also symbolize the relationship. They create value exactly because they are not earned (Hyde, 1983; Singer, 1984-1987). Even among strangers, the receipt of a gift creates trust toward the gift giver (Molm, Collett, & Schaefer, 2007; Molm, Schaefer, & Collett, 2009). The symbolic aspect of the gift is experienced as nurturance, a sign of the other's caring.

A frequent reaction of Americans (especially among American men in some social contexts) is that attachment is a kind of trap, a vulnerability that leads to our exploitation by others. But when our trust is matched by a partner's caring, when we have a relationship with someone who considers our needs as important as theirs, then we need not feel frightened by vulnerability. Our trust is a trust that they will protect us rather than hurt us, that they will nurture us rather than exploit us, because they care. From within a relationship of connection we can trust the other up to the level of the other's manifest caring. We not only "trust" the loved one to avoid giving us pain, we can also trust the other to look out for our needs as well as for their own. An immature sense of attachment, such as children experience with parents, insists that our wants be satisfied even at the expense of the other. A mature sense of attachment recognizes that the other has their own needs, but expects that our needs will be satisfied in a balance with the other's needs. This mature attachment entails our obligation to reciprocate and to support the other's needs along with our own. Because trust develops out of alter's understanding of and emotional responses to ego's caring, the extent of alter's trust depends on the extent of ego's trust. Children generally trust their parents to help them meet all of their needs. I trust the clerk at the store to give me the correct change, but not to meet my other needs.

AMAE (DEPENDING)

One of the fundamental consequences of ego's caring and of alter's resulting trust in ego is that alter can depend on ego. Dependency has a bad name in American culture and American social science. Because Westerners in general and Americans in particular exalt individualism and power, we tend to see dependency as vulnerability and weakness. In a world of selfish people, the consequence of dependency is powerlessness. When others are selfish, depending on them means that they will inevitably demand a price—a steep price—to meet one's needs. In such a world, no one would ever voluntarily choose to expose themselves to such exploitation, so dependency under such conditions must be understood as involuntary. In the self interest view, that children are dependent is simply an inherently undesirable biological fact.

Takeo Doi, however, has shown how dependency is not only a fact of childhood, it can be an overwhelmingly desirable life-long goal. The Japanese term "*amae*" (甘え)[1] denotes a desirable dependency; it has a positive connotation, indicating warmth and support. *Amae* is seen as a central concept in Japanese culture (Doi, 1981). In Japanese, *amae* is active, both grammatically and culturally: the one actor "performs *amae*" or "does *amae*" (*amaeru*) in requesting and receiving the benefits of the other's actions. Even Americans perform *amae* regularly, but English has no distinct word for positive dependency, so Americans often do not attend to this aspect of our actions. Although we do *amae*, we usually do not label it. And without a label, we often do not experience it.

Amae is the emotional intention that one's needs will be met by the other. *Amae* is thus an intention to be dependent on the other and to have one's needs met thereby. Although *amae* is not conceived here as an emotion, *amae* is emotional. We often experience it as a feeling, an intuition that the other is dependable. Like empathy and responsibility, *amae* is a goal-directed intention. Some Americans might be more comfortable with "expectation" rather than "intention" in the definition above. Such terminology would fit with the American perception of depending as passive. However, *amae* is not just an expectation that a powerful other will provide nurturance (the "stronger and wiser" partner in Bowlbian attachment); *amae* is an active intention to seek such nurturance. The feeling of *amae* is a feeling of confidence and entitlement (Doi, 1981). The dependency of *amae* is not limited to the goal of reducing fear and distress, as in Bowlbian attachment; *amae* can involve depending on the partner for any need.

Amae is a conceptual variable that varies from zero to a high positive value. At a level of zero, alter has neither expectation nor intention that ego will meet alter's needs; alter is completely independent of ego. At the highest value, alter has a complete expectation that ego will meet alter's needs. Alter feels a determined intention that alter's needs be met even if alter gives only subtle indications of need.

Although in U.S. cultural heritage "dependency" has a generally negative connotation of powerlessness, passivity, and weakness (after all, strong, self-sufficient people—real men—don't depend on anybody), there are, in fact, two meanings of the English term "dependency." While the dominant meaning equates dependency with weakness, there is a second meaning that is somewhat consistent with the concept of *amae*. This meaning is the one used in the expression, "I know I can depend on you." This expression does *not* mean "I know I am helpless with you." It means "I know I can trust you to look out for me," based on a faith in the other's dependability. The concept of *amae* in Japanese has a very positive flavor, connoting warmth and support. Unlike Western notions of dependency that focus on what alter has to give up to ego (Blau, 1986; Emerson, 1962), *amae* focuses on what alter *receives*. The connection theoretical system focuses on getting what you need through *amae* depending,[2] through actively depending on another. This approach reflects a clear awareness and acceptance of human *inter*dependence, in contrast with the intense American valuing of self sufficiency and *in*dependence.

Some authors have described dependency in a way similar to the concept of *amae*. Dependency, according to Murray (1938), is behavior which has as its goal the obtaining of nurturance from other people, or which clearly indicates the reliance upon the help of others. Murray, however, describes the concept as a global personality construct, rather than as an aspect of a specific relationship. In a similar way, Stiver (1991, pp. 160, italics removed) defines dependency as a "process of counting on other people to provide help in coping physically and emotionally with the experience and tasks encountered in the world when one has not sufficient skill, confidence, energy, and/or time." This usage also parallels a contemporary description of dependency needs (Ferguson, 1970). Bandura and Walters (1963, p. 139) define dependency as "a class of responses that are capable of eliciting positive attending and ministering responses from others." This behavioral definition avoids the consideration of alter's emotions and expectations. Sometimes this form of dependency is conceptualized as part of a self-interest-based social learning process, and thus has a strictly cognitive quality (Steinmetz, 1979). Doi suggests that Balint's concept of "passive object love" is somewhat similar to *amae* (Balint, 1965), but this psychoanalytic term overemphasizes the passivity of depending. Object relations psychologists recognize the importance of active dependency to human psychological health (Fairbairn, 1952; Winnicott, 1965b).

> **Attachment assertion 4**. The greater alter's trust of ego, the greater alter's *amae* toward ego, because alter's trust in ego's cherishing and sympathetic commitment to alter's needs produces an active expectation that ego *will* act for alter's needs.

To the extent that I have come to trust you, to feel cherished and protected by you, I can count on you. When you show evidence of caring, when I see you as having made an emotional commitment to me, then I no longer must deny my needs in self protection against an uncaring world. When no one cares about me, my unmet needs are a sources of pain, vulnerability, and loneliness. To the extent that I know you cherish me, I can be complacent and confident: I know you will take care of me. The attachment process is shown in Figure 6.3.

Amae depending is an emotional intention in that it is energized and motivated by the emotion of trust. It also includes conscious feeling, a feeling of entitlement. The actor's feeling of entitlement grows out of the actor's unbetrayed vulnerability, out of the actor's trust in the other's dependability. Doi emphasizes—and perhaps overemphasizes—that *amae* is a passive emotion (Doi, 1989). This passivity is probably often true in Japan where needs are mostly communicated through nuance and intuition. But demands for nurturance can be quite assertive. Doi acknowledges this when he notes that "it is quite possible to pursue such a passive stance actively" (Doi, 1989, p. 350). However, assertiveness is not the same as aggressiveness. Healthy *amae* tends to be well tamed and

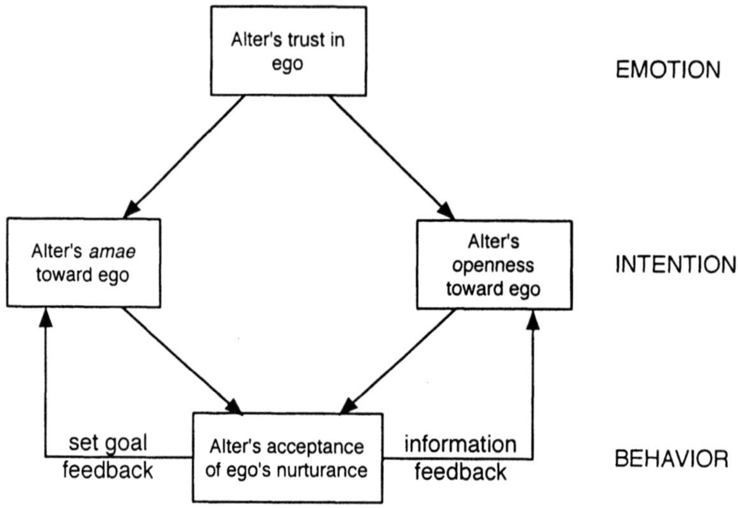

Figure 6.3. The Attachment Process

well behaved (see the next chapter). In the view of attachment proposed here, ego is a "safe haven" to the extent that alter trusts ego and depends on ego for safety and comforting. Ego is a "secure base" to the extent that alter trusts ego and depends on ego to support alter's exploration. Alter's trust means that alter can depend on ego to help meet all of alter's needs.

In a secure relationship, *amae* and acceptance have a positive, self-reinforcing association. Positive *amae* is "childlike, innocent and restful" (Doi, 1989, p. 350). However, *amae* is not always positive and trusting. One cause for negative *amae* involves the partners having different perceptions of needs. For example, the parent may have decided that the child has grown so that what used to be the child's "needs" have now been redefined as "wants." The child who needed help in buttoning her clothes may now have become an accomplished buttoner. The parent may subsequently treat a request for help with buttons as inappropriately immature. The child, however, may not have come as yet to redefine the situation in the same way. Or the child may feel accomplished in this area on some occasions, but under stress, the child may "regress" and feel this need again as a way to reactivate a nurturing relationship with the parent. In terms of attachment theory, this may be referred to as the child's "attachment behavior" as the child attempts to reestablish equilibrium after a separation (Bowlby, 1988). If the parent acknowledges the stress, the parent may see help with buttons as a need; but if the parent is not aware of the stress or sees the stress as something the child should deal with, the parent may not agree that buttoning is a need. This incongruence in the perception of need will provide the backdrop for negative *amae* from the child. The child can express *amae* either actively or passively. An example of active (and negative) *amae* is a tantrum; while passive (and negative) *amae* is exemplified in a sulk. The tantrum is grounded in the child's awareness of her special, unconditional relationship with the parent or other caregiver. There will be no tantrum unless she has a reason to assume acceptance. As the frustration continues, the child may transform the tantrum into a sulk. This sulk arises out of the child's awareness that what she wants will be denied, but it also includes her refusal to accept the denial. The sulk represents her certainty that she is right—that she deserves what she wants. Negative *amae* is generally seen as childish—whether it comes from an eight-year-old or from a business executive or a rock star.

OPENNESS

Children have to learn to keep secrets. It is natural for children to be open and self revealing. They are open when they are afraid, when they are hungry, when they are cold, when they are lonely, and when they are bored. Many terms that are used to characterize childhood, such as disingenuousness and innocence, are terms that describe the trusting openness of the child. Openness within the logic of connection, however, does not require innocence.

Openness is the emotional intention to communicate one's needs to the other. As an intention, openness includes the feeling of being opened to the other and the action of expressing one's needs. It is an intention to reveal and to be understood. At a level of zero, alter has no intention of revealing needs. At the highest value, alter intends to reveal many or all of alter's needs to ego; alter accepts the vulnerability of openness and considers such openness as an opportunity for need fulfillment. The definition of openness does not distinguish among needs. Any need can be the subject of attachment openness. However, attachment relationships differ. When we trust an attachment partner to care about all of our needs, we can reveal all of them. When we trust an attachment partner to care only about certain of our needs, then our openness will be limited to those needs.

Openness in the social context of American culture does not reflect the high level of nonverbal empathy associated with openness in Japan. American children are taught to express their ideas and their needs in words. A healthy middle class American family is one in which people share their feelings and needs openly, by which we mean vocally. American culture, with its emphasis on independence and self reliance, puts most of the burden on the actor who would do *amae* to make their wishes known. From the Japanese point of view, American childrearing practices seem insensitive.

> Inculcating children with the values surrounding individualism is of paramount importance in American culture. Telling children to "make up your mind" about what clothes to wear or what flavor ice cream to order, even when they are too young to exercise such judgment, is common. American parents seem to coax their children to become independent even before they are ready (Befu, 1986, p. 22; see also Parens & Saul, 1971).

My sons knew that if they wanted me to do something for them, they had to tell me what it is they wanted. They needed to be assertive; I couldn't read their minds. In a way this lessened the value of what I then gave. But my adopted daughter, who is Japanese, often made only vague indications of discomfort and expected me to interpret it clearly. Her view was that I am a Daddy and so she expected me to know and provide whatever is needed. Before she became more acculturated as an American, she considered it rude to say, "May I have a second helping." Instead she would gently scrape her fork over her already clean plate, or perhaps say "That was very good." The most self-assertive remark she had made (at age six) after two years in our family was, "I wonder if there is any more." I was frequently disheartened to see how my culturally ingrained habit of asking her to be more specific put an unnecessary burden on her. Why should a six-year-old child have to explain what she wants, to be direct, to be assertive? Isn't it reasonable that she should just *depend* on me? In a counterpoint to this anecdote, Roland describes the experience of a Japanese psychologist:

> [U]pon returning home after three years in New York City, he, his wife, and daughter went to a restaurant. When they sat down, he asked his eight year-old daughter what she wanted to eat. She replied, "I don't know." This was so unusual that the father asked, "Is something wrong with you, are you not feeling well?" "No," the

> daughter answered, "I am just becoming Japanese again" (Roland, 1988, pp. 190-191).

> **Attachment assertion 5**. The greater alter's trust of ego, the greater alter's openness toward ego, because alter's trust in ego's cherishing produces a feeling of safety in alter so that alter is encouraged to reveal alter's needs to ego.

Openness emerges out of trust. Because ego cares for alter, because alter has come to trust ego's emotional commitment to alter's welfare, alter can afford to be open. Because we feel trust for another and their caring, we feel not merely protected; we feel nurtured and nourished. We feel it is normal and fruitful to communicate what we need.

Telling another what we need involves risk. Unlike wants, expressing needs exposes our weaknesses. For another to reject our wants merely shows that their interests and values differ from ours. But for another to reject our needs is a basic invalidation of our character, of our value as a person (Vogel, 1963). For this reason, communicating our needs to another makes us vulnerable. But at the same time, openness enables caregiving. Emphasizing the mutuality of openness and its complementarity with empathy, Surrey notes that "'Being with' means 'being seen' and 'feeling seen' by the other and 'seeing the other' and sensing the other 'feeling seen,' which is the experience of mutual empathy" (Surrey, 1991, p. 155).

Amae and openness need not be verbal. A healthy Japanese family is said to be one where verbal sharing is not always necessary because of mutual empathy. For a Japanese man to say he takes his wife for granted is considered a compliment; it means he can count on her, she can catch his needs and wants without his needing to assert or overtly express himself (e.g., Doi, 1981). And it means that his appreciation is so apparent that it need not—indeed, should not—be overtly expressed. In a similar way, by being sensitive, a Japanese mother tries to be aware of the baby's early cues and to respond immediately, before the baby is fully aware of discomfort (Roland, 1988). The gender-relatedness of cultural expectations about openness and *amae* is captured in Stiver's description of "taking for granted":

> Wives, as caretakers and nurturers, readily respond to their husband's physical and emotional needs. . . . This is so much within the realm of the traditional wife's "job description" that the man does

> not usually need *to ask* for these things; rather he has learned to expect them (Stiver, 1991, pp. 154, italics in original).

ACCEPTANCE

Children enjoy the benefits they receive from parents. What children get to do more than anyone else is to be nurtured, to be indulged. Children get to take and consume, and they seldom are asked or expected to give anything back. Furthermore, the receiving that children do is not a passive acceptance. It is an active enjoyment of deserved satisfaction. Acceptance, like nurturance, is voluntary. It would be useless for alter to ask or demand if ego were not committed to respond. But at the same time, it would be useless of ego to nurture if alter were unwilling to accept the nurturance.

Acceptance is the behavior of experiencing and enjoying the satisfaction of one's needs by the other. The concept of acceptance seldom appears in American social science. When it appears it takes the form of "being nurtured" or "being taken care of." As such it is conceived as an inherently passive state described in the passive voice. But in the attachment process, acceptance is an active behavior. Acceptance does not just mean the infant allowing the nipple to be put in the mouth. It means sucking on the nipple, swallowing the milk, and being satisfied. It does not just mean having dinner put on the table in front of one. It means eating the dinner; it means enjoying it, appreciating it. When it rises to consciousness, it is embodied in the enjoyment that one feels when being held by a significant other. Acceptance involves the active experience and appreciation of the other's comforting, protection, and support.

Conceptually, alter's behavior of acceptance is a different variable concept from ego's nurturance of alter, although they are obviously related. If ego provides a service that is a benefit to alter, it is not nurturance unless ego is intending to fulfill alter's needs by providing the benefit. Similarly, if ego provides a benefit to alter, alter does not experience acceptance unless alter takes the behavior as meeting alter's needs. If, for example, alter believes that ego is providing the benefit to complete an exchange transaction for some action of alter's, then alter's experience is not acceptance, and alter may experience the action as a burden rather than a relief (Moody, 2008).

Acceptance is a conceptual variable that varies from zero to a high positive value. When acceptance is at a level of zero, alter is experiencing no benefits from ego that are felt to be directed toward fulfilling alter's needs. When acceptance is at a very high level, then alter is experiencing an important benefit or a large number of benefits as coming from ego directed toward alter's needs. It is not relevant to this definition whether the benefits meet some observer's judgment of alter's needs. In this process it is only relevant that the benefits satisfy alter's subjectively experienced needs, since the attachment process is one that is motivated in the mind of alter.

> **Attachment assertion 6**. The greater alter's *amae* toward ego, the greater alter's willingness to accept ego's nurturance, because alter's intention to depend on ego's responsibility leads alter to accept the nurturance that is forthcoming as fulfilling alter's needs.

> **Attachment assertion 7**. The greater alter's openness toward ego, the greater alter's willingness to accept ego's nurturance, because alter's intention to be open in expressing needs to ego's empathy leads alter to interpret ego's action as nurturance of alter's needs and thus to accept that nurturance.

Assertions 6 and 7 show how ego's perceived intentions toward alter contribute to alter's acceptance. We can see that the attachment process as described here includes the operation of what was described neurobiologically in Chapter 4 as low intensity "nondistress attachment." We see here that the attachment process does not require fear. Alter can trust and depend on ego in the face of alter's fear and distress, but alter can also trust and depend on ego to help meet other needs as well.

One way to appreciate nurturance is to say "thank you." Another way is to *show thanks* by enjoying the nurturance. When the child enjoys the gift, grandmother knows her gift provided nurturance. Acceptance is related both to the gift of the caregiver and also to the openness and *amae* of the one who receives the gift. Where *amae* expresses the expectation of nurturance and openness expresses the need, acceptance expresses the satisfaction of the need. Acceptance is thus validating to the nurturer.

Okonogi points out that acceptance "involves complex feelings of satisfaction, as well as guilt, for one's entitlement" (1992, p. 22). The balance between satisfaction and guilt depends on whether the actor has done "too much" *amae*. If ego has not had to give up ego's needs in order to nurture (or if alter is unaware of ego's sacrifice) then alter is expected to feel only satisfaction. If alter is aware that ego has sacrificed ego's needs, alter may feel guilt as well. This guilt is discussed in the next chapter in connection with the process of restraint.

Many connection relationships, especially between adults, are mutual in that each partner will do *amae* and acceptance at one time and take responsibility and give nurturance at another. In many relationships, there is a tendency toward balance that is sometimes taken as reciprocity, but neither reciprocity nor balance is a definitional requirement within the connection theoretical system because responsibility and nurturance depend on the level of need. Since caregiving involves giving someone what they need, there can be a natural imbalance when one partner has a greater need. This is especially true of parent-child relationships where the parent mostly nurtures and the child mostly performs *amae* and accepts nurturance. Traditionally in the husband-wife relationship, there has also been an imbalance in *amae*. In the United States, as in Japan, the nurturing role falls much more frequently and more heavily on women than on men. In traditional U.S. and Japanese culture, the husband is often seen as a dependent within the family at home, relatively helpless and cared for by his wife. The nurturance that he receives is what makes the house a "haven" for him (Lasch, 1977). A Japanese husband once explained that his staying away from home was a sacrifice in support of his wife and children. If he were at home, his wife would have to devote time to care for him, too, adding stress for her and taking her away from nurturing the children. From the standpoint of contemporary American values, we are likely to interpret the imbalance of marital roles as exploitation, as husband's power and wife's submission. There is certainly some truth to this; women can experience a lack of economic alternatives and a legal and moral system geared to a male-dominant status quo. However, in Japan, as in earlier U. S. society, women are often seen as powerful, as fully dominant in the one sphere they share with men—the family. My mother during the 1940s and 1950s did not strike me as weak and submissive, for all the attention she gave to providing for her husband and children. She seemed to experience—and in later life reported that she experienced—feelings of satisfaction and self worth that are not allowed for in the exchange and power models that social scientists have often used to try to account for her behavior. Thus, an imbalanced *amae* relationship does not imply exploitation.

One aspect of traditional marital relationships is what Japanese call *hohitsu*, "shouldering all actual responsibilities while conceding all apparent authority" (Doi, 1981, p. 58). A number of authors have noted wives' competence and strength in supporting a myth of husband dominance in Japan (Lebra, 1984; Salamon, 1986) and elsewhere (Segalen,

1983). These observations suggest that, whatever the actual level of power difference, some part of the perceived power difference may well be a myth. Dr. Doi points out (personal communication, 1988) that the *amae* and acceptance of men in Japan is not so much *less* than that of women, rather more *visible*. The less visible acceptance of women relates to their receiving more protection than overt nurturance. "Dependability," he notes "is what women look for in men" (see also Diamond, 1995). This view is consistent with life in Japan in the 1980s or in the United States before the 1960s. Of course, both societies are evolving. As the husband's economic role has declined (absolutely in terms of the increasing instability of employment during economic downturns, and relatively in terms of the loss of the husband's monopoly on external employment), his "dependability" in the public arena has become less important. But even with increasing employment by wives, their nurturant role shows little evidence of decline. As women have increased their occupational contributions to the family, men have been slow to significantly increase their level of housework and parenting (Knudson-Martin, 1993).

In the adult, trust, *amae*, openness, and acceptance are not restricted to family members. One can do *amae* with almost anyone, but to do so activates a set of obligations and responsibilities. In Japanese, to respond to another's kindness (i.e., when one has engaged in acceptance by receiving from the other), one may say, "*sumimasen*," which means literally, "It is not finished," indicating a continuing relationship (Doi, 1981, pp. 31-32) or obligation (Benedict, 1954). Westerners think of "Thank you" as a punctuation mark; the "thank you" completes the cycle of giving and receiving. In Japan, the equivalent of "thank you" (*"arigato"*) is frequently replaced by "*sumimasen*": implying that the cycle cannot be completed by mere words (see also Bell, 1989). Because I feel the nurturance I receive from you as a reflection of your emotional caring for me, I respond without calculation and with a desire to nurture you.

ATTACHMENT STYLES

Although the attachment process described in Figure 6.3 is quite straightforward and direct, it is also somewhat misleading. Alter's experience of acceptance, of being taken care of, is at the end of a long causal chain that depends on ego's caring and caregiving. The full process of a connection relationship is somewhat more complex and indirect than this simple causal chain because of the double contingency of caregiving and attachment. The logic of the double contingency is expressed in Figure 6.4. Neither ego's caregiving or alter's attachment operate alone; each depends on the other. Ego's responsibility and empathy determine ego's willingness to nurture (caregiving assertions 3 and 4). Ego's nurturance not only depends directly on ego's level of responsibility and empathy to turn ego's willingness into effective action, but also indirectly on alter's level of *amae* and openness. If alter has not openly expressed alter's need, the behaviors that ego offers as nurturance may not be well directed, and they may not be perceived as nurturing by alter. At the same time, alter's conscious or unconscious awareness of ego's responsibility and empathy enables alter to correctly interpret ego's nurturance and accept it. Alter's *amae* and openness are results of alter's trust in ego. The effectiveness of alter's *amae* depends fully on alter's ability to activate ego's responsibility. Alter's *amae* (alter's willingness to depend on ego) can only be fulfilled if ego has the intention to meet alter's needs (ego's responsibility). Similarly, alter's openness depends fully for its effectiveness on ego's empathic accuracy. We can conceive patterns among these contingent responses in terms of attachment styles.

The double contingency of caregiving and attachment expressed in Figure 6.4 help to understand the nature of attachment styles. Building on the themes of the three volumes of Bowlby's masterwork (Bowlby, 1969/1982, 1973, 1980), attachment researchers have identified three basic patterns of attachment, referred to as "attachment styles:" security, attachment avoidance, and attachment anxiety (Ainsworth, et al., 1978). The nature of these styles can be seen as responses to the double contingency of dyadic relationships.

Attachment security

The expression of both *amae* and openness are influenced by the mutuality of the double contingency. *Amae* can only be fulfilled to the extent that ego is willing to take responsibility to help meet alter's needs. In a similar way, openness (alter's expression of needs to ego) can only be fulfilled if ego has the intention to understand alter and alter's needs (ego's empathy). From alter's point of view this depends on alter's expectations: alter's *amae* and openness develop out of alter's trust which in turn develops out of alter's experience and perception of ego's caring. Having inferred ego's caring, alter can anticipate a comparable level of responsibility and empathy in ego. This expected responsibility in turn facilitates alter's *amae*, while the expected empathy facilitates alter's openness. If alter's openness is overt, intentional and explicit, ego's em-

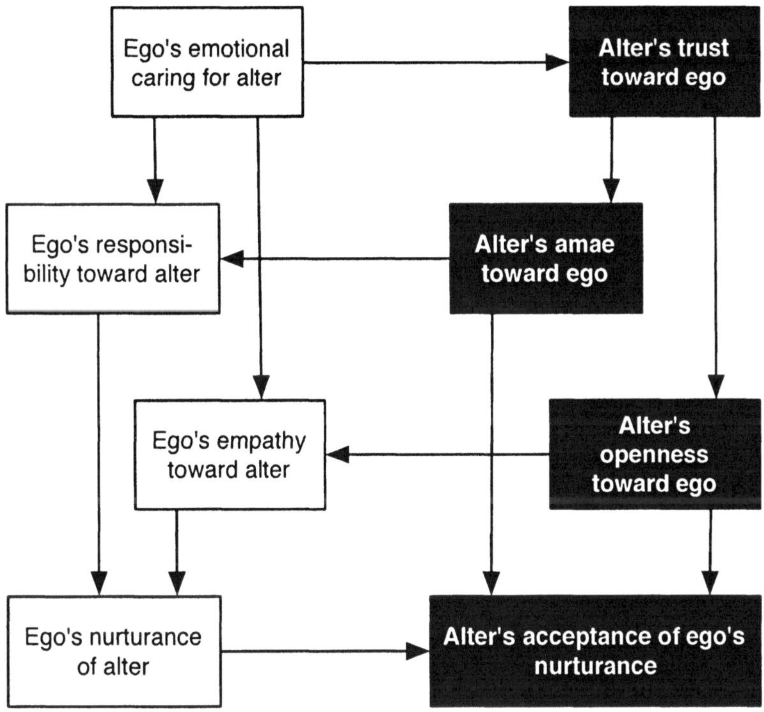

Figure 6.4. Interdependence of Caregiving and Attachment

pathy will be more easily achieved. Thus high *amae* and openness in alter are found to go with high responsibility and empathy in ego. "Active *amae*" refers to the situation where alter's high intention of being nurtured (high *amae*) is supported by a correspondingly high level of communication of alter's needs (high openness) (Doi, 1981). This pattern is described in the attachment literature as "attachment security." Over time, as a significant relationship shows high levels of nurturance, alter will come to create an expectation of such behaviors, so that alter comes to have a general internal working model that anticipates a secure attachment relationship with subsequent partners.

Attachment anxiety

When alter perceives that ego's level of caring is low, but not *very* low, alter may anticipate a low to moderate level of responsibility in ego. Low to moderate responsibility may have been expressed in ego's lack of enthusiasm for meeting alter's needs or else in ego's temporal inconsistency: high responsibility at one time and low responsibility at another. To activate this responsibility, alter activates elicitation behaviors at a high level to try to convince ego to respond to alter's need. Note that alter's *amae* is low to moderate (alter has a low to moderate willingness to depend on not-very-dependable ego): but the behaviors that express the low to moderate *amae* are high energy behaviors. In the language of Bowlbian attachment theory, alter uses an anxious hyperactivation strategy toward ego (Mikulincer & Shaver, 2007). In this anxious relationship, alter's openness will also sometimes be expressed at a very high level (when it is expressed) because alter is convinced that ego's empathy will be difficult to activate—strong action is required to "break though" against ego's reluctance to respond to alter's needs. At the same time that alter expresses openness at high energy and perhaps high volume, the actual content of the openness is limited by alter because of the risk of vulnerability when ego is not experienced as trustworthy.

When attempts to achieve nurturance are unfulfilled, *amae* and acceptance take a negative form. Doi calls this negative *amae* a "convoluted" *amae* that is "childish, willful and demanding," asking for too much (Doi, 1989, p. 350). Groves (1978) refers to "dependent clingers" experienced by therapists as "hateful patients." The negative aspects derive from the feeling that we can—we should be able to—depend on someone, but that the other has failed in their responsibility to provide the nurturance in the manner that we intend. It is always deeply wounding to rely on someone (feel *amae*) but then to have our needs unfulfilled. There is some evidence (Roland, 1988) that the problem of negative *amae* is especially acute in Japan, where there is a tradition of not overtly expressing one's needs.[3] In this situation, even when the other wants to nurture us, the difficulty of accurately determining our only-hinted-at needs can compound the problem. Negative *amae* is sometimes described as a "dependent personality" (Bornstein, 1993). Bornstein traces dependency to parental overcontrol as a form of failed nurturance.

From the perspective of the model presented here, the failure of the other to provide the nurturance that we have opened ourselves up for provokes an intense disappointment and possibly rage that lies behind anxious hyperactivation. By opening ourselves we have made ourselves vulnerable, so there is a strong component of pain in this reaction (we saw in Chapter 4 that this can be literal as well as metaphorical pain). Rage can also be seen in a child's temper tantrum. The frustration and rage of this negative *amae* process are heightened by a sense of weakness and powerlessness. Negative *amae* is not a low level of *amae*. It must, almost by necessity, grow out of a high degree of positive *amae*. It is only by experiencing the other's expression of caring that we can develop the trust that allows us to open up to be nurtured, and to feel the *amae* of depending on another. If one has never experienced another's caring and nurturance, the logic of attachment in the connection theoretical system suggests that one will never develop a high level of trust or *amae*. In such a case there can be no negative *amae*. But once we have experienced *amae* at a high level, the actual or perceived loss of the other's caring and nurturance can be deeply wounding. The effort to regain the enjoyment of the other's nurturance, to restore the emotional security of *amae*, can lead to the demanding behaviors of negative *amae*.

If alter's perception of ego as having low responsibility is accurate, then alter's expectations will be upheld and little nurturance will occur. But the double contingency is important here. If ego does in fact care for alter, then alter's passive amae and resulting lack of openness create a problem for the relationship. To the extent that alter engages in passive *amae* and resists openness, the effectiveness of the caregiving-attachment relationship depends on the competence and effectiveness of ego's empathy: ego will need to achieve successful empathy through reading indirect cues in body language or facial expression, through previous knowledge of alter, or through cultural expectations. For example, in conversation, one might seek a response from another even though he is quiet.

Attachment avoidance

In a pre-existing connection relationship where alter perceives that ego has a very low level of caring toward alter, alter anticipates very low responsibility and very low empathy from ego. If ego does not take responsibility for alter's needs, then any attempt by alter to depend on ego will be unfruitful. If ego has low empathy, then alter will anticipate that openness about alter's needs will not be heard. There is no reason to demand much if there is no reason to expect much response, and the resulting level of alter's *amae* will be low. In the language of Bowlbian attachment theory, alter uses an avoidant deactivation strategy toward ego (Mikulincer & Shaver, 2007). This creates what Doi calls "passive *amae*" (Doi, 1989). With low trust, alter will express low openness. There is little point in exposing one's vulnerability when it is unlikely to be supported. Alter's openness will be low with ego because of alter's conviction that ego will not respond with empathy.

Although both *amae* and openness both emerge from trust, they need not result in equivalent levels because of the operation of other processes besides connection. Discrepancies between openness and *amae* put different kinds of burdens on a relationship. Passive *amae* occurs when a high level of *amae* is not supported by a high level of openness. Passive *amae* depends almost exclusively on the partner's empathy, unsupported by the actor's active openness. The actor who sits quietly while waiting to be invited into a group discussion is displaying passive *amae*.

Non-attachment

There are also dyads within which no attachment systems and no caregiving systems are active at all. These non-connection relationships include dyads in which the partners are strangers as well as dyads in which the partners are acquaintances and even friends, but neither caregiving nor attachment systems have been consolidated. Non-connection dyads can also include actors about whom a normative expectation of attachment is held, such as partners in a marriage of convenience or parents who, coming out of unloving or abusive homes, have never learned to love or to trust. There is significant evidence from studies of institutionalized children (Chisholm, 2000; Chisholm, Carter, Ames, & Morrison, 1995; Zeanah, et al., 2005) that under some circumstances attachment circuits do not form. Such children do not have a *de*activated attachment system (Mikulincer & Shaver, 2007): they have little or no attachment system at all. Human children with little or no physical or emotional contact with a caregiver appear to develop very sparse and unconsolidated attachment circuits, as indicated by low production of both vasopressin and oxytocin (Fries & Pollak, 2004; Fries, Ziegler, Kurian, Jacoris, & Pollak, 2005). Behaviorally, there may be little detectable difference between an avoidant attachment relationship and a non-attachment relationship.

REFLECTIONS ON CAREGIVING AND ATTACHMENT

Both the caregiving and attachment processes within the connection theoretical system are active. The caregiving process emphasizes the active giving to another, sometimes reactively in response to a direct signal or request from the other, but often proactively in anticipation of the other's as yet unexpressed needs. The attachment process in turn describes the active receiving of benefits from another, sometimes in response to the other's autonomous proactive behavior and sometimes as a result of one's own direct action to stimulate or request nurturance.

The connection theoretical system, consisting of the caregiving and attachment theoretical orientations, builds on Bowlby's original attachment theory in the light of the evolutionary and neurobiological analyses described in the previous chapters. This theoretical system has several features that mark an explanation of the original model. Of course, attachment theorists have already expanded the scope of Bowlby's proximity attachment theory to include security attachment (Chapter 2). What I am proposing here is a further expansion to include nondistress attachment.

Many of the contributions of the model I propose relate to the caregiving system. First, this analysis gives specific neurological meaning to the affectional bond described by Bowlby and describes its correspondence in the caregiving system to the caring emotion. Second, this analysis describes the psychodynamic and social psychological processes of caregiving and thus explains not only parental caregiving but also caregiving in other relationships. Third, the caregiving theoretical orientation gives explicit attention to the caregiver's nurturance in association with multiple motivation systems in alter. In addition, I propose an expansion of Bowlby's model of the attachment system. The connection theoretical system builds on the neurobiological evidence to construct a view of attachment that is separate from the fear system so central to Bowlby's formulation, and then explores the association between this attachment system and the fear system. In addition, the expanded model of attachment proposes a wider range of goals than have been considered in traditional attachment theory.

The connection theoretical system has other conceptual advantages. It allows us to explore relationships that many attachment theorists exclude from consideration by definition. Many authors have asserted that the term "attachment" should only be applied to those relationships with enduring and irreplaceable bonds (Ainsworth, 1989; Berman & Sperling, 1994; Bowlby, 1969/1982; Main, 1999; Simpson & Rholes, 2000) or to partners who are "stronger and wiser," who exhibit greater strength and wisdom (Bretherton & Munholland, 1999; Cassidy, 1999; Main, 1999; Shaver, et al., 1988). In contrast, I note that ego does not have to be stronger and wiser to breastfeed an infant, to encourage a child to develop a new skill, or to comfort a partner who is sad. I believe that in making these conditions for attachment and caregiving, attachment authors have restricted the meaning too much.

The connection theoretical system conceptualizes variable concepts: that is, it focuses on the *level of* caregiving and the *level of* attachment within a relationship. Within this theoretical system, the caregiving motivation system can be activated in a given relationship at any level from zero to some practical maximum level set by the level of consolidation of caregiving neurons. The attachment motivation system similarly can be activated in a given relationship at any level from zero to its maximum level. This is a significant departure from Bowlbian attachment. In the attachment literature, an "attachment relationship" is defined by the existence of an attachment bond. That is, a relationship with an attachment bond is an "attachment relationship," while a relationship without an attachment bond is not. This view makes it very difficult to study the development of a relationship involving attachment because attachment logic by definition cannot describe what happens in a relationship before the attachment bond forms. The connection theoretical system takes the concepts describing caregiving and attachment as variables and thus can track changes from zero.

Empirical, lived behavior involves multiple motives not entirely discernible by an observer. Providing rewards to someone because they have power over you, and nurturing them because you cherish them are not necessarily differentiated in the mind of the actor, nor empirically distinguishable by an outsider. The imbalance of caregiving in marital relationships has led some authors to claim that caregiving by wives is always a sign of powerlessness (for example, Chafetz, 1990; Knudson-Martin, 2000). That there is some truth in this argument is undeniable. But until we are able to recognize caring, nurturance and connection in these marital relationships, we will not be able to compare the relative importance of these power and connection processes for understanding relationships, across time, across and within cultures.

Having described the causal effects of caregiving and attachment as a linear process, it is time to talk more about the circular causal logic of connection. At the same time that ego's caregiving is affecting alter's attachment, alter's attachment is affecting ego's caregiving. And vice versa: both parties in a relationship can both give and receive nurturance. Even the parent-child relationship does not start with the parent's full-blown caring, and it does not end with the child's acceptance. These circular causal relationships are the subject of the next chapter. In addition, although the internal logic of connection describes a closed system in which each conceptual variable in the system depends causally on other system variables, there are always other variables outside the connection processes that affect and are affected by connection variables. Connection processes, when considered alone, can appear to be a logically closed system. However, other logics also operate in any given empirical situation, so the processes can be seen to operate as an open system. I turn to these now.

Notes

1. Three syllables, with an accent on the second syllable in the English pronunciation (ah-MΛH-eh); the vowels are pronounced as in Spanish or Italian, each vowel being pronounced separately. The verb form, *amaeru* (甘える), has 4 syllables, with a soft accent on the second.

2. I occasionally use the redundant "*amae* depending" as an aid to readers who might find it hard to remember what the unfamiliar term "*amae*" means.

3. The Japanese have a cultural myth of homogeneity. They are "one nation, one people, one language." In our research on 60 Japanese families, virtually every family apologized at least once during the interview that they were "not a typical Japanese family." Because of the myth of homogeneity, Japanese believe that empathy is easily achieved. It is my unsupported and anecdotal observation that, because of the actual wide differences among Japanese, empathy frequently fails. But because of politeness and restraint (next chapter), empathic inaccuracy is seldom acknowledged.

Chapter 7. Interconnections

This chapter discusses connection processes between the caregiving and attachment systems as well as effects from other systems. First are various feedback processes by which caring increases as a consequence of other factors. Second are other processes which influence the caregiving system. Last are processes which influence the attachment system.

The connection theoretical system has been described so far primarily as a unilinear causal process driven by ego's caring for alter and ending with alter's acceptance of nurturance from ego. The caregiving theoretical orientation explains in a straightforward way how ego's caring leads to ego's nurturance of alter, and the attachment theoretical orientation explains in a similar straightforward way how alter responds with trust, openness, and depending. In that process, each conceptual variable has effects on one or more conceptual variables that come later in the sequence and has no effects on those that come before it in the sequence. At the end of the last chapter we began to look at some of the interconnections between the two systems (Figure 6.4). In this chapter, we look at processes by which other factors affect the caregiving and attachment systems.

Ego's caregiving process that we discussed in Chapter 5 and alter's attachment process that we discussed in Chapter 6 together describe less than half of the connection relationship between ego and alter. There are, in addition, alter's caregiving process toward ego and ego's attachment process toward alter. While each caregiving-attachment complementarity can be conceived of as one-way, the relationship as a whole consists of two such caregiving-attachment processes. Thus, although the logic of connection that we have explored to this point is unidirectional, the way relationships operate is bidirectional and circular. Relationships may be uneven, as in a parent-young child relationship, but each relationship has the potential to operate from both sides.

The connection processes of caregiving and attachment described so far give the impression of an unending positive spiral, consisting of largely positive, affirmative processes. This is of course a simplification. I have abstracted out of multiplex reality a well behaved theoretical fiction. This unilinear approach has made it possible to present the connection processes with a high degree of clarity. This approach, however, presents only part of the story. We have not yet looked closely at any processes that will naturally lead to a decrease in caregiving or attachment. Several processes that operate on the connection theoretical system can be identified that augment or limit caregiving and attachment (Figure 7.1).

Caregiving and attachment relationships are not inevitable, invariably flowing from positive emotions and feelings. One of the reasons conflict models of the family (including most self interest theories) have been popular is that in-depth studies of families have long revealed a great deal of conflict (Seeley, Sim, & Looseley, 1956; Sprey, 1971). When conflict is interpreted from the point of view of self interest, conflict is seen to be a power struggle as each family member attempts to take what they want. Within connection, the "constant struggle" can be seen as a struggle to be understood, to do *amae*, to depend on the support of those we love. Within an exchange or power theory of the family, one is gratified to receive what one wants. Within a connection theory of the family, one is gratified by receiving what one needs, especially when we perceive it to be given voluntarily out of the partner's caring.

I organize this chapter around those factors that affect caregiving and those that affect attachment. These factors include "feedback" and "feed-forward" causal processes that operate between the elements of the connection theoretical system, as well as causal factors outside of the connection theoretical system.

EFFECTS ON CAREGIVING PROCESSES

In Chapter 5, the emotion of caring was described as the "engine" that drives the caregiving process. We have seen that caring is neurobiologically connected to memory, attention, decision, and reward circuits in the brain. It is through these neurological connections that caregiving emerges as a psychological system. Emotional caring is not, however, an

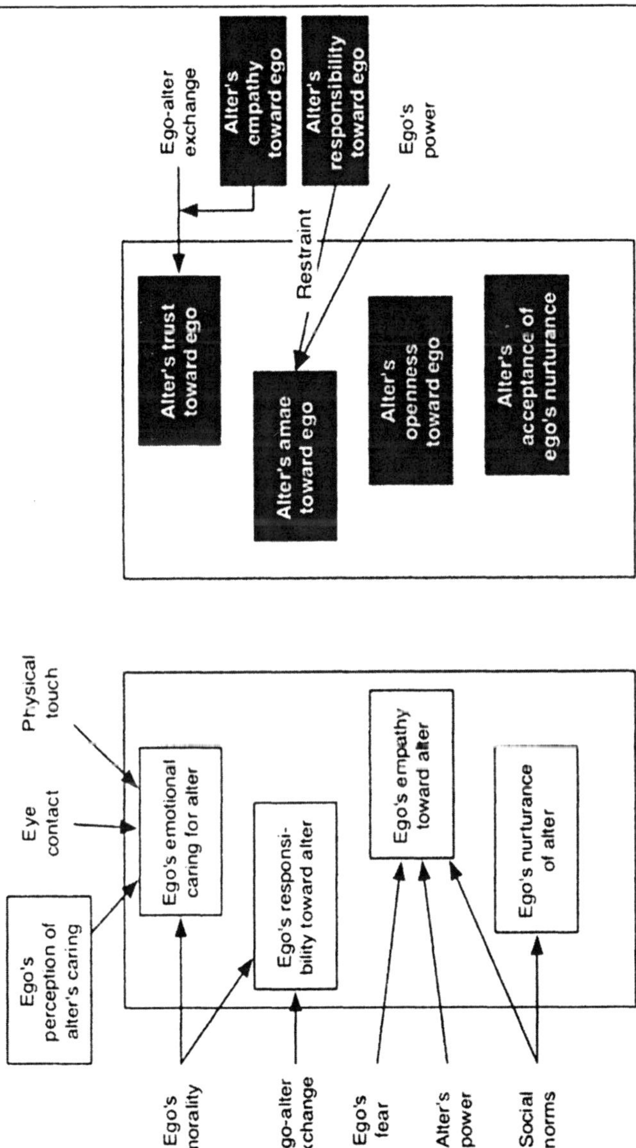

Figure 7.1. Other Connections

independent, exogenous concept. Caring is inherently dyadic, directed to a specific partner within a relationship. We turn now to a circular effect within the connection process. Concepts that were previously outcomes of caring from a partner will now be seen to be, also, causes of caring for the partner. Previously we have seen that ego's empathy, responsibility and nurturance, along with alter's trust and *amae* depending, are *effects* of ego's emotional caring for alter. These same processes in alter are also among the psychological *causes* of ego's emotional caring for alter (see Figure 7.1).

Caring as a response to experiencing caring

There appear to be several causal effects contributing to the growth of ego's caring for alter. The first psychological source of ego's caring seems to be ego's direct emotional contact with alter. When ego experiences alter's caring, ego responds to alter and comes to care emotionally for alter. I do not hold, however, that this response is a direct "contagion of emotion" (Gaylin, 1979) or a necessarily "congruent" emotional state (Batson, 2002). Nor do I accept Thomas' (1989, p. 83) hydraulic model in which the child's love "replenishes the emotional outlay that comes with caring for a child." Rather, I see a more conventional process of perception and interpretation based on a perception of caring, a perception that is both "seeing" and "feeling." To the extent that ego perceives that alter cherishes him/her, ego will respond emotionally by cherishing alter in turn.

Ego's response to alter's caregiving nurturance is both directly emotional and (indirectly) cognitive. The direct emotional response is probably neurochemical. What may be a major component in this automatic response is that the neurotransmitter oxytocin is central to both the attachment and caregiving brain systems. The oxytocin-based caregiving bond that is the biological foundation of the caring emotion is related to, but probably not identical to, the oxytocin-based attachment bond. Although there is not yet evidence on the amount of overlap of—or connections between—these two circuits, we can hypothesize some degree of natural overlap or influence. Thus, ego's attachment response to alter's caregiving augments the neurochemical basis for ego's caring. The cognitive response is more indirect. Ego perceives alter's empathy from alter's behaviors of listening and paying attention. As ego becomes aware of alter's nurturing behaviors, ego infers that alter cares, and as a result ego comes to feel closer to alter. This effect is a relatively direct emotional reciprocity: I care for you in response to my awareness of your caring for me.

Let us look more closely at the process of inferring alter's caring. Alter's caring is, at base, an unconscious emotional experience within alter. Ego probably becomes aware first of alter's nurturance behaviors. But alter's caring also produces observable intentions from alter (empathy, responsibility). The process of perceiving alter's caring is thus based both on these observable actions and on an intuitive awareness of alter's caring behind them. A discussion of this perceptual inference process was given with attachment assertion 3 (Chapter 6). But although the inference about alter's caring from observation of alter's behavior is cognitive, ego's response to this inference is emotional. Because alter loves and nurtures ego, ego responds by coming to develop an emotional contact with alter, to cherish alter in turn (Hyde, 1983; Mauss, 1967; Moschetti, 1979).

That this process is cognitive can be seen in ego's potential susceptibility to manipulation. It is not necessary that alter's caring be real—only that ego has a perception of alter's caring. If alter provides an "account" (a proposed interpretation of alter's action) that defines alter's action as directed toward the fulfillment of ego's needs, then to the extent that this account is persuasive, ego may decide that alter's action is a manifestation of alter's caring (Orbuch, 1997; Scott & Lyman, 1968). This may be manipulation by alter, a "con job" that is directed toward exploiting ego. Or it may be a matter of alter's self deception so that alter believes that the action is directed toward ego's needs even though it is actually directed toward alter's self interest. Discipline of children, in this way, can involve both connection and power processes. For example, for an insecure parent, discipline may be manipulative, an expression of power, but for the child who believes the parent's account, the discipline may inferentially be taken as caregiving. Children are likely to believe that parental discipline is for their own good, whatever parental motives truly are (Miller, 1984).

However, this is not an automatic response. If ego is unable to perceive alter's caring, ego will not reciprocate. If ego is insecure and unable or unwilling to trust, then ego may discount all evidence of alter's caring. Or if ego is a victim of abuse by people who claimed to care, then ego may be unable to respond positively to alter's caring (Bowlby, 1988).

From the point of view of the exchange orientation, an empirical correlation between alter's nurturance and ego's caring is interpreted as exchange reciprocity: ego's caring is seen to be alter's reward for providing nurturance. This causal effect involves a kind of normative reciprocity proposed by authors such as Gouldner (1960) and Blau (1986). A weakness of normative reciprocity theory is that it claims that ego's caring is a strategic choice in order to get more nurturance from alter. This explanation might make sense if ego's caring is taken in isolation. However, when we recognize that ego's caring emotion is focused on alter's needs rather than on ego's interests, we see the shallowness of this explanation. At a personal level, ego's neurochemical and cognitively constructed caring response to alter's caring may be experienced as reciprocity. And ego's caring response to alter's caring reinforces alter's caring. Because this reciprocity is common, it may, over time, lead to the emergence of a social norm within society as people come to expect it to occur. As people observe the regularity with which family members love and nurture one another, such reciprocated love becomes expected (a descriptive or emergent custom). In cases where family members do not exhibit reciprocated love and nurturance, such as child abuse, elder abuse, or spouse abuse, legal and other social forms of coercion can attempt to enforce nurturance. Nevertheless, reciprocity of caring is not generally the result of social norms, but rather the result of a person's experience of receiving care. As a matter of fact, as a methodological principle, all norms should be considered as emergent customs until direct evidence is presented that the norms are prescriptive or proscriptive (discussed in Chapter 9).

We have already seen in Chapter 4 how alter's caring leads alter to physical contact and interaction with ego. On ego's side, this physical touch and the eye contact of interaction stimulates ego's oxytocin production and thus contributes to the growth of ego's caring. The pervasiveness of this oxytocin-based direct emotional response creates an expectation (an emergent social custom) that it will (almost) always occur, and perhaps that it *should* always occur (a social norm). Thus, as ego begins to respond emotionally, ego may also feel a sense that this response is appropriate morally. To nurture the relationship in which alter has cared for ego, ego may feel a moral obligation to reciprocate the feeling of caring in the name of the relationship. However, the process that I am describing is not caused by these customs and norms. However much the emotional response is ratified by a moral expectation, within the connection theoretical system, this reciprocity is grounded emotionally in caring. Failure to reciprocate emotionally, especially among adult partners but also in parent-child relationships, can damage the relationship. The damage is not caused by social sanctions for failure to follow a norm. The damage from a failure to reciprocate emotionally is a weakening of the emotional connection. Ego's caring response is validation of alter's dedication to the relationship (e.g., Moschetti, 1979). Americans usually think of obligations as more a matter of thought than of emotion. However, the obligation of connection is not an abstract norm or exchange obligation; it is a concrete human emotional response to the other's caring. To the extent that I come to see that I can depend on you, you become a more and more special person to me. The very genuineness of your nurturance awakens an emotional reaction in me, a feeling of love toward someone who loves me. You are a person who cares for me, and I respond by caring for you.

The voluntary nature of nurturance is of critical importance to the relationship. The fact that a person in a connection relationship voluntarily chooses to nurture the other ratifies their connection. It sends the clear message that the partner and the relationship are important. By supporting the other person it sustains and empowers the ongoing relationship. When we move from an exchange theoretical orientation to the connection theoretical system, what used to be an "offer" or a "reward" becomes a "favor." Each favor from the other then becomes a symbol of our intensely personal connection, commitment, and trust. And we respond by caring back.

Limits on caring

Although caring can increase in response to the partner's caring, caring does not always increase. One way that the elements of the caregiving and attachment processes can decline is with time, or more accurately, with lack of attention. Caring and the various connection processes that stem from caring require effort. Because human beings have a finite budget of time and attention, there is an upper limit to the number of connection relationships that can be sustained (Dunbar, 1996). Since the initial formation of a connection relationship takes more attention than maintaining an existing relationship, people living in a stable community can be expected to have the potential to build larger numbers of strong connections than those in a mobile society. Furthermore, when two connected people lose touch, as when friends move apart, there is a gradual but inevitable loss of emotional contact. Without periodic activation, the strongest of connections will decline over time.

Because a relationship involves two actors, every relationship depends in part on the unique properties of the individuals and on the corresponding uniqueness of the "fit" that they construct. When two actors form a connection relationship they usually construct a bond (exceptions will be discussed in Chapter 8). At base, developing a bond is an unconscious emotional process of oxytocin-producing neural circuit growth and consolidation, so that a dyadic preference bond can at least partially form without awareness, especially the first childhood connections to parents, parent figures, and siblings. However, among humans, an emotional caring bond usually evokes conscious feelings of emotional contact and commitment. As a caring bond develops, the feeling is initially fragile. The "warmth" of this emotional contact leads the one to want to engage the other. As two actors explore their feelings and learn about one another, they may create a shared understanding out of those things that make them special to one another. To consolidate a mutually caring relationship generally requires a great deal of effort. Furthermore, the effort to create such a connection works against the abandonment of a relationship once it is created, and the unconscious neurochemical processes of the caring bond are only partially under conscious control, so that one cannot "just stop" a caring bond at will. The loss of a bond other than by a gradual process of nonrenewal produces feelings of grief (Bowlby, 1980).

Caring, disappointment, and betrayal

A connection relationship is a relationship of touching, of warmth. But the warmth is not always the warmth of "chestnuts roasting on an open fire." In a relationship energized by needs, there is no reason to assume harmony and agreement. In relationships of high connection, and more frequently in relationships of low connection, there will not be perfect correspondence between need and nurturance. And if ego believes that ego's needs are greater, while alter believes that alter's needs are greater, the connection relationship can become angry and painful.

A critical disjuncture in a connection relationship can be the discrepancy between *amae* behavior, based on expectations of what we intend to receive, and acceptance behavior, based on what we gladly receive. The discrepancy between *amae* and acceptance involves a cognitive perception and evaluation. But its effects are emotional. Disappointment (often felt as "frustration") is an emotional response to the perception of the discrepancy. Anger can be another.

For convenience I will distinguish three levels of disappointment: "not disappointed," "disappointed," and "betrayed." At low levels of attachment (low levels of trust, openness, *amae* and acceptance in a relationship of non-attachment or avoidant attachment), one's needs are not an issue in the relationship, because one does not expect this relationships to meet one's needs, so disappointment is low. Even if the other exploits us we feel little disappointment because we have no reason to expect better. At moderate levels of attachment, needs may be frequently unmet and we can characterize the actor as "disappointed" and probably angry. This can lead to the kind of hyperactive expression seen in anxious attachment. At the highest levels of attachment, all three levels of disappointment are possible. If all needs are substantially met, there is no disappointment. If needs are only moderately met, the actor may feel disappointment and may protest vigorously. But when the actor has a firm sense of *amae*, when there is a firm expectation that the actor's needs will be and should be met, then a substantial failure to meet the actor's needs is experienced as betrayal. Those things that we perceive as our needs are of fundamental importance to us. When our needs are met, we feel a pervasive warmth and contentment. When our needs are frustrated, we can feel coldness and resentment toward the person we expected to help us. Disappointment and betrayal are experiences of loss and fear of loss. Because we know intuitively that the nurturance we receive comes from the other's caring, failure to receive the nurturance we expect—and deserve and crave—is a sign that we may have lost the other's affection. In an anxious attachment relationship, the loss has already occurred over and over, so the protest is immediate, if perhaps forlorn. In a previously secure attachment relationship, the lack of nurturance, if other than momentary, is unexpected, and can be quite painful. Disappointment and betrayal can produce a decay of caring.

If we see the other as emotionally caring for us and committed to us, then escalating trust deepens the relationship and increases our caring response. But if the other should betray us—seemingly ignoring the relationship and sacrificing our needs for their own self interest or for some other illegitimate reason—we feel that as a betrayal, and we are angry at them. They have rejected our needs; they have rejected *us*. We have seen the tantrum and sulk of children; children are generally more open than adults. But adults also feel the disappointment when someone we are connected to fails to give the nurturance we feel we deserve. Betrayals of trust sometimes result in extreme behavior: temper tantrums, fights, even suicide or homicide. Solomon interprets some of these betrayals as "misunderstandings":

> misunderstandings, perceived as attacks, leave each partner feeling wounded, leading to a series of escalating retaliations and to defensive walls (Solomon, 1989, p. xiii).

Betrayal, or the (possibly misunderstood) perception of betrayal, threatens the relationship. Caring, with its deep emotional core in limbic neural circuitry, is apparently relatively robust to occasional betrayals, but openness and *amae* are likely to respond immediately by declining in value. We are less likely to be open about our needs when the partner has just been shown to be undependable. *Amae*, which represents our intention to depend on the other, is also damaged to the extent that the partner is discovered to be undependable. Furthermore, our caring itself will decline if disappointment and betrayal continue.

Responsibility and exchange

When two self interest seeking individuals with approximately equal resources enter into a relationship, an exchange relationship is created in which the two parties can make mutually agreeable voluntary trades. In a normal exchange both parties benefit because either one can refuse to consummate any exchange that does not give them profit. Under certain circumstances a self-interested actor may be willing to forego current benefits to achieve greater future benefits. And a person can have multiple interests that conflict. In order to maximize rewards (and minimize the costs of having to continually reassess one's choices), a person may sometimes choose to constrain one set of interests (usually short term) in order to maximize total rewards. Brickman (1987) defines commitment as "a force that stabilizes individual behavior under circumstances where the individual would otherwise be tempted to change that behavior" (1987, p. 2). Commitment is seen as a resolution of ambivalence. A self-interested person takes a risk in making a promise to the partner. Even if a promise is made in order to achieve selfish outcomes, changed circumstances might lead to a loss. A commitment is a promise to carry out the action whatever the circumstances. In this view, parents are seen to accept the sacrifice of taking responsibility for children because they believe long term benefits *for the parents* outweigh short term sacrifices.

The most positive view of commitment in this form is given by Becker (1960). For Becker, commitment is seen as a gradual process by which a person comes to conclude that a relationship will give positive net rewards. At each step of the commitment process, ego chooses to stay in the relationship with alter and forego potentially more rewarding short term profits from other relationships. Each of these choices is a "side bet" that the ongoing relationship will pay off. The side bets are the opportunity costs of relationships given up (the rewards from alternate relationships that now cannot be received). To the extent that ego has made a commitment, ego is constrained—by ego's own choice—from leaving the relationship, even if more attractive alternatives appear. For Blalock & Wilken (1979), making such a commitment only makes sense if one's choices are already limited by dependence on the relationship so that there are few opportunity costs. They describe no positive reasons why commitment should form. Commitment for them is strictly a self-protective response. Applying this argument to parenting, social penalties on child abandonment are what constrain parents to take responsibility for children.

For Blau (1986), like Becker, a commitment is an investment. Ego gives rewards to alter, risking their loss, in order to show that ego trusts alter and desires to develop the relationship. The resources ego has put into the relationship represent ego's commitment because they make it disadvantageous to ego to withdraw from the relationship. Making a commitment has opportunity costs in the relationship, but these very costs convince alter of ego's trustworthiness. Commitment is thus a behavioral act that serves to restrain ego's short term selfish desire to be able to terminate the relationship at will. By restricting ego's choices and convincing alter of ego's trustworthiness, ego thus promotes ego's own long term self interest in continuing rewards from the relationship.

Scanzoni and his colleagues (1989) use a slightly less individualistic approach. For Scanzoni, ego is concerned with alter's interests as well as ego's own interests. One of the dimensions of "intrinsic commitment" is "a sense of how much Other is (or is not) concerned with maximum *joint* profit instead of primarily his or her own interests" (Scanzoni, et al., 1989, pp. 112, italics in original). This notion of commitment assumes some sort of merger which creates a bilateral corporate actor whose interests are the sum of ego's and alter's interests. This approach allows for some form of cooperation or even sacrifice. Related exchange views of commitment are given by Elster (1989), Coleman (1990), and Kanter (1972).

Responsibility and morality

Morality differs from social norms in that, while norms are coercive on the unwilling actor, morality is voluntary. There is a suggestion of coercion in morality, but it is a voluntarily accepted internal coercion, a commitment to moral principle. Unlike the oversocialized view of society (Wrong, 1961), which holds that the actor once and for all fully internalizes norms in childhood, the morality orientation views the actor as making continuous voluntary decisions to act on the basis of moral principles. While normative power orientations emphasize the constancy of the social norm as a standard of action, the morality orientation gives voice to the ongoing ambivalence of the actor between self interest and other standards (Brickman, 1987).

The concept of obligation has been described as "the key and the problematic concept" of the morality tradition (Baier, 1993, p. 22). Moral obligation is a commitment to respond to others' unmet needs (Thomas, 1989). Morals may develop from the internalization of external criteria, something one may learn from observing others' values, such as philosophers or parents. Or morality may develop out of personal experience and thought. For Noddings (1984), it is empathy that creates responsibility. It is our knowledge of another's needs that activates our responsibility. Work by Batson and his colleagues (Batson, et al., 1989; Batson, et al., 1988) proposes a direct causal link from ego's knowledge of alter's needs to ego's sense of responsibility.

In the last chapter, I will explore the source of moral norms. I do not find the source in philosophical reasoning and speculation. Instead, I find the source in the caregiving and attachment processes of the previous chapters.

Empathy and weakness

Within connection, empathy comes from caring. We want to know the other because we love them. From a power perspective, however, empathy is defensive. We want to know the other in order to decrease our exposure to punishments. It is the Bob Cratchits of the world who must understand the Ebenezer Scrooges in order to avoid punitive results from the exercise of arbitrary power. In this view, when we are dependent on someone, the only way to control our own rewards is to be able to predict the powerful one's behavior (Goode, 1982; Thorne & Yalom, 1982). If we know in advance that a certain behavior of ours might provoke the other's anger, that knowledge can be used to avoid punishment (Bornstein, 1993; Goode, 1982; Lakoff, 1990; Miller, 1986; Wrong, 1988).

Empathy and fear

We saw in Chapter 4 that the fear system can activate the attachment system, motivating a person to seek nurturance from a partner. In addition, the operation of the attachment system in collaboration with a caregiving partner down-regulates the fear system (Bell, 2009a). The person's trust in the partner contributes to security, the low-fear state. An actor who feels loved develops high levels of trust, openness, *amae*, and acceptance. These attachment concepts, in turn, generate a sense of security. When the level of security thus produced is high, then caregiving and attachment processes are unhindered. We saw in the previous chapter how low trust/security resulting from the partner's inconsistent or inadequate caregiving produce low levels of attachment openness, *amae*, and acceptance.

Fear also has an effect on the caregiving system. Fear for the partner can activate the caregiving system proactively or reactively. We saw in Chapter 5 how empathy, the intention to know the other, comes from caring. Thus in the general case, we expect caring to be followed by empathy at the same level. However, self-focused fear can have a down-regulating effect on the caregiving system, particularly on empathy. When ego is frightened, for example, when ego feels a need for protection, or when ego is worried about role performance, or when ego worries about what will happen in a relationship, then the focus of ego's attention will be on the self. Ego will have less ability to give attention to alter. Miller observes:

> I cannot listen to my child with empathy if I am inwardly preoccupied with being a good mother; I cannot be open to what she is telling me (Miller, 1984, p. 258).

When basic protective needs are fully gratified, they recede to the background and focus shifts to other less basic needs (Maslow, 1987). Secure persons are able to give love, experience self esteem and seek self actualization (Bowlby, 1988; Maslow, 1987; Stern, 1985).

Fear thus inhibits high levels of empathy. Because less secure people must provide for their own needs, the outside world tends to be interpreted strictly in terms of the availability of means of achieving those needs. For such people, to relax is to fall behind, to be close is to be vulnerable. In the absence of empathy, ego's self interest has free rein. This may lead to ego's use of alter to meet ego's needs. One way can happen is through fantasy, whereby ego sees alter in ways that allow ego to meet his or her needs unilaterally. Parents' fantasy has consequences for children.

> Fantasy is reverie designed to protect the psyche from pain, self-induced blindness designed to protect it from insight. It is the dreams one invents or is driven by to assuage pain and achieve desires, irrespective of the intentions and projects of others. Fantasy creates children to meet a mother's desires; creates an abstract plan for their lives that will fulfill a family's or nation's aims; creates a mind for the child that embraces a mother's world and a will that satisfies her desire (Ruddick, 1989, pp. 120-121).

Empathy and social norms

Fear and lack of power are not the only factors contributing to empathy within the power perspective. The more subtle coercion of social norms is also held to cause empathy. There are two ways that norms can lead to empathy. In the first place, there are certain roles that contain norms that mandate empathy. Roles of service providers, such as flight attendants, may mandate punishments (or loss of rewards) for failure of empathy (Hochschild, 1983). Under this view, there are clearly defined and widely accepted social norms that mandate empathy in other roles, such as the role of parent. Parents are required by social norms to show empathy toward their children. In this view, parents exhibit empathy as a defense against punishment by society.

The second way that social norms are said to promote empathy is through a process of role-taking. When relationships are interpreted as socially mandated and socially sanctioned roles, then empathy involves imaginatively taking the role of the other (Turner, 1962). "Through role-taking, one can see the line of action that gives direction, coherence, and meaning to another's acts" (Stets, 1992:166). In order to facilitate smooth social interaction, ego needs to be able to predict alter's behavior and alter's response to ego's behavior.

Nurturance and social norms

Society has a functional interest in cooperation and nurturance among its members, and so there are social norms that require nurturance, such as the normative requirement that parents feed, clothe, and provide a home for their children. Within this view, parents are coerced into providing nurturance either by the threat of social punishment or by deeply internalized attitudes and values. Parents nurture their children to avoid social sanctions applied by their neighbors or others (Bernstein, 1983a; Blake & Davis, 1964; Brickman, 1974; Coleman, 1990; Gecas, 1976; Greenberg, 1980; Hill, 1971; Homans, 1950; Lamb, 1978; LaRossa & LaRossa, 1981; Nye, 1980, 1982; Ruddick, 1989; Scanzoni, et al., 1989; Turner, 1985). In addition, parents can be seen to nurture in order to avoid self punishment. Social norms of nurturance may be so deeply internalized in childhood that a failure to nurture causes feelings of guilt (Bahr, 1982; Burgess, et al., 1971; Cahill, 1983; Caspi & Elder, 1988; Dager, 1964; Kagan, 1977; Katz, 1979; LaRossa, 1986; McDonald, 1977; Nye, 1979; Parens & Saul, 1971; Parsons & Bales, 1955; Parsons & Shils, 1951; Rollins & Thomas, 1979; Smith, 1970; Steinmetz, 1979).

EFFECTS ON ATTACHMENT PROCESSES

Trust and exchange

When others are selfish, we are always at risk. When we expect others to be selfish, we can minimize our risk by protecting ourselves. In exchange transactions, we make offers but we are always prepared to backtrack and renegotiate. We provide information to the other to facilitate agreement, but the information is generally guarded. Too much information may enable them to exploit or manipulate us. Some exchange theorists (e.g., Blau, 1986) see trust as based on enlightened self interest. Alter trusts ego to the extent that alter calculates that it is in ego's interest to continue the relationship. If alter sees ego as basically selfish, then each time alter escalates the level of trust—each time alter becomes vulnerable—alter is tempting ego to betray that trust. From an exchange perspective, alter is calculating that ego will find future rewards from alter more valuable than current exploitation. The success of alter's exchange-trust in ego depends on alter's ability to predict ego's contingencies.

Exchange-trust is founded on predictability—a predictability based on a knowledge of the source of ego's corresponding rewards (Lederer & Jackson, 1968). Rationally self-interested alter can only trust ego's nurturance if alter can successfully manage the situation to generate continued benefits from ego. Alter trusts ego's provision of benefits because alter is aware of ego's calculation of rewards and benefits, and alter expects to be able to continue to provide the rewards that ego expects. Under such an arrangement of self interest, trust requires that alter's focus remain on ego to monitor ego's probability of continuing to provide benefits.

Amae and power

One of the most consistent definitions in the social analysis of relationships is that dependency is powerlessness (Aldous, 1978; Blau, 1986; McDonald, 1980). Power-dependency in this view involves receiving something one needs from someone else who will not give it to you except at a price. In a world of self interest, everything has a price, and the price of depending on someone else for what one needs is one's vulnerability to exploitation. Alter's power-dependency on ego is defined as ego's control over rewards that alter desires (1962). To be dependent is to be a target. Dependency is vulnerability.

The involuntary nature of dependency is emphasized by McDonald (1980). No rational, self-interested person will voluntarily put themself in the position of having to pay another. It is preferable to depend only on oneself. Thus dependency is always to be avoided. Ego's power thus reduces alter's willingness to depend on ego.

Even a child must learn self-reliance.

> Equating passivity with subservience, we have seen the child as helpless. Thus becoming an adult involves a struggle, a conflict, to outgrow this relation of subservience into the spontaneity of adult love, at once free and equal (Sampson, 1965, p. 280).

Blalock & Wilken (1979) see dependency as invariably involving a component of deprivation. They expect that power-dependency will constrain the person from pursuing more attractive alternatives:

> whichever spouse is relatively more dependent on his or her partner will be more likely to develop a commitment to the marriage relationship and thus will forego the option of seeking relationships with others that potentially might offer greater goal fulfillment than the relationship with the spouse. Over time this spouse's degree of dependence is therefore likely to increase (Blalock & Wilken, 1979, p. 202).

Although for Blalock & Wilken it is dependency that leads to commitment, for Blau it is commitment that creates dependency:

> . . . any commitment to a social relationship entails a degree of dependency by excluding alternatives. An employee presumably remains in a job either because alternative employment opportunities are less attractive to him or because his investment in this job is so great that moving to another would be too costly for him. Whatever the reason, this lack of equally preferable alternatives makes him dependent on his employer (Blau, 1986, p. 119).

Turner (1970) also discusses dependency in terms of deficits. He argues that interdependence means a division of roles so that if one person takes on a job, others will suffer a deficit because they will lose or not learn the skills associated with the job. In a family where roles are specialized, family members become weak outside their own areas of specialization.

Over time, power-dependency affects the self concept (Bornstein, 1993). An overcontrolling parenting style creates a self concept in the child as powerless and ineffectual. For Bornstein, it is this cognitive component of the self concept that leads the actor to pursue "one central goal"—"obtaining and maintaining nurturant, supportive relationships" (Bornstein, 1993, p. 166).

Restraint of *amae*

Whereas feelings of disappointment and betrayal can lead to an escalation of *amae* demands, there are other feedback processes that provide constraints on *amae* behavior. In a strong attachment relationship, if you love me, if you have said or indicated that you will nurture me, then there is little need for me to monitor my requests: I can ask for whatever I need. This is the essence of *amae*. Because I feel that I deserve what I need from you, it is inconceivable that you would let me down. Because of my sense of unlimited acceptance, I need feel little restraint. In a one-way relationship, *amae* has no limits. "In the parent-child relationship," Doi notes, "there is no *enryo* [restraint]" (Doi, 1981, p. 38). However, such unlimited demands by older children or by adults can lead to a feeling of exploitation: "it frequently happens that discord between parents and children, or the estrangement of close friends, is attributed to a lack of *enryo* between the parties concerned" (Doi, 1981, p. 39). Thus, a value is placed on restraint.

In Japan, a person who fails to show restraint is seen as childish (Okonogi, 1992). The person who exhibits too much *amae* behavior is described colloquially as "*ombu ni dakko*," literally "carry [the baby] on the back [and] in the arms." For this child it is not enough always to be with the mother (carried on her back); he insists on restricting her intercourse with others by monopolizing her arms as well. This is a connection equivalent of the power expression, "give him an inch and he'll take a mile." Being sensitized to connection behavior, the Japanese are also aware of its potential costs and abuses.

Limits to the demands of *amae* are thus created by restraint. Japanese

> families solidly dislike extended mutual exploration of emotion, particularly the more primitive sentiments of love and hate, and consider it best for each to control his feelings and to limit his expression of personal demands (Vogel, 1963, pp. 196-197).

Restraint is particularly important in a mutual relationship. In a relationship of equals, I will generally monitor my demands and will try to make reasonable requests. I can act childish or spoiled now and then, and you will indulge me. But this does not mean I can act spoiled all of the time. This would put too much strain on our relationship because it would indicate that I am not appropriately committed to the relationship, that I lack appropriate concern for *your* needs. It would be seen as "too much *amae*." By monitoring requests and limiting myself to important needs I can help maintain our special relationship.

Restraint is the reduction in *amae* that results from the person's caring for and responsibility to the other. Unlike some views, particularly in the United States, that wants and needs are infinite. The connection theoretical system shows how the sense of responsibility that grows in a developing relationship serves to limit *amae*, to limit demands for nurturance within the relationship. The American fear of "spoiling" a child may be based in part on an American belief that children will not spontaneously learn restraint (out of responsibility toward the parent). This may reflect—and be reflected by—the Bowlbian attachment view that caregiving is a one-way relationship from parent to child. In economics, the lack of restraint among beneficiaries is known as the Samaritan's Dilemma (Becker, 1991; Bruce & Waldman, 1990). If we assume that people who ask for help have unlimited wants, how can we rationally decide how much help to give? What if giving them help makes them dependent on our help and thus discourages them from trying to meet their own needs?

Japanese parents, in contrast, expect children to naturally develop restraint as they become aware of their effects on parents. In a very close-knit family such as is particularly common in Japan, "too direct assertion of one's views becomes disruptive to family and group functioning" (Roland, 1988, p. 189). Because connections are very strong, family members are open to one another. This makes them mutually vulnerable to anger and disapproval. Anger is immediately and deeply felt; and it is normatively suppressed (Roland, 1988). To allow for communication under these conditions, the Japanese have developed the art of sensitivity and empathy to a fine degree: a "subtle sensing of each other's feelings and mind that is pervasive in normal Japanese social relationships" (Roland, 1988, p. 194).

> When a person asks someone to do him or her a favor, the request is based on the assumption that it will be honored. To have a request refused means a loss of face. The favor-seeker should be able to divine what the other person is willing and able to do, given their particular degree of mutual commitment. Demands should not be made that the other person would feel uncomfortable meeting or be unable to carry out. The person from whom a favor is requested is, of

> course, aware of the consequences of refusal and will normally try to honor the request, even if it results in inconvenience, diminution of privacy, or loss of time (Befu, 1986, p. 23).

Emphasizing the empathic role of the listener in Japanese communication, Lebra notes:

> In conversation the speaker does not complete a sentence but leaves it open-ended in such a way that the listener will take it over before the former clearly expresses his will or opinion. This is possible because, in Japanese, the verb expressing the speaker's will comes at the end of the sentence. By letting a sentence trail off before coming to the verb, the speaker can avoid expressing and imposing his ideas before knowing the listener's response (Lebra, 1976, pp. 38-39).

The infant's demands are unlimited and unrestrained. The infant wants what it wants, now, immediately. Learning to moderate demands, however, is a prerequisite for social living. As the child grows, to the extent that the child's empathy and responsibility grow, the child will grow more restrained toward the parent. As adults, we can count on few people who have committed to nurture us. We grow to appreciate the other's effort and to understand the limits to their resources. In Japan this understanding is taught indirectly by giving in to the child's demands and then letting the child observe the effects that unreasonable demands put on the caregiver. In the dominant middle class culture in the United States, we attempt to instill this understanding by refusing to nurture excessively and by ignoring or punishing unreasonable demands.

Self monitoring and restraint are not the same as equity. The amount of nurturing in any connection relationship will depend on a complex adjustment of need, responsibility and restraint. There is no reason to expect that the partners will take equal roles. Children, for example, "exploit" and "take advantage" of their parents' forbearance, forgiveness and acceptance. Children do not monitor their demands to the same extent that parents do. My son complains to me when he does not have enough money for the toy he wants, but I do not complain to him that I cannot afford the sports car—admittedly a toy—that I want, just because he needs to go to college. Just as parents are generally more self-monitoring and self-denying than children, wives tend to be more self-monitoring and self-denying than husbands, in both Japanese and U. S. cultures.

We have seen above how restraint out of responsibility can limit *amae*. There are also adult contexts in which restraint can be minimal, for either personal or cultural reasons. In the culture of India, there is less of a felt need for restraint. Relationships are seen to progress quickly to a level of *amae* where demands can be made.

> Conversations with a number of Americans who have had contact with Indians frequently elicit their sense of annoyance at the degree of asking, since Americans experience this as a profound infringement upon their autonomy. Indians, on the other hand, usually experience this as a confirmation of intimacy and caring, and of according the other respect—unless it is another with whom there are no ties, in which case it can be manipulative (Roland, 1988, p. 198n).

In Japan, however, this level of *amae* is seen to be harder to achieve and thus more rare.

> Japanese who have contact with Indians also react negatively to this overt expression of wishes in non-intimate relationships: Japanese strongly reserve the same kind of dependency to a closed inner circle of relationships, showing considerable self-restraint in extra-familial ones (Roland, 1988, p. 228).

We have noted that, while the logics of self interest and connection are different, they are not mutually exclusive. In fact, of course, all theoretical orientations are logically true rather than factually true and thus both self interest and connection theoretical orientations are potentially applicable in any empirical situation. This is where scope rules and practical application come into play. There is every reason to expect that *both* self interest and connection motivations are simultaneously active in a wide variety of situations. Simultaneous operation of multiple motivations can lead to complexity in our analyses, but this is the price we pay for trying to study the real world.

Chapter 8. A Connection Theory of Adult Relationship Formation

The connection theoretical system is used to construct a theory of adult relationship formation. The theory describes the initial formation of an exchange relationship and its gradual transformation into a connection relationship. This analysis identifies a critical imbalance that can be created in such a transformation during which the probability of power and violence may be elevated. The theory also describes some of the ways that close relationships can end.

The logic of the connection theoretical system may be used to construct theories in a number of empirical domains. Most of the examples of applying connection logic in this book have focused on the connection relationship between parent and child. This is the prototypical nurturing relationship, and it is where Bowlby began in developing the logic of attachment. However, when most Americans first think of connection, especially when we describe a relationship in the terms of love, we think about romantic love. Almost all philosophical and sociological accounts of love describe romantic love; most do not discuss parental love.

All theories apply the logic of a theoretical orientation within some empirical scope (Bell, 2008). Because most of the literature I will cite describes close relationships in middle class American culture in particular and Western culture in general, I propose here a theory of close relationships within European-American middle class culture. In this chapter I use the connection theoretical system to examine the creation and maintenance of close relationships. I do not create a complete connection theory of close relationships, but I suggest the form such theory might take.

FROM EXCHANGE . . .

There appears to be solid agreement among American social scientists that most voluntary close relationships begin as exchange relationships (e.g., Blau, 1986; Brickman, 1987; Levinger, 1983 and others described below). During the exchange process at the beginning of the relationship, each person offers rewards to the other in order to receive rewards themselves. I (attempt to) make my conversation charming and you make an effort to be agreeable. I give gifts or make gestures I expect you to enjoy and I anticipate receiving reciprocal efforts from you.

At some point, however, the relationship shifts. Brickman, for example, refers to "the point at which people switch from rational processing to something else" (Brickman, 1987, p. 18). For most sociological observers, the "something else" is usually more of the same. From one exchange point of view, this shift is a weakness. As Lederer & Jackson see it, self-interested sexual attraction becomes so strong that all other self interest is overpowered and rational thought becomes impossible.

> Courtship—the time of ecstatic paralysis—has been cleverly designed by Nature to lure members of the species into reproducing themselves. Courtship is a powerful manifestation of sexual excitement. In Western culture, it has well-defined rituals; these are simple steps leading up to the ultimate goal—legal breeding. The man and the woman are in a trance. By the magic of Nature, they have become wonderfully attractive to each other (Lederer & Jackson, 1968, pp. 42-43).

For other sociologists, the shift is more under personal control. For Blau (1986) and especially for Scanzoni (1982), it is purposive and calculated. Each partner uses their knowledge of the other's self interest to get what they want. Waller, an early student of the process, gives a somewhat cynical description:

> The affair begins with the lightest sort of involvement, each individual being interested in the other but assuming no obligations as to the continuation of the affair. There are some tentatives of exploitation at the beginning; "the line" is a conventionalized attempt on the part of the young man to convince the young woman that he has already at this early stage fallen seriously in love with her—a sort of exaggeration, sometimes a burlesque, of coquetry—it may be that each person, by a pretense of great involvement, invites the other to rapid sentiment-formation—each encourages the other to fall in

> love by pretending that he has already done so. If either rises to the bait, a special type of interaction ensues; it may be that the relation becomes exploitative in some degree and it is likely that the relationship becomes one in which control follows the principle of least interest, i.e., that person controls who is less interested in the continuation of the affair (Waller, 1937, p. 733).

Not much has changed in over seventy years. Contemporary theories of relationship formation, as we shall see, are not very different.

The standard account of relationship formation is built on a strategic form of the implicit social exchange process (Bell, 2008). Knowing that you will be at least somewhat bound by the social norm of reciprocity, I make small offerings (for example, revealing my feelings) that are at the same time my vulnerabilities. These revelations serve to convince you of my (at this point, at least, false) commitment. These offerings also serve as tests that tell me whether I can trust you (i.e., predict your behavior). Each step in this dance of growing intimacy is a small step because neither partner has more than a shallow belief in the norm of reciprocity. By a continuing incremental process of unfolding trial and commitment, we each come to judge that the rewards of an ongoing exchange relationship will outvalue the rewards from short term defection and exploitation (Blau, 1986; Rubin, 1973). In this way we both come to calculate the long term advantage of commitment. Our initial short term exchange relationship becomes "something else": a long term exchange relationship. "This ongoing process is labeled 'social exchange' and is the basis for the formation and *maintenance* of *any* social relationship including love and marriage." (Scanzoni, 1982, pp. 50, italics in original).

There are certain problems with this exchange theory of relationships. The primary one is that this theory assumes that we calculate, that we compute long- and short term rewards. The evidence appears to be strong that people frequently do make such calculations when they initiate interaction. But it appears to be a largely unexamined assumption that such calculations continue to fully underlie all relationships as they develop. The *experience* of love and friendship relationships is that of commitment rather than exchange, and the strongest love and friendships involve a commitment regardless of outcome ("for richer or for poorer" in marriage vows) that makes these relationships special.

Another problem with exchange theories of love and friendship is that they are based exclusively on interests, on wants. The difference between new and ongoing relationships is seen to be in the time focus. New exchange relationships are seen inevitably to focus on short term self interest, while continuing relationships are seen to shift focus to a long term stream of rewards that satisfy self interest.

A more developmental approach to the establishment of relationships is given by Murstein (1970). He sees the relationship as developing from a "stimulus" stage through a "value" stage to a "role" stage. Each stage adds new criteria on which partners test for mutual reward. The stimulus stage is seen as based primarily on first impressions: physical, reputational, and behavioral cues make each person attractive to the other. In the value stage, the persons explore one another's interests and values; to the extent that they have similar values, they are attractive to one another and the relationship continues to develop. In the role stage the partners explore deeper aspects of personality and character (temperament, responsibility, ability at vocational roles, for example). In part this exploration is designed to uncover deception during the value stage; in part it uncovers deeper compatibility. A major change occurs at the role stage. This change is the process of internalizing a new role vis-à-vis the partner.

> A primary feature of the role stage is the evaluation of the perceived functioning of oneself in a dyadic relationship in comparison with the roles one envisages for oneself, and the perceived role functioning of the partner with respect to the roles one has envisaged for him (Murstein, 1976, p. 126).

In the courtships that Murstein studies, the primary role is the role of spouse. As the person begins to internalize the role of spouse, "the feeling of personal commitment for the marriage partner becomes stronger" (1976, p. 113).

For Murstein, the developmental course involves changes in an exchange relationship. At each stage the partner is evaluated in terms of the ability to provide rewards, but the rewards emphasized change from the superficial to the deeper and longer term. In his theory he conceptualizes the entire process as exchange, but in his empirical work Murstein acknowledges that the end of the process may be something different. In Murstein, Cerreto & MacDonald (1977), evidence is presented that suggests that marriages are *less* successful when they are based on exchange. Marital adjustment scores are higher for a spouse who is "nonexchange-oriented," that is, "who is not concerned with keeping a mental balance sheet on just what he has done for others and what they have done for him" (1977, pp. 543-544).

For Clark & Mills, changes as the relationship progresses are more qualitative than quantitative. They distinguish the exchange relationship of friendship from the later "communal" relationship of marriage. A communal relationship is one "in which each person has a concern for the welfare of the other" (Clark & Mills, 1979, p. 12). This new relationship is focused on the needs of the partners, and it does not involve exchange or even reciprocity.

> In a communal relationship, the receipt of a benefit does not create a specific debt or obligation to return a comparable benefit, nor does it alter the general obligation that the members have to aid the other when the other has a need. In a communal relationship, the idea that a benefit is given in response to a benefit that was received is compromising, because it calls into question the assumption that each member responds to the needs of the other (Clark & Mills, 1979, p. 13).

If this is not an exchange relationship any longer, where do Clark & Mills find the motivation? Although they conceptualize a communal relationship as non-exchange, they still hold to the assumption of self interest.

> The rules concerning the giving and receiving of benefits are what distinguish communal and exchange relationships, rather than the specific benefits that are given and received (Clark & Mills, 1979, p. 13).

Thus the shift from an exchange to a communal relationship is seen as a change in social norms around the relationship rather than a change in the self interest basis of the relationship itself.

Another approach is found in Schwartz & Merten (1980). Their account of the dating experience documents the importance of exchange in the behavior of both participants. But in addition they document the simultaneous (and growing) importance of what they call the "solidarity perspective."

> In the solidarity perspective, people tend to think of individual interests as common interests. This does not mean that everything that matters to me matters to you, and vice versa. Nor do lovers pool all their resources all the time. Rather, this sense of commonality arises from sharing those things that are very important to both of us. In the solidarity perspective, we recognize that what happens to each

> of us individually affects both of us because these events gain much of their meaning from the fact that our lives are interdependent (Schwartz & Merten, 1980, p. 32).

We associate with many people in the course of our lives. A few of these associations pass a point beyond which we begin to feel that a "relationship" exists. Within the connection theoretical system, at the point where a "relationship" exists, we may say that the two people are "connected," they share a "connection." This connection exists because the partners have come to see one another as special, to feel that they "belong," to feel that they "touch" one another. This belonging may be tentative and fragile at first, and many potential connections are not made as one or both persons' tentative moves toward emotional contact do not meet with success—or are met with misunderstanding, exploitation, or rejection. From this point of view we see that the counterfeit displays of affection that Blau and Scanzoni describe are not likely to be effective exactly because they are part of an unfolding exchange relationship. These displays become ineffective if they are not found to be genuine. Schwartz & Merten emphasize that, to be "genuine," interpersonal revelations must not be based on exchange. These displays of affection are effective only to the extent that they reveal a new kind of relationship, a relationship based on connection.

As we look at the transformation of an exchange relationship to a connection relationship, we will see that the connection relationship does not so much replace the exchange relationship as it grows out of it—and outgrows it. The very behaviors of face-to-face exchange (and sometimes exchange at a distance), because they involve contact, contribute as well to the emergence of caregiving and attachment processes.

. . . TO CONNECTION

The connection theory of relationships proposed here suggests that the development of a close relationship from its initial stage to an ongoing nurturing relationship involves a change from an exchange process (an anticipation of staying in the relationship to achieve greater rewards) to a connection process (an intention to stay in a relationship to express one's caring and experience the other's). In the very process of pursuing my self interest through exchange, I come to learn about you and to trust you. As described in Chapter 7, the exchange view considers trust to be a cognitive matter of prediction—I come to trust you because your failure to exploit me helps me predict your future cooperation. In the connection view, my understanding of your feelings is what transforms the relationship. As we engage in exchange behaviors over time, I come to notice that I am valued—that my behavior is experienced as nurturing by you. It comes to give me satisfaction to see you pleased by what I give. And to the extent that you avoid opportunities to exploit me, I come to infer and feel your caring and thus come to trust your emotional commitment to me and to my needs. Your caring strengthens the trust building in me toward you. I feel cherished. What used to be a "reward" has become nurturance. I come to care how you are, to be concerned about your happiness. My character and personality come to be invested in our relationship. My motivation shifts from staying in the relationship because it works, to making the relationship work because I want to be in it, because I feel warmly connected to you. As caring increases and responsibility deepens, the focus on my wants and your wants shifts to a focus on your needs and my needs. As more nurturance is given and received by each of us, and as trust strengthens, the focus evolves from a primary concern with what I can get to a growing focus on what I can give. The relationship becomes, not necessarily more rewarding, but closer and deeper.

Exchange relationships are partial relationships. Each transaction deals with a limited number of interests, and a given exchange relationship tends to specialize in a given set of interests: commodities for money; or advice and information for gratitude and status; or dinner for sex. But when two people interact, even in an exchange relationship, the whole person can get involved. Even if there is a focus on one set of interests, the rest of the body and the rest of the self may become involved. When you sell me a product, you may also smile. Or we may hold a conversation.

Thus, along with the stream of (instrumental, interest) rewards that I am receiving from you, I am also making human contact with you. Your smile and your conversation are helping to meet some of my needs for approval and contact. Many, if not most, continued face-to-face exchange relationships (with regional, class and gender variations) develop some level of connection, sometimes a more formal connection in the form of civility and sometimes a more personal connection in the form of real friendship. Of course, most exchange relationships never develop more than a small degree of connection. But some do. And other relationships, such as dating relationships in those cultures that adopt the practice, intentionally anticipate or test the possibility of deeper connection.

As described by the attachment theoretical orientation and discussed in Chapter 6, the growth of our trust in our partner depends cognitively on an inference of their caring, and perhaps also directly and emotionally on the oxytocin production associated with caring. The process of cognitive inference depends on our expectations and assumptions. If we assume that the clerk's smile is because she is following a norm of civility, or if we assume that the server is helpful simply because he wants a larger tip, then we are unlikely to infer that they are sincere. The attribution process is, of course, highly complex, and influenced both by the social context and by the psychology of the individuals involved, particularly by attachment and caregiving internal working models that record our relationship history and current expectations.

It may be largely because of hope and optimism from our internal working models that we look for caring and commitment in dating relationships. This optimistic and hopeful outlook makes us vulnerable. Waller (1937), Scanzoni (1982), Freie (1998), Badcock (2000) and others have pointed out the self-serving benefits and techniques of counterfeiting caring, of pretending concern to elicit trust. A little later we will examine imbalanced relationships, but for now the focus turns to genuine, reciprocal caring and contact, however limited.

We can use the connection process to examine the formation of a relationship between two people. Let us call them "Boy" and "Girl," using Blau's (1986) terminology from his excellent exposition of a social exchange theory of dating. As we construct this example, we will become aware of some of the problems of working at the level of theory. In a gendered theory such as this one, we will find ourselves importing a number of assumptions, many of them easily unrecognized. These assumptions are inescapable at the level of theory. When Boy is pursuing Girl, our American cultural mind's eye is inclined to see his ill-concealed leer and her downcast eye. When Girl is pursuing, we will see her coquettish flashing of eyelashes and his attempt to remain aloof. The logic of connection presented here, however, is not gendered, so it can be applied to same-gender relationships as well as to cross-gender relationships.

In this example, following cultural stereotypes, Boy will be described as active, while Girl will be described as reactive. Boy and Girl have up to now carried on a mutually satisfactory exchange relationship. But now their relationship is about to change. Each person is rewarding the other, by agreeing with the other's tastes or laughing at the other's jokes. If they each stay at this superficial reward level, the relationship will not progress (except perhaps to decline when they begin to get tired of the other's repertoire of jokes and stories). A new dimension in the relationship begins to emerge as the partners begin to reveal more of themselves. This corresponds to Murstein's "value" and "role" stages. Murstein, however, sees only the attempt to receive a widening range of rewards.

The increasing revelation of history and values not only provides new rewards from the other's understanding. It also provides emotional contact. These behaviors reveal not only the partners' continuing willingness to reciprocate rewards. They also reveal the beginnings of warmth and caring. Blau (1986, p. 98) describes this process using exchange terms: "His commitment, which would make it disadvantageous for him to abandon the partnership in favor of another, gives the other additional reasons to trust him not to evade his obligations in their relationship." This is undoubtedly true: Boy and Girl do not cease being self-interested.

It is possible that Boy's revelations are counterfeit and designed to manipulate, and it is possible that Girl may take Boy's talk as a "line." But to the extent that Girl takes his revelations as genuine, she will infer some, initially minimal, level of caring. To the (limited) extent that Girl perceives Boy's caring, she will develop a (limited) level of trust. This trust will facilitate (limited) openness and *amae* as she begins to reveal herself and to expect his continued (limited) nurturance. To the extent that her revelations, her vulnerabilities, are met with nurturance—that is, to the extent that she learns that she can depend on Boy to meet her (minimally) revealed needs—her trust will grow. This involves a series of cognitive processes. Murstein interprets the final "role stage" as involving the attempt to verify the partners' mutual ability to follow through on rewards into the future. For Murstein the main element in the ability to reward is the partner's role performance (Murstein, 1976). How well can Boy perform the roles that will reward Girl, and simultaneously, how well can Girl perform the roles for Boy that will reciprocate and sustain the relationship? From the point of view of the developing connection relationship, we can reinterpret Murstein's role stage in terms of the expansion beyond verbal indicators of caring, empathy, and responsibility to less manipulable behavioral indicators. He has verbally agreed with her values, but does he act in ways that she can approve? He says he cares, but does he actually nurture her? As the Japanese say, words are "just words" (Bell, 1989; Lebra, 1976). Words alone cannot sustain the developing connection relationship.

Alongside the cognitive process of evaluation and assessment in the developing relationship are emotional processes. As social interaction continues, especially when involving physical contact but also in face-to-face interaction and eye contact, oxytocin production increases and emotional caring is enhanced. In an evolving cycle of caring and trust, a connection relationship will begin to develop alongside the continuing exchange relationship. As we explored in Chapter 4, oxytocin is released both as a response to physical touching and as a response to social interaction. Thus, the interaction involving the early exchange of information begins low levels of oxytocin production. If the first feelings of caring are consistent with Murstein's value consensus, then touch, kissing, and other physical contact will contribute to building of and consolidating dyadic caring circuits. Increased oxytocin production in turn motivates increasing touching and social interaction. As caring grows, the conscious and unconscious awareness of the partner's caring creates trust. Connection may then grow in an increasing spiral if no countervailing processes intercede.

Within Murstein's role stage we can see a transformation within the connection relationship from a more negative trust that the other will not embarrass us or hurt us to a more positive trust that the other's emotional commitment is such that they will positively seek to satisfy our needs. The importance of trust in this process is discussed by Schwartz & Merten:

> Trust means more than loyalty to another person. It also means fidelity to our relationship and respect for its integrity. Anything that tends to diminish the relationship threatens both of us. Similarly, while I accept your independence as a person and you accept mine, both of us feel that neither of us should do anything which would jeopardize our trust in each other. What we do on our own can shake the spirit of cooperation and mutuality if it forces our love to doubt our intention to put the continuance of the relationship before our individual interests (Schwartz & Merten, 1980, p. 32).

We see that, as each person comes to love the other and begins to take responsibility for the other's needs, trust deepens. Because Girl sees Boy as caring, Girl comes to trust Boy to look out for her needs (as well as his own). Because Girl trusts Boy, she becomes more willing to open herself and reveal her needs. Her trust also activates her *amae*, as she comes to expect and insist that Boy will meet her needs. This is not an instantaneous process: it occurs over repeated iterations of the cycle into deeper and deeper connection. At the same time as Girl is feeling more freedom to ask that her needs be met, her own caring and commitment are growing from the associated social and physical contact.

The growth of Girl's caring leads her to focus her empathy on Boy. She begins to increase her level of listening and observing; no longer from the formal connection of politeness but from a more personal emotional connection. Because she cares about Boy, she wants to know him. Girl's caring also leads her to take responsibility for meeting Boy's needs. As Boy becomes more special to her, Girl's responsibility for Boy's needs comes to rival her responsibility for her own. Girl becomes prepared to sacrifice her own needs when Boy seems to have greater needs. Traditionally, of course, in many cultures Girl has learned to value Boy's needs as more important as her own. Using her empathy to know him and his needs, and expressing her sense of responsibility for his needs, she nurtures him. And finally, as Girl comes to feel more responsible for Boy, her concern for Boy leads her to restrain somewhat her expression of *amae*, counterbalancing the expectation of Boy's nurturance that her trust has released.

And of course, while these internal and dyadic changes are occurring in Girl, corresponding changes are occurring in Boy.

The exchange theory of relationships sees this transitional time of relationship development as a time of intense if implicit bargaining. I want to get the best long term bargain I can achieve, but I have to give you enough (but as little as possible to increase my profit) to make the relationship worthwhile to you. This is one reason why the increments in trust can be small. Connection theory, on the other hand, sees this period as one in which bargaining has begun to be replaced (or eclipsed) by a sense of connection, caring, and nurturance.

When the two partners have an equal exchange relationship, the relationship can develop only by mutual increase in rewards. Only if I am willing to give you more will I be able to receive more from you. There are two ways to increase rewards: I can give you more rewards (more and larger presents, for example) or I can give you more personal "rewards." The first choice will continue the exchange relationship but at a higher level of mutual rewards. No change of motivation will necessarily occur. But the second choice will change not just the level of the relationship but its nature as well.

Instead of giving you another gift, I might "reward" you by listening to you. For exchange theorists like Homans, Blau, Scanzoni or Murstein, listening is an "intrinsic" reward, but functionally just another reward. But from the point of view of connection, listening is partially a reward (it makes you feel good if anyone, even a stranger listens to you), but it is also more. Empathic listening is an outgrowth of caring. By listening, I learn about you. I've always been paying attention to what you said, but I was looking for clues about how best to maximize my rewards. But if I begin listening—to *you*—I begin to learn who you are. You begin to be differentiated from others, and not just in terms of my awareness of the classes of rewards that might activate your rewarding of me. Now you are becoming unique, a valued and cherished other, a partner.

By listening I learn more about you, about your strengths and your weaknesses. I have a choice here. I can choose to use this new information to exploit you. Knowing more about your weaknesses, I can find ways to threaten you so that I get more and give less. This behavior will probably end up, at least eventually, in the termination of the relationship, but in the meantime I can increase my profits. However, I have another choice. By listening to you I not only make you unique in that I know things that differentiate you from all others. I also make you special.

IMBALANCE OF COMMITMENT

The early stage of the transition from an exchange process to a connection process is particularly volatile. As the partners begin to construct their caring and trust, the shift from surface wants to inner needs leads to particular sensitivities and vulnerabilities. Furthermore, because the grammar of needs is much less developed than the grammar of wants (especially, perhaps, in American society), the communication of needs is particularly liable to miscommunication. This difficulty with the vocabulary of needs is compounded by the tentativeness in attempting to express needs during the incremental revelation process of the developing relationship.

Another major source of vulnerability in the development of new relationships is a result of timing. Because people differ in their temperament, their emotional history, and in their skills, there will frequently be imbalance in the degree to and speed at which each person comes to care emotionally and to trust. If relationship development depends on change—on changing from wants to needs, on changing from an emphasis on rewards to an emphasis on caring and nurturance—then there is no reason to expect that partners will make the transition either smoothly or simultaneously. Even though this process of relationship development involves innumerable small changes, it is likely that at any given time, one partner will have comparatively more of an emphasis on connection while the other has comparatively more of an emphasis on exchange. If Boy continues to have an exchange motivation and Girl has come to have a connection motivation, this is the best of all possible worlds—for Boy. Both partners are in agreement: Boy wants what is best for himself and girl wants what is best for Boy. It is an exploitative relationship, and from an exchange perspective, Boy has no reason to want to change it. The relationship is, however, highly artificial and unstable. Over time, Girl is likely to reevaluate her options.

Girl's responses to imbalance

Assuming Girl is dissatisfied with this unbalanced relationship, she has three basic choices.

(1). Girl can unilaterally reduce her level of caring and thereby reduce her risk of exploitation. This is a choice that returns the relationship to an exchange basis. This is a probable choice if she judges that Boy is not (yet) ready to increase his caring and responsibility. The most extreme version of this choice is to reduce her responsibility to zero and leave the relationship. Termination of the relationship is more likely if she estimates that Boy will never make a commitment comparable to her own.

(2). Her second option is to try to increase Boy's caring. This usually takes the form of a challenge to Boy, a demand for an accounting of his behavior. To make this effective, Girl must reveal her caring to some degree. Boy is asked to put up or shut up: does he really care about Girl (and the relationship) or is he only concerned with his own self interest? If Boy does not give a satisfactory account, the Girl may adopt the first option above. Boy's account may seek to reframe his behavior to show that it actually represented his caring and responsibility, or it may take the form of an apology and a promise of change.

Both of these responses to imbalance given by Girl can be accounted for by exchange theory. The first is seen as a reduction of risk. By reducing her commitment, Girl reduces her risk of exploitation. The second can be seen as a matter of revaluing or recontracting to achieve better future outcomes. If Boy revalues his estimation of Girl's rewards upward, then he must give her greater rewards in the future, restoring the balance in the relationship. But there is a third option for Girl that is considered irrational within exchange theory.

(3). Girl's third option is to increase her connection responsibility for Boy unilaterally. From the point of view of exchange, this behavior involves the irrationality of throwing good commitment after bad. Only a fool would make herself more vulnerable to a person who has shown his untrustworthiness. But from the point of view of connection, an increase in commitment makes sense. It may not work to restructure the relationship, but it follows logically from Girl's belief that there is a connection, or at least the potential for a mutually nurturing relationship. If Girl believes that Boy's failure to make a corresponding commitment is because of his fear and distrust, then by increasing her caring and responsibility she seeks to induce greater trust in Boy.

If Girl is skilled at interpersonal perception, she may see Boy's (limited) caring and come to trust him. At the same time, Boy's perceptual ineptitude may mean that he does not see Girl's (greater) caring and responsibility and is too insecure to increase his own level of trust and caring. Because caring is not directly observable, Girl may be aware that Boy has not correctly perceived her caring. Option 2 where Girl tells him of her caring, or Option 3 where she increases her nurturance and makes her caring more visible and thus less liable to be misperceived, may help her to make Boy more aware of her emotional commitment. This additional information may overcome Boy's fear and/or lack of perceptual skills and finally make him aware of her caring and thus able to develop the trust to increase his own caring. As Boy sees Girl's caring, his distrust and fear may be reduced. Within the logic of the attachment theoretical orientation, Boy's increased awareness of Girl's caring will lead to an increase in his trust and ultimately to an increase in his caring.

From within the connection theory of relationship formation, we can identify criteria that allow us to predict which of the three choices Girl will make when she experiences Boy as unequally committed. If Girl sees boy as unconnected and uncaring, and thus interacting only by exchange processes, then the first choice of reducing her emotional commitment is the only safe alternative. Creating his caring from zero is much more problematic than increasing an existing caring. If she perceives no real caring, then asking for an account or increasing her own nurturing will likely have no effect on Boy's caring. This does not mean that Girl will never choose the last two options if she sees Boy as unconnected. If her own connection is strong, and/or if her self confidence is strong, she may be willing to make rather intense efforts to induce Boy to become connected. We will touch on this again below when we examine Boy's response.

If Girl believes that Boy is connected, but at a lower level then herself, then the last two options are ways within the connection theoretical system to increase Boy's trust and caring. Option 2 is a cognitive approach. By describing her commitment and asking Boy to examine his feelings, intentions and behaviors, Girl attempts to induce Boy to recognize and acknowledge his connection. Option 3 is based on an implicit understanding of connection logic. By increasing Girl's caring (and especially increasing Boy's *perception* of Girl's caring), Girl senses that she can improve Boy's trust, and thus Boy's caring and responsibility. Increased trust and security in Boy will act to make Boy better able to see Girl's real caring clearly. Girl anticipates that this increased clarity of perception will also make Boy more aware of Girl's needs and, within a developing relationship of connection, will increase both his empathy and his sense of responsibility for her.

Boy's responses to imbalance

Let us turn now to Boy. We are examining a relationship in which Girl has a greater sense of caring and has made a greater emotional commitment than Boy (this stereotypical gendered example may reflect a common script in American middle class culture, but the theory is symmetrical: the same logic applies when Boy is the more emotionally connected). If Boy has achieved no emotional contact, then he is still motivated strictly by his self interest motivation. Girl's Option 1 is probably the most effective strategy for developing the relationship. In Option 1, Girl reduces her commitment to Boy's level and continues the initial exchange relationship. By bargaining at an equal level with Boy, she communicates to him that he must increase his rewarding behavior if he wants to increase the rewards he receives. If he chooses to increase the depth of his rewards rather than just their quantity, then Boy may begin to develop caring for Girl. If Boy decides that the price is too much to pay, he may continue at a lower level of change—if Girl is willing—or he may terminate the relationship.

However, Boy may no longer be exclusively oriented toward exchange. At this point in the relationship, Girl's greater caring has already led to her greater empathy and responsibility, and thus to her nurturance of Boy. Girl's caring and its behavioral indicators are likely to have increased Boy's trust, openness and *amae*, maybe just at an unconscious level. Boy's attachment may thus be activated before his caregiving develops. He may come to trust her before he comes to care, even though his conscious focus is still on exchange.

But if Boy has developed some proactive caring for Girl, he has yet other choices. If Girl has chosen Option 1 (reducing her responsibility), he may accept this reduced level if he is uneasy about increasing his caring. Or he may use Option 2 himself (demanding an accounting) as a way of mutually clarifying and perhaps balancing caring.

Boy may have limited perceptual skills. Or he may be afraid. A most sought-after gratification, feeling cherished, also creates vulnerability. And previous insecure attachment relationships may have been associated with pain. We take a chance when we let another see our vulnerabilities—the ability to cherish us goes hand in hand with the ability to devastate us. If he is afraid, then Option 2 by Girl (asking for an accounting) is likely to result in denial and defensiveness. Occasionally Boy can be talked through his defensiveness. But if Boy is afraid, he may respond by attacking Girl's weaknesses instead of acknowledging his caring and vulnerability, thus creating mutual pain and defensiveness. In the case of strong fear in Boy, even Option 3 (Girl increasing her commitment) may be ineffective. Girl's increased responsibility—and concomitant vulnerability—may simply exacerbate Boy's fears. After all, in American society, depending on someone is often taken as weakness—especially for men.

There are two other responses that Boy can choose if he enjoys the results of Girl's greater caring but is afraid to make a corresponding commitment of his own. The first is an exchange option; the second is a power option. The exchange option for Boy is to expand the initial exchange relationship. Boy may attempt to "buy" Girl's exchange-commitment. He reasons that if he can give enough "safe" rewards—perhaps only monetary, but with no acknowledged emotional commitment—he can exchange them for the deeply satisfying nurturance from Girl. If Girl is optimistic, or desperate, she may agree to this bargain. This creates one of those anomalies that make social science so exciting—and often so frustrating. A relationship now exists that is an exchange relationship from the point of view of Boy and a connection relationship from the point of view of Girl.

The discrepancy between the relationship experienced by Boy and that experienced by Girl emphasizes that a relationship is not a "thing," not a "social fact" except in a metaphorical sense. There is no *singular* relationship. Instead, the "relationship" involves a unique experience within each partner (Bernard, 1982; Tannen, 1990). While the two "relationships" may become similar over time, this is not a logical or empirical necessity. In the case described here, they are quite different. Boy experiences the relationship as exchange, and thus as competitive and conflictual. He sees his reticence as self-protection and her nurturance as enjoyable but threatening. At the same time, Girl experiences this relationship as connection, and thus as interdependent and cooperative. She sees his reticence as shyness and her nurturance as facilitative. Human beings are amazingly adept at self-deception, so this relationship of mutual misunderstanding can continue for some time (Safilios-Rothschild, 1976). On the other hand, over time, the lack of commitment from Boy is likely to erode Girl's trust and result in a formal, perfunctory form of nurturance. A cooperative relationship may develop which is essentially hollow, lacking a core of real affection.

Violence

Boy has another option to try to continue a relationship without making an emotional commitment to Girl. In a relationship in which caring has reached a moderate or high level for Girl, but a low level for Boy, Boy may choose to transform the exchange relationship into a power relationship.

An extreme form of power in a relationship is physical violence. However, "milder" forms of psychological or emotional abuse are similar in effect if not so overtly brutal. The purpose of the violence is to sustain Girl's side of the connection relationship while allowing Boy to avoid or deny a caring commitment on his side of the relationship. If Boy can make Girl afraid enough, he can guarantee that she will not cease her nurturance of him. And if she is appropriately afraid of him, she will not try to exploit any weaknesses she has discovered in him. This approach has the further advantage for Boy that if his emotional caring increases over time, the violence will protect him from the inevitable vulnerabilities that he will develop with greater openness and greater emotional contact. On the other hand, because of the violence, Boy will find it difficult to believe that Girl's nurturance comes from her caring rather than from her fear.

Forward uses similar ideas to understand misogyny, a general hatred of women, and the physical and emotional abuse that comes with it:

> This man needs, as we all do, to feel emotionally taken care of, to be loved, and to feel safe. As adults we fulfill these yearnings through physical intimacy, emotional sharing, and parenting. But the misogynist finds these yearnings terribly frightening. His normal needs to be close to a woman are mixed with fears that she can annihilate him emotionally. He harbors a hidden belief that if he loves

> a woman, she will then have the power to hurt him, to deprive him, to engulf him, and to abandon him (Forward & Torres, 1986, p. 99).

Abusive power is not just a rationally planned strategy for assuring that Boy's needs are met by Girl. Abuse can also be an emotional response to pain. A self-interested person gets frustrated: their wants are not being met. The connected person is betrayed when needs are not met as expected (*amae*). When someone you love has failed to give you what you need and deserve, the result is not anger derived from frustration; it is rage as a result of betrayal. When you don't trust, you construct defenses so the other can't reach you. If you don't trust someone, they can't hurt you. Attacks from outside hit your shield. But if you open up, if you let them in, then you are vulnerable. The abuser may not in fact intend to become emotionally unprotected. However, the neurobiological process of oxytocin release associated with physical contact and social interaction may subvert this intention and create the unwanted emotional response and vulnerability. This growing attachment and its accompanying vulnerability can be a source of fear that motivates abuse.

To the extent that Boy's sense of betrayal and the resulting anger focuses his attention solely (or at least primarily) on self needs and self interests, Boy comes to orient to Girl primarily in terms of Girl's failure to nurture. An unfortunately common occurrence is for Boy to conclude that Girl should ("needs" to) be able to nurture him. Violence may then be selected as an effective way to force Girl to meet Boy's needs. In this case, Boy's violence is self-defined as an attempt to restore what is perceived as a failed connection.

Violence can be highly effective in the short run. But, in the long run violence fails. First, because of the violence, Boy cannot finally attribute any achieved nurturance to caring, so that Boy's trust and security cannot increase. This may prolong the violence, often in an increasing spiral, guaranteeing that it cannot achieve its ultimate goal of satisfying nurturance. Second, violence eventually reduces Girl's caring, and Girl becomes increasingly unwilling to satisfy Boy's *amae* dependency.

The violence that is found in families with embarrassing regularity may thus often be a negative result of connection process (Gilgun, 1995). Usually we do not want to consider that love might have negative consequences. However, people whose *amae* is frustrated can become desperate to achieve nurturance of their needs. The person who is insecure in his or her self worth can be extremely sensitive to the slightest sign of a failure of nurturance. Relationship and marital violence can be seen, at least in part, as an attempt to use power to "restore" the actual or fantasized prior nurturance and acceptance.

We see that abuse may occur in the context of self interest, or connection, or both. It may be, at least in part, an outcome of love. However, violence has obvious, and often severe, negative consequences for the victim. The abuser's violence is physically painful for the victim. It also undermines her self confidence. Gelles & Straus (1988, p. 137) note that violence "leaves victims depressed, demoralized, despondent, and in despair."

The violence also has negative consequences for the abuser because it fails subjectively to secure the nurturance that the abuser desires. But as Boy's violence undermines Girl's caring and responsibility, it results in a decrease in his trust. Boy's sense of vulnerability grows. A late dinner that once was just a late dinner may now be experienced as a lack of nurturance. With the erosion of trust he is less able to tolerate ambiguity. Any behavior that might indicate caring but might also indicate something else is unsatisfying. There can be no "benefit of the doubt" in such a state of insecurity. The occasion for Boy's violence is usually some action of Girl's that he has interpreted as her not caring for him. Because of the erosion of his trust, his attribution of blame to Girl may end up having little relation to her actual behavior or motives. Battered women routinely report "walking on eggshells" around a violent man who explodes over some minor "transgression." Furthermore, because the victim continues to feel connected, she still feels responsible: battered women routinely accept the incident as being their fault (Forward & Torres, 1986; Gelles & Straus, 1988). Often they continue to love and feel love in return. The abuse may be seen as a failure, an aberration, not as a reflection of true feelings.

Both a man who "buys" a woman's commitment in an exchange/connection relationship and the one who uses control or violence in a power/connection relationship may lack the ability to change the relationship. If they come to develop a connection, change in the relationship will almost certainly occur gradually. The man may eventually discover that the woman has come to mean something special to him, or that he wants to assume a responsibility to care for her. Empirically, I know of no evidence of the frequency of such epiphanies. But subjectively, the hope for such a transformation seems to be a motivating factor for many women who remain in such "economic" or violent relationships.

From the self interest point of view, there are only negative reasons for the victim to remain in an abusive relationship—she must have no other viable alternatives (she may be economically dependent), or she must be a masochist (she must pathologically enjoy pain) or she must be unable to escape. A connection theory, however, is based on the conception that emotional caring for the other person is a positive motivation. Just as people in an exchange relationship can misinterpret genuine nurturance as "merely" part of an exchange transaction, people in a connection relationship can misinterpret abuse as an attempt at nurturance: "He's doing it for my own good"; as a sign of weakness in a failed attempt at nurturance: "He loves me, but he can't help himself" or maybe "I did something to set him off." Violent relationships are usually not constantly abusive. The violence is often seen as a "temporary" aberration in a generally nurturing relationship. Hope, however misguided in the view of an outsider, can be sustaining (Armstrong, 1978).

It is clear that frightened people can succeed in forming connections. Whatever the disadvantages from childhood, relationships continue to form throughout life. The gradual awakening of trust, openness, caring and responsibility can potentially occur in any relationship. Justice & Justice (1990, p. 156) describe "the impact one loving person can make in the life of a child in an abusive family." A person who is emotionally insecure because of childhood experiences might meet someone with whom they can feel secure, perhaps a teacher or a friend's parent. A good therapist might help. Patience and nondefensiveness on the partner's part seem to be an important component.

In this description of exchange/connection relationships, I have placed the male in the exchange and power positions and the female in the connection position. This is certainly the empirically most common situation, but the process is not based on sex or gender. In some male-female relationships, the man will be emotionally more secure than the woman, who is emotionally insecure and unwilling to make an emotional commitment. Some of these relationships will develop and the men will experience a greater connection and make a greater commitment. In these cases, we may expect the emergence of an exchange/connection or power/connection relationship with the "normal" positions reversed. Same gender relationships may show the same patterns.

ENDING THE RELATIONSHIP

It is reasonable to propose as a testable hypothesis that all relationships are motivated both by self interest and by connection. In most instrumental relationships the role of connection is small, although there are clearly some such relationships in which connection grows to high levels. In the "ideal" close relationship—marital and family relationships in particular, love relationships in general—the level of connection is high and the level of self interest may be either high or low. But human relationships are seldom ideal.

One place where we may be able to see with some clarity the workings of multiple motivations is in the breakup of a relationship. Divorces in particular often show the effects of power, exchange, caregiving, and attachment processes. We have seen how connection leads to vulnerability. Our own openness and the other's empathy contribute to our vulnerability. An unsatisfied want may cause frustration, but this frustration is limited to the want. A need is experienced as fundamental, so an unmet need is emotionally more painful. In a divorce the two caregiving and two attachment relationships are formally ended. The disengagement from a connection is experienced as a loss. A grieving process often occurs with divorce (Wiseman, 1975). Many people experience the grief before the divorce actually occurs so that they are able to start letting go of the emotional connection before the legal rupture occurs. But others can experience some level of connection for years past divorce, especially if a co-parenting relationship continues.

For those people who are emotionally connected but no longer legally connected, vulnerability can still be acute. Because they are still connected at some level, they are still open and vulnerable. When a ex-spouse begins to engage exclusively in exchange transactions, the loss of nurturance may be painful to a former partner who still cares. The partner may then choose to switch to exchange because it appears to be the only viable choice and/or may choose power out of revenge ("I'll show him/her"). While emotional connection exists, the other's lack of nurturance will still cause disappointment and pain. This pain is exacerbated by the other's increasing lack of connection and caring. Since the two people are now formally individuals and formally only self-interested, the formal expectation is that their relationship will be governed by exchange and reciprocity. This reciprocity can take a rather perverse form in many divorces, becoming a reciprocity of pain.

In more amicable divorces, without rancor or mutual reciprocal punishment, the connection relationship is not replaced by an exchange—or power—relationship. Instead, the (now unmarried) partners continue their connection relationship, albeit at a different level. In these "successful" divorces, the partners cycle down their connection. Caring decreases, but is not revoked. Each partner recognizes a continuing, though diminished, empathy and responsibility. Though the couple has rejected a marital relationship, they can continue to care and to help one other through the transition to lower levels of caring and connection. Because the partners continue to nurture one another (again, at decreasing levels), they continue to respond to the other's needs. Thus while they each go through the grief work of accepting the loss of their marriage, they do not have to deal with deeply painful behaviors from the former spouse. This process can be protective of children and form the basis of successful coparenting.

All theories are time- and space-bound. The theory that I have just outlined above is a theory of dating and marital relationships in contemporary middle-class European-American culture. It does not claim to describe relationships in other cultural contexts, such as arranged and semi-arranged marriages in Japan (White, 1993), or among the American upper-upper class (e.g., Domhoff, 1970). Arranged marriages do not begin with the mutual exchange relationship described above. An arranged marriage begins with a formal rather than a personal connection. This is generally a mutual normative commitment based on loyalty to family (this loyalty can be seen to reflect the responsibility emerging from connection relationships within the family).

Because of the normative commitment, each partner originally feels a formal responsibility (usually described by sociologists as a motivation to perform their marital role), achieved by performing role-defined behaviors. This provides the opportunity for an (initially formal) trust. Knowing that you will give me role-prescribed nurturance, I can open up and do *amae*. I am protected by your initial normative commitment. In such a relationship of formal connection, *amae* will grow before openness. From the beginning I expect you to meet my role-defined needs. Over time, perhaps, I come to perceive that you not only will care behaviorally for me, but I come to believe that you *emotionally* care for me. As the connection grows, I will develop a more personal level of trust and will develop a willingness to reveal more personal needs. With the growth of personal trust comes the growth of my openness. And as I come to trust your concern for my personal needs as well as my formal needs, I develop a more personal *amae*, an expectation that you are motivated to meet my deeper needs. As my *amae* and openness thus expand and as you come to nurture my more personal needs, I come to develop greater trust. The relationship may become reciprocal.

In an arranged marriage, the connection relationship must develop, if it does, after the marriage ceremony. Bernstein quotes a Japanese informant's description of the development of his marriage.

> "In your twenties you feel passion," he philosophized, echoing sentiments voiced by others in the countryside. "In your thirties you work toward cooperative effort with your spouse. In your forties you learn forbearance. In your fifties you are finally resigned to each other. And in your sixties you feel *kansha*, gratitude, which is the expression of love" (Bernstein, 1983b, pp. 55-56).

There is reason to believe that the connection relationship that potentially develops in an arranged marriage will be similar to the connection relationship that can develop from a dating environment. The connection process itself is expected, over time, to replace the remnants of the prior relationship. Whether initiated in a "love match" or an arranged marriage, the processes of caring and empathy, responsibility and nurturance, trust and openness, *amae* and acceptance, develop according to their own logic.

Chapter 9. Reconsidering Families

> *The connection theoretical system adds some important elements to Bowlbian attachment theory, especially in terms of its ability to describe the logic of caregiving. The caregiving and attachment processes of the connection theoretical system embody the central theoretical meaning for what constitutes a family. The connection theoretical system goes beyond exchange and social norms in being able not only to account for family nurturance, but also to explain the origin of family norms.*

Bowlby's conceptualization of attachment was a brilliant achievement of synthesis and speculation. His work both transcended and was limited by the milieu in which it was created. Bowlby transcended Freudian ideas of reinforcement. Instead of asserting that the child is gratified only by the satisfaction of bodily needs and thus responds only to feeding and changing and such comforts, Bowlby realized that the child responded directly to being held and comforted. Furthermore, Bowlby rejected the model of child as passive. Unlike Freud's infant, overwhelmed by environmental stimulation and desensitized to the overstimulation of the world, Bowlby saw a child who was open to the world, who was protected and comforted by caregivers, who reached out to the world where wonderful and interesting things occurred. The child that Bowlby saw was not only active in exploring the world, but also active in attracting and demanding protection and comfort.

While Bowlby transcended the limited understanding of children in his day and created a new model of relationships that has guided child and adult relationship research to this day, the model that he developed was also limited by the research and tools available to him in his time. In particular, his understanding was limited by the available research on evolution and neurobiology during the 1940s and 1950s.

The connection theoretical system and associated theories of parent-child and adult relationships that I have presented here continue the work Bowlby began over fifty years ago. In the course of his work, Bowlby proposed that caregiving and attachment are complementary brain systems that evolved in the "environment of evolutionary adaptation" (Bowlby, 1969/1982). The proposed connection evolutionary model and the enhancements of the caregiving and attachment processes that I have proposed here extend Bowlby's model in a number of ways.

Bowlby's evolutionary theory of attachment showed how an attachment motivational system could provide survival advantages for the earliest humans within the environment of evolutionary adaptedness. The attachment evolutionary model thus gave primacy to the attachment system over the caregiving system. However, the neurological underpinnings of the connection theoretical system suggest that the evolutionary advantages of attachment can only be realized if there is a pre-existing caregiving system. Crying, one of the prototypical attachment behaviors, would be an evolutionary *disadvantage* if there were no caregiver to respond, because crying can attract predators. Offspring do not cry in species where parents do not provide protection. Crying is only an advantage to the extent that it usually attracts the caregiver faster than it attracts the predator. Furthermore, I have extended Bowlby's evolutionary model in time by showing how the caregiving and attachment systems evolved well before humans, in the earliest mammals.

Not only does the connection evolutionary model explore the survival advantages of parental caregiving, but the connection neurobiological model also describes the emotional motivation by which caregiving is produced. By acknowledging caring as a partner-focused emotion that both comes from and increases physical contact and social interaction, the connection theoretical system identifies a mechanism that can account for the earliest intense parental caregiving that promotes the survival of offspring. Caring as a dyadic emotion goes beyond explaining caregiving/attachment in biological parent/child dyads. It also accounts for parent-adoptive child caregiving, for adult pair bonding, and for child-parent caregiving. Adoption is a very important species survival mechanism when adults are at risk from predators alongside children. With the death of a parent, other group members who have been in proximity to the child and have developed feelings of caring toward the child can step forward in response to the child's need. Even if the feelings are initially weak, the very processes of contact will likely lead to the development of (unconscious) emotions and (conscious) feelings and thus to continued caregiving. Furthermore, the very generality of the caring motivation accounts for the ability to love non-human animals, an ability with no demonstrated evolutionary advantage (Archer, 1997).

Attachment researchers frequently describe "affectional" bonds between caregivers and dependents. Unfortunately, these casual references to affect in the bond(s) are seldom explicit as to the nature of the emotion in the bond. The caregiving theoretical orientation explicitly identifies the emotion of caring with the caregiving bond itself; embodied in specific oxytocin producing circuits in the brain. It is the emotion of caring that provides the ongoing motivation for the caregiving process. This caregiving motivation also serves to identify the caregiving set goal, to see that the needs of the partner are met.

The sign of a significant theoretical advance is that it not only accounts for what is already known, but also suggests new understandings (Lakatos, 1978; Popper, 1965). There are a number of implications of a dyadic caring motivation that suggest some new understandings.

The connection view of caregiving oriented toward the partner's needs has extended Bowlby's original view by showing the functional equivalence of some activities that Bowlby sometimes viewed as separate from attachment, such as feeding the child, clothing the child, holding a nondistress child, playing with the child, and so on. The caregiving theoretical orientation suggests that these various subsystems all respond to the same emotional motivation. It thus provides a parsimonious and comprehensive emotional foundation for understanding parental caregiving.

Another innovation of the connection theoretical system has been the explicit conceptualization of all of the connection concepts as variable. The emotion of caring, for example, is seen to vary across caregivers, as does nurturance, the primary overt caregiving behavior. Different levels of caring and nurturance are thus accounted for within this orientation. For example, it was noted that there are at least three conditions under which a low level of caregiving behaviors will be performed. First, a caregiver may have a low level of caring (such as a severely depressed parent who has little emotion to direct outside the self). Second, a caregiver may have a high or medium level of caring while alter has a low level of need. Third, a caregiver may have a high or medium level of caring but be unable to offer effective nurturance because of incompetence or interference (a lack of skill, or competing forces or pressures that interfere with the performance of a learned skill).

Caregiving follows an emotional logic that is quite different from the calculating logics of exchange and power. Caregiving is focused on partner needs rather than own interests, on love rather than personal gain. The connection theoretical system is methodologically individualist. It describes the process of interaction of individuals, connected individuals who respond to one another and construct unique caring relationships with one another. The connection is not something bigger than a person, nor is it a merging of two persons. It is a self-transformation that reflects an individual's proactive response to another that is both intentional and emotional, associated with specific neurological processes that are also variable in strength. The connection is described as an internal response that is other-regarding. It is expressed in a person's nurturing contact with another.

There are several advantages to conceptualizing the set goal of caregiving as meeting the needs of the other. In the first place, the proximity and security attachment set goals are both needs to which parents respond (Feeney & Noller, 1996). In the second place, it uses a meaning of caregiving that is congruent with cultural understandings. Meeting the needs of the child is what we *mean* by good parenting and how we judge the qualities of good parenting (Wilson, 1993). A parent who gives food, shelter, proximity, safety, even security, but who does not give love and respect or permit independence would be judged a "bad parent" by most in American society and deficient in caregiving. In the third place, research has shown that attachment styles measured in terms of proximity in the Strange Situation (Ainsworth, et al., 1978) are related to actions in many arenas other than proximity (Ainsworth, 1982; Feeney & Noller, 1996). The dyadic emotion of caring for the child emerges from the parent's contact and interaction with the child. Male and female birth parents, adoptive parents, stepparents, siblings, daycare caregivers, teachers, and even readers or viewers of a story about the child may respond with concern and caring to the child and become committed to meeting the child's needs.

If the idea of a dyadic caring motivation had application only to adult caregiving toward children, it would be of little interest except to specialists in parent-child relationships. However, children usually feel as much caring as parents. This observation is controversial only for attachment theorists who equate caregiving with protection and safety. Many attachment theorists have noted that attentiveness and responsiveness are characteristic of "good parents" who become attachment objects for children (Bowlby, 1969/1982; Sroufe & Waters, 1977; Stern, 1985). If attachment logic is consistent, then just as the parent's experience of attentiveness and responsiveness leads to nurturance of the child, the child's caring, attentiveness and responsiveness toward the parent similarly ought to lead to the child's nurturance of the parent as well. Because the caregiving that parents direct to children is so obvious, most researchers have been slow to observe the caregiving that children ordinarily direct to parents, from saying thank you and offering food to "playing quietly while Daddy takes a nap" to giving hugs and love. For Bowlby, the child's caregiving is only visible in the case of pathologically insecure parents (actually, he only talks about mothers) who turn children into caregivers through "role reversal" (Bowlby, 1979, 1988). However, Bowlby does not ask why children would become caregivers under such conditions because he is interested in other problems. The connection theoretical system provides the answer in the parent's and child's mutual caring, and the set goal of meeting the partner's need. Children usually have greater needs than parents, leading to the usual preponderance of nurturance from parents to children. In some clinical cases that Bowlby describes, however, "needy" mothers evoke the voluntary caregiving of their children. Much nurturance of needy parents by children is successful in the sense that it enables family functioning and continuity. It is also true, however, that the limited developmental level of such children often contributes to their "failure" to meet all the needs of their parents and thus sometimes leads to physical abuse (Justice & Justice, 1990). However, the unsuccessful caregiving of some children should no more be dismissed by attachment theory than the unsuccessful caregiving of some parents.

The dyadic emotion of caring can account for the caregiving motivation system and for its evolutionary advantage. Because of its wide applicability (to parent-child and child-parent caregiving, to group cooperation, and to adult-adult caregiving), the dyadic caring emotion is not necessarily efficient in any particular relationship. Boorman and Levitt (1980) have shown the evolutionary advantages of such inefficiency. In fact, it is the very inefficiency of the caregiving system that makes attachment necessary at all. Because of competing motivations, most parents do not give full attention to their children. When they do give attention to their children, other motivations are still operating. Thus, parents are not always proactively aware of children's needs, or adults of their partners' needs. The attachment motivation system in the child has an important role in "reminding" parents (or other partners) to provide nurturance.

DEFINING FAMILY

In this book I have frequently contrasted connection with self interest, showing that connection helps to understand a series of sociological problems—especially in the family—better than they can be understood in terms of self interest. Just as self interest alone is not sufficient to understand social behavior, neither is connection alone sufficient. Both motivations—and certainly others—are necessary for a full appreciation of social behavior.

Furthermore, the motivations of self interest and connection are variable. In some contexts, we are strongly motivated to achieve our self interests; we carefully calculate the relative personal benefits of our alternatives and select the one with the greatest personal profit. In other contexts, self interest is not a major motivation. We are not calculating profits. These contexts include when we are asleep, when we are with someone we love, sometimes when we are alone, and when we are angry or when we are apathetic and do not care about ourselves. The range of the self interest motivation from low to high is depicted in Figure 9.1, where a "market" describes those contexts in which the strength of the self interest motivation is at a maximum for all actors. Within the concept of a market, a "pure market" occurs when self interest is the only nonzero motivation. A pure market as a system of actors motivated only by self interest would be a cold place lacking trust, where actors are unconcerned with the feelings or outcomes of other actors.

In addition to the motivation of self interest, there are the connection motivations of caregiving and attachment. The caregiving and attachment motivations of the connection theoretical system are also variable. In some contexts, we are strongly motivated to achieve connections; we are caring and we trust and we make decisions so as to meet the needs of those we love and to depend on them for help with our needs. We know empirically that there are unhealthy families where people are not caring, where abuse and other forms of violence occur. But healthy families are characterized by high levels of connection, where people care and where they trust. A "pure family" occurs when connection is the only nonzero motivation. The pure family, like the pure market, would be a strange and unfamiliar place, where actors without a self interest motivation are only focused on helping one another.

Because the self interest motivation and the connection motivations are independent, orthogonal dimensions, they can vary independently: both strong, both weak, or only one strong. We can have a strong motivation to meet our family's needs along with a strong motivation to meet

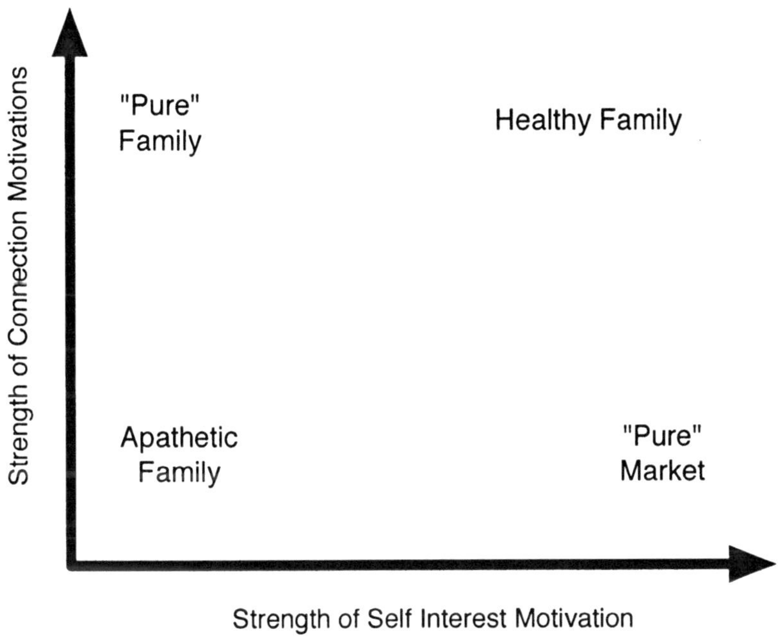

Figure 9.1. Self Interest and Connection as Orthogonal Motivations

our own individual wants. I want my family to be happy and secure, but I also want the various gadgets and accessories that make me personally happy. A healthy family is one where caregiving behaviors provide support for family members' attachment needs for protection and comfort, as well as provide support for individuation needs to explore and grow independently.

And there are contexts in which self interest and the motivation to nurture are both low. These contexts include situations where we are apathetic and unconcerned, where our energy level is low. They include situations where we are acting out of habit or convention. Just as important as it is that we acknowledge that human beings have more than the single motivation of self interest, we need to acknowledge the multiple motivations we already know about (including fear, anger, lust, and play), as well as being open to the existence of other motivations as well.

In the preceding discussion, I have given an implicit definition of family. It is time to move toward an explicit definition. First, let us look at some of the definitions proposed in the family literature.

- "The term *nuclear family* refers simply to two adults of opposite sex living in a socially approved sexual relationship and living with their own or adopted children" (Leslie & Korman, 1985, p. 12, emphasis in original).
- A family is "one or more adults related by blood, marriage, or affiliation who cooperate economically, share a common dwelling place, and *may* rear children" (Strong & Vault, 1989, p. 6, emphasis in original).
- "The family is a relatively permanent group of persons linked together in social roles by ties of blood, marriage, or adoption, who live together and cooperate economically and in the rearing of children" (Brinkerhoff & White, 1988, p. 335, emphasis in original).
- "The family may now be defined as a group of persons united by ties of marriage, blood, or adoption; constituting a single household; interacting and communicating with each other in their respective social roles of husband and wife, mother and father, son and daughter, brother and sister; and creating and maintaining a common culture" (Burgess, et al., 1971, p. 7).

Each of these definitions is an empirical definition, an operationalization. Each defines the family in terms of its usual empirical referents. As such, they capture our historical observations of the family. These definitions, therefore, give rules for classifying observed households into "family" and "not family" categories. They tell what most families look like. They do not tell *why* we classify households in this way. There clearly are cases for each of these definitions where entities are classified in ways that do not correspond to what we mean by "family." The first definition excludes families without children or with children away at school. The second, third, and fourth definitions say that non-residential parents are not part of a family. The last two exclude unmarried parents with children. The first, third, and fourth exclude same sex couples raising children. Empirical definitions such as these suggest how to recognize something as a family when we see it, but do not thereby help us to understand what "family" means.

None of the textbook definitions above mentions love (although the Strong & DeVault definition refers rather vaguely to "affiliation" as an alternative to blood or marriage). And yet love is at the heart of what we *mean* by the family. When each of us thinks of a family, we do not think of a biologically linked, socially sanctioned marital group where members exploit and abuse one another. We think of a family as a group, however constituted, where members love one another, where they understand one another and are committed to one another's welfare, where they trust and depend on one another. It is where, in Frost's expression, "when you go there, they have to take you in." This is the "normal" family of our conceptualization (Strong & Vault, 1989).

This analysis suggests a theoretical definition of the concept of family that recognizes that it is connection that makes a group a family. Furthermore, since the concepts of connection are variable concepts, the concept of family is also a variable construct (Figure 9.1).

> **Theoretical definition.** A group of actors is a family to the extent that the connection motivations, caring and trust, are at a high level among the actors.

Using this variable conceptualization, a group of actors becomes a family as connection motivations and processes increase, or ceases to be a family as these motivations and processes decrease. If we are willing to set a threshold for the amount of connection that is required to consider a group to be a family (dichotomously defined), then we could define the family as a place where connection processes predominate. In so doing, we solve many of the problems of empirical definitions. Marital status, sexual relationships, genetic relationship, presence of children make no difference to this definition, although they are clearly associated. Actors who cohabit without marriage can be a family—if they have a strong connection. By this definition, actors who share living quarters and perhaps even child rearing for reasons of profit—but not connection—are not a family in the conceptual sense, even if the adults are married. By this definition a business establishment that is run "like a family," where people care about and respect and trust one another, where *amae* depending and nurturance are high, *is* a family.

In this analysis, both the social acknowledgment of marriage and adoption and the biological relationship of family members are secondary to caregiving and attachment. It is the operation of the emotional processes of connection that create the caring and trust, empathy and openness, responsibility and *amae*, and nurturance and acceptance of the family. The family as defined here corresponds to the "family realm" of Beutler et al. (1989), who describe the family in terms of emotionality, altruism, nurturing, and an orientation toward the whole person.

Once we have a theoretical definition of the family, we will still need empirical definitions to conduct research. We will still need to define what a family is "on the ground." But now our empirical definition needs to be justifiable within its context. For example, the Leslie & Korman definition ("two adults of opposite sex living in a socially approved sexual relationship and living with their own or adopted children") or the Brinkerhoff & White definition ("a relatively permanent group of persons linked together in social roles by ties of blood, marriage, or adoption, who live together and cooperate economically and in the rearing of children") are defensible if we are studying parent-child relationships (so we insist on families with children) in a stable community of long term marriages (where there are few single-parent households), but Leslie & Korman's requirement of two parents would make this definition highly problematic for the general study of parent-child relationships in contemporary U. S. society. The Burgess et al. definition ("a group of persons united by ties of marriage, blood, or adoption; constituting a single household; interacting and communicating with each other in their respective social roles of husband and wife, mother and father, son and daughter, brother and sister; and creating and maintaining a common culture") would probably be adequate for this more general study as it will include parents without children and single parents with children, although it would exclude non-residential parents and families with children away at school.

Outside of doing research, it doesn't make too much difference how we define the family. We can do just fine with our "common sense" imprecise definitions. In our daily lives and in our teaching of undergraduates, "family" has implicit meanings based on life experiences that are untouched by formal definitions. It may make little difference in our lived lives to distinguish "connected families" from "unconnected families." It makes no difference whether we define cohesive organizations as "like families," or even as "families."

And yet, when family scientists talk to one another, when we work at the level of theoretical orientation and theory, definition is important. For theoretical understanding, precision and clarity are necessary. What matters is that we apply exchange, power, and connection theories when they are appropriate and helpful, and do not apply them when they are not appropriate and not helpful. The connection theoretical system makes visible the processes by which family members—and others in close relationships—connect with one another. I would argue that it is in these processes that the family is special. These processes, in fact, make the family *theoretically* a family. The processes of connection are what gives the family its special feeling.

INSTITUTIONALIZED AVOIDANCE

I am going to round out this discussion of the family by giving a critique of two of the most common attempts to account for parenting.

The study of parenting in the social sciences has often been characterized by a kind of institutional avoidance. People in general, and social scientists in particular, have often decided that some topics related to families are not worthy of study. I want to be clear what I am claiming here. It is not that parenting has not been studied. Parenting has been extensively studied. But studies of *why* parents nurture are virtually nonexistent. There are innumerable studies of the forms of parenting (e.g., parenting styles), the consequences of these forms (e.g., abusive parenting), and the predictors of these forms (e.g., predictors of attachment style). There are hundreds of studies of why parents parent in a particular way, but virtually no studies of why parents parent at all. Theories of evolution and of social norms have filled the gap.

The evolution argument

Parenting is natural: parenting is an evolved behavior, so there is no need to study it further. Parental nurturance of children is fundamental to the species. If parents did not nurture at all, virtually all children would die and the human species would disappear. If parents nurtured only physically, providing only food, clothing, and shelter, many children would still die without any comforting; and the rest would never develop the ability to care for others, so the next generation would get even less parental nurturance. Contemporary human parents provide physical nurturance, normative training, and affection to their children. Three reasons have traditionally been given for using evolution as an excuse not to study parenting. First, there is the "nature" approach. Since parenting clearly occurs and has "always" occurred, parenting must be a natural phenomenon (and thus sacred and dangerous to study: Hinde, 1982). Women, after all, have a "need" to nurture (Solomon & George, 1996).

A second reason for not trying to understand why parenting occurs is that it is an evolved phenomenon (Mann, 1992; Tooby & Cosmides, 1992). Parenting occurred even before the growth of civilization as we know it so it must be innate and biologically based. There might exist a motivation for parenting, but this is a "proximal" cause of parenting and not as important or as interesting as its "ultimate" cause in evolution (Cassidy, 2000; Geary, 2000). Of course, many evolved conditions and behaviors are considered worthy of study, such as cancer, HIV, and violence, but the motivation for parenting has not been.

A third reason for institutional avoidance is that the motivation of parenting has not been considered important. Parenting has traditionally been done by women, those members of society who have "always" been "behind the scenes" and thus unstudied and understudied (Epstein, 1988; Harding, 1991; Millman & Kanter, 1987). It is important to note that this reason has become much less prevalent in the last couple of decades: fathers in the United States have been observed to have taken an increasing role in parenting. So now researchers want to understand why fathers would stay home and be active and sometimes primary caregivers (Doherty, Kouneski, & Erickson, 1998; Dollahite & Hawkins, 1998; Hawkins & Dollahite, 1997).

The social norms argument

There are social norms for parenting, so even though we do not know where the norms come from, we can feel confident that we know why parents nurture children. Within the social sciences, a second explanation for parental nurturance has been to trace it to social norms. Most normative discussion of parenting has been parallel to the "natural" explanation above—it makes a casual reference to "norms" or "roles" in a way that assumes that the problem has already been solved. This approach assumes that prescriptive norms determine parental nurturance.

It is important to distinguish between *emergent* customs (also called "descriptive norms," which describe what people ordinarily do, and are thus descriptions of "normal" behavior), *prescriptive* norms (which describe what people are supposed to do *and* thus cause the behavior to occur), and *proscriptive* norms (which describe what people are not supposed to do *and* for which they are punished). The "and" in the definitions of prescriptive and proscriptive norms is intentional and critical. If norms are not shown to *cause* behavior, then claims that norms *explain* the behavior are unjustified.

A strong case can be made that proscriptive norms have a causal impact on parenting. There are proscriptive norms against infanticide or child abandonment. There are proscriptive norms against child abuse or neglect (as well as against spouse abuse and elder abuse). These are norms that are enforced by legal mechanisms. Such proscriptive norms may contribute to good parenting practices to the extent that they inhibit disapproved practices. Some additional proscriptive norms appear to be widespread, but are not (yet) universally enforced by the law enforcement establishment. These include norms discouraging parental spanking and parental smoking, both of which tend to be widely, but not universally, disapproved. A significant limitation of proscriptive norms as an explanation of parental nurturance is that nurturing a child well is not just a matter of not doing the wrong things. Good parenting requires performing the right behaviors, behaviors that change over the development of the child. If the surveillance required for the enforcement of proscriptive norms is only activated for a small number of parents who come to the attention of enforcement authorities, then proscriptive norms are not likely to explain parenting practices of most parents—and if they do, they will only explain the control of extreme behaviors.

The most common normative explanation of parental nurturance, though, relies on prescriptive social norms. This approach has an extremely long and pervasive history in sociology and other social sciences. Normative theories assert that husbands and wives, fathers and mothers, have roles built out of prescriptive norms that define their rights, obligations, and expected behaviors toward one another and toward their children. These roles are said to include norms prescribing nurturance and other behaviors that mothers and fathers are expected to perform. Some theorists see these norms as negotiated in day-to-day interaction (Heiss, 1981; Hewitt, 1988; Turner, 1962). Other theorists see them as authoritatively imposed by society (Blake & Davis, 1964; Brickman, 1974; Burns, 1973; Coleman, 1990; Ferree, 1990; Gecas, 1976; Greenberg, 1980; Hill, 1971; Homans, 1950; Lamb, 1978; LaRossa & LaRossa, 1981; Nye, 1980, 1982; Rodgers, 1973; Ruddick, 1989; Scanzoni, et al., 1989; Scheff, 1990; Turner, 1985). Still others see norms as somehow absorbed in childhood and still active and remembered when persons become parents (Bahr, 1982; Burgess, et al., 1971; Cahill, 1983; Caspi & Elder, 1988; Dager, 1964; Kagan, 1977; Katz, 1979; LaRossa, 1986; McDonald, 1977; Nye, 1979; Parens & Saul, 1971; Parsons, 1951; Parsons & Bales, 1955; Rollins & Thomas, 1979; Smith, 1970; Steinmetz, 1979). In all cases, these views assert that prescriptive norms are in some way causative of parenting actions. It has been almost half a century since Wrong (1961) rigorously critiqued this "over-socialized" conception of norms in sociology. But family theorists, with great frequency, continue to characterize parental behavior as caused by norms.

One telling argument against prescriptive norms as the source of parenting is the observation that lots of non-human species without any known systems of social norms exhibit parental nurturance (see Chapter 3). Furthermore, prescriptive normative explanations treat parental nurturance as externally caused and therefore discourage examination of the *experience* of the nurturing parent. Explanations that trace parental nurturance to prescriptive norms assume that parents will not spontaneously nurture their children in the absence of such norms (if parents nurture spontaneously, why bring up norms at all?).

Furthermore, the normative account is not parsimonious. It depends on an unwieldy superstructure of assumptions. Given the wide variations reported in human parenting practices: permissive, authoritarian, authoritative parenting approaches (Baumrind, 1968) or secure, preoccupied, dismissing, fearful caregiving styles (Bartholomew, 1990), it is not at all clear how these disparate parenting practices are produced by prescriptive social norms. Do all parents know all the social norms? If so, how do they choose which ones to follow? Or do different parents learn different social norms? If so, who enforces these different social norms on different parents? The normative account must assert that others are prepared to issue sanctions for parental behavior, especially the previous generation of parents, whose reinforcements and sanctions must be asserted to have been so overwhelming that their effects continue for a generation.

To assert that parental nurturance is caused by social norms begs the question of what these social norms are, as well as where they came from. Some theory is required that is capable of explaining how such social norms come to exist and, of course, what actions they are to prescribe. In spite of the assumed consistency of parental norms, sociologists have failed to propose, much less agree on, any list of parental norms. Family researchers have described lists of extra-family expectations that are derived from, and in fact phrased as, societal functions, such as "to train children to make them available for community roles" (Pitts, 1964, p. 57), and "socialization of children for adult roles in the family and in other social groups" (Hill, 1971, p. 16). These "norms," however, are so vague as to provide none of the imputed guidance for parents (Brim, 1959). Furthermore, none of the lists even mentions such a relevant topic as "love" or "caring." Lacking a list of parental norms, sociologists have failed to provide direct evidence that parents either know or follow these alleged norms. A major reason for any general lack of impact of prescriptive norms of parenting is that prescriptive norms for parents are essentially unenforceable, because no one with the ability to assess sanctions is ordinarily present when the behaviors in question are enacted.

Emergent customs. In the caregiving orientation, the case is made for neurobiologically based emotional processes as causes of nurturance behaviors and thus as a cause for the emergence of descriptive norms of parenting. What is "normal" is what caring parents spontaneously do. Emergent customs of parenting describe this normal, spontaneous action. The connection theoretical system thus provides an explanation of the origins of parental norms as well as their content. If we look at the positive end of each of the dimensional concepts of the caregiving and attachment theories of parent-child relationships, we find the following customs:

- (Caring). Highly connected parents love their children.
- (Empathy). Highly connected parents pay attention to their children and learn about their needs.
- (Responsibility). Highly connected parents take responsibility for their children's needs.
  - (Attachment responsibility). Highly connected parents are committed to protecting their children and helping them to feel secure.
  - (Individuation responsibility). Highly connected parents are committed to encouraging their children's exploration and growth.
- (Nurturance). Highly connected parents nurture their children and meet their needs.
- (Trust). Highly connected children trust their parents.
- (Openness). Highly connected children freely reveal their needs to their parents.
- (*Amae*). Highly connected children depend on their parents.
- (Acceptance). Highly connected children are appreciative of their parents' nurturance.

These behaviors are natural behaviors. They are produced by the logic of human connection. They occur naturally when parents and children are connected and connection processes are operating at high levels. To the extent that connection processes operate in families, the regularity with which these patterns are observed, both in personal experience and vicariously, will create expectations about the actions of good parents. Such expectations are what sociologists mean by social norms. The actions presented here are thus emergent customs and descriptive norms of parent-child relationships.

Prescriptive and proscriptive norms. The emergent customs described above, it must be emphasized, are associated with connection concepts as they exist in healthy families. But in some families, connection processes operate at a low level. When connection is low, caring, empathy and responsibility are also at a low level. As a result, nurturance, trust, openness, and *amae* will also be low, and the actions in such families will not spontaneously conform to the emergent norms. To the extent that low connection families wish to be "good citizens," they can try to "act like" high connection families, to act as they "should," or to so present themselves to others. This is accomplished by turning the observational statements above into moral expectations:

- (Caring). Parents should love their children.
- (Empathy). Parents should pay attention to their children and learn about their needs.
- (Responsibility). Parents should take responsibility for their children's needs.
    - Parents should be committed to protecting their children and helping them to feel secure.
    - Parents should be committed to encouraging their children's exploration and growth.
- (Nurturance). Parents should nurture their children and meet their needs.
- (Trust). Children should trust their parents.
- (Openness). Children should freely reveal their needs to their parents.
- (*Amae*). Children should depend on their parents.
- (Acceptance). Children should be appreciative of their parents' nurturance.

The preceding statements can be taken as prescriptive social norms of family nurturance.

But some families either do not care to be "good citizens" by conforming to the expectations of the society, or have psychological, cultural, economic, or other resource deficits that prevent them from living up to the ideals of "good enough" families. It is in these families that society often will not let nature "take its course." It is in these families that society has an interest in forcing or supporting the family to act as if connection were at a high level. Because high connection is approved, and low connection disapproved between parents and children, we can also recognize the origin of some proscriptive norms of family life that society has created to regulate the actions of families with unacceptably low levels of connection:

- (Caring). Parents should NOT be indifferent to their children.
- (Empathy). Parents should NOT fail to pay attention to their children and learn about their needs.
- (Responsibility). Parents should NOT neglect their children's needs.

- (Nurturance). Parents should NOT fail to nurture their children and meet their needs.
- (Trust). Children should NOT distrust their parents.
- (Openness). Children should NOT hide their needs from their parents.
- (*Amae*). Children should NOT avoid depending on their parents.
- (Acceptance). Children should NOT dismiss their parents' nurturance.

What is not clear, because it is not generally studied, is to what extent either prescriptive or proscriptive norms actually affect parental or child behavior in particular cases. How many parents nurture their children well because of high levels of caring? How many have low levels of caring and nurture well anyway because of prescriptive norms? In such cases, who provides the sanctions that motivate the nurturance? How many parents nurture well or adequately because their tendency to neglect or abuse their children is curbed by proscriptive norms? These are empirical questions to be answered by research. Most parents, I expect, are influenced directly by a caring motivation and also indirectly by a concern for what others might think. I anticipate that research will show that caring, because it is immediate, will have a stronger effect than norms.

I expect that when research is conducted, we will learn that proscriptive norms against abuse and neglect have substantial effects only for a limited number of people, in particular those whose brain circuits for caring and empathy are not fully developed, probably mostly because of their own limited early childhood experience of supportive caregiving. Furthermore, there seems to be a clear role for the causal effectiveness of some prescriptive parenting norms that are sure to be of interest for sociologists of fashion (cloth diapers and paper diapers; Nancy Drew and Harry Potter).

The case made in this book is that actions of parental and other caregiving are usually voluntary. In most cases, parents voluntarily give good care to their children from the motivations that I've discussed in detail throughout this book. High quality care, of course, is relative to knowledge. When people have believed that spanking is good for the child, then spanking has been common, whatever our current sensibilities on this issue. Spanking, strenuous beatings, feeding by schedule, letting children cry themselves to sleep, swaddling, "hardening," and the like have been performed toward children because parents believed these actions were best for the child (deMause, 1974). In contexts provided by socially shared beliefs about children's needs, parents nurture in patterned ways motivated by their caring. Alongside these parents motivated by connection, there will have been other parents with low levels of caring, empathy, or responsibility who may have performed similar behaviors because they felt constrained by their social networks to follow prescriptive or proscriptive norms. The extent to which such behaviors may have been socially coerced by norms or otherwise socially influenced by cultural preconceptions is an empirical question.

Altruism

Altruism is most often discussed in the context of evolution or social norms. In Chapter 3, I showed why the usual conceptualization of altruism toward strangers views it the wrong way around and thus does not provide an adequate basis for understanding nurturance in close relationships. Here I want to reverse the question and ask what the caregiving theoretical orientation can contribute to an understanding of altruism. The connection theoretical system in general, and the caregiving theoretical orientation in particular provide unique insights into the phenomenon of altruism. "Altruism" is a term that has been used to describe behavior to meet the needs of strangers as well as behavior to meet the needs of partners in close relationships. Once one understands how caring leads to nurturance for a special other, one can recognize occasions where this same mechanism operates at lower levels of nurturance for strangers and other non-special others. Thus we can see altruism toward strangers and acquaintances as caregiving in non-enduring relationships.

To the extent that we care about someone, to that extent we are motivated to feel a responsibility to respond to their needs and to nurture them. As a general rule, we do not nurture those who are not emotionally important to us. In this book I have emphasized the kind of responsibility that derives from personal emotional caring developed over time. However, it is clear that limited forms of responsibility can also be expressed. We sometimes see responsibility directed toward strangers, such as the person who risks his/her life to save another person in danger. Unlike the proactive nurturance that is produced by the caring emotion in relationships with a caregiving bond, a more reactive and limited form of nurturance can be produced by caring induced in a quiescent or even previously nonexistent relationship. As Batson has shown in a series of experiments (Batson, 2002) learning about another's need can make us care about the other and take some responsibility for helping them to meet that need. We can sleep untroubled in spite of the hunger of hundreds of homeless children in our city. But a media story about a single hungry child can make us feel caring. Our caring, however temporary, expresses our emotional contact and raises the salience of the needs of this child and by extension of the homeless in general. This can lead to a sense of increased responsibility and thus to donations and voluntary action. But the emotional contact is usually episodic and thus so is the responsibility. Tomorrow, as the memory of our emotional sense of caring fades, we will sleep easy again even as the hunger continues. "While I care for my children throughout our mutual lifetimes, I may care only momentarily for a stranger in need" (Noddings, 1984, p. 16).

The ability to respond altruistically outside of ordinary connection relationships should depend, as does all caring, on the prior establishment of caregiving circuits. Thus our caring and other-oriented responsibility begin in our earliest relationships and depend on the physical and emotional contact of these frequent interactions (Gillath, et al., 2005; 1988). This account of altruism helps to understand the evolutionary correlation of altruistic behaviors with kinship, as was discussed in Chapter 3. The interaction in these early relationships is most frequently with those who are kin to us. That caregiving behaviors are frequently associated with kinship relationships has provided an evolutionary pathway for the propagation of these nurturing outcomes. But we also have such frequent interactions and resulting caring with non-kin, as in adoptive and step-parent relationships and relationships with close friends, dating partners, and spouses.

Index

References

Ainsworth, M. D. S. (1972). Attachment and dependency: A comparison. In J. L. Gewirtz (Ed.), *Attachment and dependency* (pp. 97-137).

Ainsworth, M. D. S. (1982). Attachment: Retrospect and prospect. In C. M. Parkes & J. Stevenson-Hinde (Eds.), *The place of attachment in human behavior* (pp. 3-30). New York: Basic.

Ainsworth, M. D. S. (1989). Attachments beyond infancy. *American psychologist, 44*, 709-716.

Ainsworth, M. D. S., Blehar, M. C., Waters, E., & Wall, S. (1978). *Patterns of attachment: A psychological study of the strange situation*. Hillsdale, NJ: Erlbaum.

Aldous, J. (1977). Family interaction patterns. *Annual review of sociology, 3*, 105-135.

Aldous, J. (1978). *Family careers: Developmental change in families*. New York: Wiley.

Alexander, J. C. (1988). *Action and its environments: Toward a new synthesis*. New York: Columbia.

Allen, S. M., & Hawkins, A. J. (1999). Maternal gatekeeping: Mothers' beliefs and behaviors that inhibit greater father involvement in family work. *Journal of marriage and the family, 61*, 199-212.

Altman, J., & Bayer, S. A. (1997). *Development of the cerebellar system: In relation to its evolution, structure, and functions*. Boca Raton, FL: CRC Press.

Altmann, M. (1963). Naturalistic studies of maternal care in moose and elk. In H. L. Rheingold (Ed.), *Maternal behavior in mammals* (pp. 233-253). New York: Wiley.

Apter, T. (1990). *Altered loves: Mothers and daughters during adolescence*. New York: St. Martins.

Archer, J. (1997). Why do people love their pets? *Evolution & human behavior, 18*(4), 237-259.

Aristotle (1952). *The works of Aristotle* (W. D. Ross, Trans.). Chicago: Great Books.

Armstrong, L. (1978). *Kiss daddy goodnight: A speak-out on incest*. New York: Hawthorn.

Arnold, M. B. (1960). *Emotion and personality (Vols 1 & 2)*. New York: Columbia University Press.

Arnold, M. B. (1970). Perennial problems in the field of emotion. In M. B. Arnold (Ed.), *Feelings and emotions: The Loyola Symposium* (pp. 169-185). New York: Academic.

Ashton, P. T. (1978). The role of the attachment bond in effective parenting. In Joseph H. Stevens, Jr. & M. Mathews (Eds.), *Mother/child, father/child relationships* (pp. 31-49). Washington, DC: National Association for the Education of Young Children.

Aube, M., & Senteni, A. (1996). Emotions as commitment operators: A foundation for control structure in multi-agent systems. In W. Van de Velde & J. W. Perram (Eds.), *Agents breaking away* (pp. 13-25). Berlin: Springer.

Aune, B. (1977). *Reason and action*. Dordrecht, Holland: Reidel.

Axelrod, R. (1984). *The evolution of cooperation*. New York: Basic.

Babbie, E. (1989). *The practice of social research*. Belmont, CA: Wadsworth.

Bachrach, P., & Baratz, M. (1963). Decisions and nondecisions: An analytical framework. *American political science review, 57*, 632-642.

Badcock, C. (2000). *Evolutionary psychology: A critical introduction*. Cambridge: Polity Press.

Bahr, S. J. (1982). Exchange and control in married life. In F. I. Nye (Ed.), *Family relationships: Rewards and costs* (pp. 81-95). Beverly Hills: Sage.

Baier, A. C. (1993). What do women want in a moral theory? In M. J. Larrabee (Ed.), *An ethic of care: Feminist and interdisciplinary perspectives* (pp. 19-32). New York: Routledge.

Bakan, D. (1966). *The duality of human existence*. Chicago: Rand McNally.

Balint, A. (1965). Love of the mother and mother love. In M. Balint (Ed.), *Primary love and psycho-analytic technique* (pp. 91-108). New York: Liveright.

Bandura, A. (1977). *Social learning theory*. Englewood Cliffs, NJ: Prentice-Hall.

Bandura, A., & Walters, R. H. (1963). *Social learning and personality development*. New York: Holt, Rinehart & Winston.

Barash, D. (1979). *The whisperings within*. New York: Harper and Row.

Bardwick, J. M. (1974). Evolution and parenting. *Journal of social issues, 4*, 39-62.

Bargh, J. A., & Barndollar, K. (1996). Automaticity in action: The unconscious as repository of chronic goals and motives. In P. M. Gollwitzer & J. A. Bargh (Eds.), *The psychology of action: Linking cognition and motivation to behavior* (pp. 457-481). New York: Guilford.

Baron-Cohen, S., & Wheelwright, S. (2004). The Empathy Quotient: An investigation of adults with Asperger Syndrome or high functioning autism and normal sex differences. *Journal of Autism and Developmental Disorders, 34*(2), 163-186.

Bartholomew, K. (1990). Avoidance of intimacy: An attachment perspective. *Journal of social and personal relationships, 7*, 147-178.

Bartholomew, K., & Horowitz, L. M. (1991). Attachment styles among young adults: A test of a four-category model. *Journal of personality and social psychology, 61*, 226-244.

Batson, C. D. (1990). How social an animal? The human capacity for caring. *American psychologist, 45*, 336-346.

Batson, C. D. (1991). *The altruism question: Toward a social-psychological answer*. Hillsdale, NJ: Erlbaum.

Batson, C. D. (2002). Addressing the altruism question experimentally. In S. Garrard (Ed.), *Altruism and Altruistic Love: Science, Philosophy, and Religion in Dialogue* (pp. 89-105). Cary, NC: Oxford University Press.

Batson, C. D. (2009). These things called empathy: Eight related but distinct phenomena. In J. Decety & W. Ickes (Eds.), *The social neuroscience of empathy* (pp. 3-15). London: MIT Press.

Batson, C. D., Batson, J. G., Griffitt, C. A., Barrientos, S., Brandt, J. R., Sprengelmeyer, P., et al. (1989). Negative-state relief and the empathy-altruism hypothesis. *Journal of personality and social psychology, 56*, 922-933.

Batson, C. D., Dyck, J. L., Brandt, J. R., Batson, J. G., Powell, A. L., McMaster, M. R., et al. (1988). Five studies testing two new egoistic alternatives to the empathy-altruism hypothesis. *Journal of personality and social psychology, 55*, 52-77.

Baumrind, D. (1968). Authoritarian versus authoritative parental control. *Adolescence, 3*, 255-272.

Becker, G. S. (1991). *A treatise on the family* (Enlarged ed.). Cambridge: Harvard University Press.

Becker, H. S. (1960). Notes on the concept of commitment. *American journal of sociology, 66*, 32-40.

Befu, H. (1986). The social and cultural background of child development in Japan and the United States. In H. Stevenson, H. Azuma & K. Hakuta (Eds.), *Child development and education in Japan* (pp. 13-27). New York: Freeman.

Bell, D. C. (2001). Evolution of parental caregiving. *Personality and social psychology review, 5*(3), 216-229.

Bell, D. C. (2008). *Constructing social theory*. New York: Rowman & Littlefield.

Bell, D. C. (2009a). Attachment without fear. *Journal of family theory and review, 1*, 177-197.

Bell, D. C., Brown, V., & Montoya, I. D. (2004). Motivations for parenting: Lessons from neurobiology. Unpublished manuscript.

Bell, D. C., & Richard, A. J. (2000a). Caregiving: The forgotten element in attachment. *Psychological inquiry, 11*(2), 69-83.

Bell, D. C., & Richard, A. J. (2000b). The search for a caregiving motivation. *Psychological Inquiry, 11*(2), 124-128.

Bell, L. G. (1989). Song without words. *The family therapy networker, 13 (2)*, 48-53.

Bell, L. G. (2009b). Mindful psychotherapy. *Journal of spirituality in mental health, 11*, 126-144.

Bell, L. G., Bell, D. C., & Nakata, Y. (2001). Triangulation and adolescent development in the U.S. and Japan. *Family process, 40*, 173-186.

Bell, R. Q. (1974). Contributions of human infants to caregiving and social interaction. In M. Lewis & L. A. Rosenblum (Eds.), *The effect of the infant on its caregiver* (pp. 1-19). New York: Wiley.

Bellah, R. N., Madsen, R., Sullivan, W. M., Swidler, A., & Tipton, S. M. (1985). *Habits of the heart: Individualism and commitment in American life*. New York: Harper & Row.

Belsky, J. (1984). The determinants of parenting: A process model. *Child development, 55*, 83-96.

Belsky, J., & Isabella, R. A. (1988). Maternal, infant, and social contextual determinants of attachment security. In J. Belsky & T. Nezworski (Eds.), *Clinical implications of attachment*. Hillsdale, NJ: Erlbaum.

Benedict, R. (1954). *The chrysanthemum and the sword*. Tokyo: Tuttle.

Bengtson, V. L., Olander, E. B., & Haddad, A. A. (1976). The "generation gap" and aging family members: Toward a conceptual model.

In J. F. Gubrium (Ed.), *Time, roles, and self in old age* (pp. 237-263). New York: Human Sciences.

Berman, W. H., & Sperling, M. B. (1994). The structure and function of adult attachment. In M. B. Sperling & W. H. Berman (Eds.), *Attachment in adults: Clinical and developmental perspectives* (pp. 1-28). New York: Guilford.

Bernard, J. (1982). *The future of marriage (2nd Ed.)*. New Haven: Yale.

Bernstein, D. (1983a). The female superego: A different perspective. *International journal of psycho-analysis, 64*, 187-201.

Bernstein, G. L. (1983b). *Haruko's world: A Japanese farm woman and her community*. Stanford: Stanford University Press.

Berscheid, E. (1983). Emotion. In H. H. Kelley, E. Berscheid, A. Christensen, J. H. Harvey, T. L. Huston, G. Levinger, E. Mc-Clintock, L. A. Peplau & D. R. Peterson (Eds.), *Close relationships* (pp. 110-168). New York: W. H. Freeman.

Berscheid, E. (1999). The greening of relationship science. *American psychologist, 54*, 260-266.

Berscheid, E. (2006). Seasons of the heart. In M. Mikulincer & G. S. Goodman (Eds.), *Dynamics of romantic love: Attachment, care-giving, and sex* (pp. 404-422). New York: Guilford Press.

Berscheid, E., & Peplau, L. A. (1983). The emerging science of relationships. In H. H. Kelley, E. Berscheid, A. Christensen, J. H. Harvey, T. L. Huston, G. Levinger, E. McClintock, L. A. Peplau & D. R. Peterson (Eds.), *Close relationships* (pp. 1-19). New York: W. H. Freeman.

Beutler, I. F., Burr, W. R., Kathleen S. Bahr, & Herrin, D. A. (1989). The family realm: Theoretical contributions for understanding its uniqueness. *Journal of marriage and the family, 51*, 805-816.

Bierstedt, R. (1974). *Power and progress: Essays in sociological theory*. New York: McGraw-Hill.

Blackburn, S. (1994). *The Oxford dictionary of philosophy*. Oxford: Oxford University Press.

Blake, J., & Davis, K. (1964). Norms, values and sanctions. In R. Faris (Ed.), *Handbook of modern sociology* (pp. 456-484). Chicago: Rand-McNally.

Blalock, H. M., Jr., & Wilken, P. H. (1979). *Intergroup processes: A micro-macro perspective*. New York: Free Press.

Blau, P. M. (1986). *Exchange and power in social life* (Expanded ed.). New Brunswick: Transaction.

Blood, R. O., Jr (1969). *Marriage* (2nd ed.). New York: Free Press.

Blumberg, M. S., & Wasserman, E. A. (1995). Animal mind and the argument from design. *American psychologist, 50*, 133-144.

Blustein, J. (1982). *Parents and children: The ethics of the family*. New York: Oxford.

Boorman, S. A., & Levitt, P. R. (1980). *The genetics of altruism*. New York: Academic.

Borgatta, E. F., & Borgatta, M. L. (1992). *Encyclopedia of sociology*. New York: Macmillan.

Bornstein, R. F. (1993). *The dependent personality*. New York: Guilford.

Bowen, M. (1978). *Family therapy in clinical practice*. New York: Aronson.

Bowlby, J. (1969/1982). *Attachment and loss, Volume 1: Attachment* (2nd ed.). New York: Basic.

Bowlby, J. (1973). *Attachment and loss, Volume 2: Separation: Anxiety and anger*. New York: Basic.

Bowlby, J. (1977). The making and breaking of affectional bonds. I. Aetiology and psychopathology in the light of attachment theory. *British journal of psychiatry, 130*, 201-210.

Bowlby, J. (1979). *The making and breaking of affectional bonds*. New York: Methuen.

Bowlby, J. (1980). *Attachment and loss, Volume 3: Loss*. New York: Basic.

Bowlby, J. (1988). *A secure base: parent-child attachment and healthy human development*. New York: Basic.

Bradley, M. M. (2000). Emotion and motivation. In J. T. Cacioppo, L. G. Tassinary & G. G. Berntson (Eds.), *Handbook of psychophysiology* (2nd ed., pp. 602-642). Cambridge: Cambridge University Press.

Brazelton, T. B., & Cramer, B. G. (1990). *The earliest relationship: Parents, infants, and the drama of early attachment*. Reading, MA: Addison-Wesley.

Bretherton, I. (1978). Making friends with one-year-olds: An experimental study of infant-stranger interaction. *Merrill-Palmer Quarterly, 24*, 29-52.

Bretherton, I. (1980). Young children in stressful situations: The supporting role of attachment figures and unfamiliar caregivers. In G. V. Coelho & P. J. Ahmed (Eds.), *Uprooting and development* (pp. 179-210). New York: Plenum.

Bretherton, I., & Ainsworth, M. D. S. (1974). Responses of one-year-olds to a stranger in a strange situation. In M. Lewis & L. A. Rosenblum (Eds.), *The origins of fear* (pp. 131-164). New York: Wiley.

Bretherton, I., & Munholland, K. A. (1999). Internal working models in attachment relationships. In J. Cassidy & P. R. Shaver (Eds.), *Handbook of attachment: Theory, research, and clinical applications* (pp. 89-111). New York: Guilford.

Brickman, P. (1974). *Social conflict.* Lexington, MA: Heath.

Brickman, P. (1987). *Commitment, conflict and caring.* Englewood Cliffs: Prentice-Hall.

Brim, O. G., Jr (1959). *Education for child rearing.* New York: Russell Sage.

Brinkerhoff, D. B., & White, L. K. (1988). *Sociology* (2nd ed.). St. Paul: West.

Broderick, C. B. (1993). *Understanding family process: Basics of family systems theory.* Newbury Park, CA: Sage.

Bruce, N., & Waldman, M. (1990). The rotten-kid theorem meets the Samaritan's dilemma. *Quarterly journal of economics, 105,* 155-165.

Buckley, W. (1967). *Sociology and modern systems theory.* Englewood Cliffs: Prentice-Hall.

Burgess, E. W., Locke, H. J., & Thomes, M. M. (1971). *The family: From traditional to companionship* (4th ed.). New York: Van Nostrand Reinhold.

Burns, T. (1973). A structural theory of social exchange. *Acta sociologica, 16,* 188-208.

Burr, W. R., Hill, R., Nye, F. I., & Reiss, I. L. (Eds.). (1979). *Contemporary theories about the family, Vol. 1: Research-based theories.* New York: Free Press.

Buss, D. M., Haselton, M. G., Shackelford, T. K., Bleske, A. L., & Wakefield, J. C. (1998). Adaptations, exaptations, and spandrels. *American psychologist, 53,* 533-548.

Buss, D. M., Haselton, M. G., Shackelford, T. K., Bleske, A. L., & Wakefield, J. C. (1999). Interactionism, flexibility, and inferences about the past. *American psychologist, 54,* 443-445.

Cacioppo, J., & Berntson, G. G. (1994). Relaitonships between attitudes and evaluative space: A critical review with emphasis on the separability of positive and negative substrates. *Psychological bulletin, 115,* 401-423.

Cahill, S. E. (1983). Reexamining the acquisition of sex roles: A social interactionist approach. *Sex roles, 9,* 1-15.

Cancian, F. M. (1987). *Love in America: Gender and self-development.* Cambridge: Cambridge University Press.

Cannon, W. B. (1929). *Bodily changes in pain, hunger, fear and rage.* New York: Appleton.

Caporael, L. R. (1997). The evolution of truly social cognition: The core configurations model. *Personality and social psychology review, 1*(4), 276-298.

Carpenter, E. M., & Kirkpatrick, L. A. (1996). Attachment style and presence of a romantic partner as moderators of psychophysiological responses to a stressful laboratory situation. *Personal relationshps, 3*, 351-367.

Carter, C. S. (1998a). Neoroendocrine perspectives on social attachment and love. *Psychoneuroendocrinology, 23*, 779-818.

Carter, C. S. (2003). The developmental consequences of oxytocin. *Physiological behavior, 79*, 383-397.

Carter, C. S. (2005). Biological perspectives on social attachment and bonding. In C. S. Carter, L. Ahnert, K. E. Grossmann, S. B. Hrdy, M. E. Lamb, S. W. Porges & N. Sachser (Eds.), *Attachment and bonding: A new synthesis* (pp. 85-100). Cambridge, MA: MIT Press.

Carter, R. (1998b). *Mapping the mind.* Berkeley: University of California Press.

Caspi, A., & Elder, G. H., Jr (1988). Emergent family patterns: the intergenerational construction of problem behaviour and relationships. In R. A. Hinde & J. Stevenson-Hinde (Eds.), *Relationships within families: Mutual influences* (pp. 218-240). Oxford: Clarendon.

Cassidy, J. (1999). The nature of the child's ties. In J. Cassidy & P. R. Shaver (Eds.), *Handbook of attachment: Theory, research, and clinical applications* (pp. 3-20). New York: Guilford.

Cassidy, J. (2000). The complexity of the caregiving system: A view from attachment theory. *Psychological inquiry, 11*(2), 86-91.

Cassidy, J., & Shaver, P. R. (Eds.). (1999). *Handbook of attachment: Theory, research, and clinical applications.* New York: Guilford.

Chafetz, J. S. (1978). *A primer on the construction and testing of theories in sociology.* Itasca, IL: Peacock.

Chafetz, J. S. (1990). *Gender equity: An integrated theory of stability and change.* Newbury Park: Sage.

Chisholm, K. (2000). Attachment in children adopted from Romanian orphanages: Two case studies. In P. M. Crittenden & A. H. Claussen (Eds.), *The organization of attachment relationships: Maturation, culture, and context* (pp. 171-189). New York: Cambridge University Press.

Chisholm, K. M., Carter, M. C., Ames, E. W., & Morrison, S. J. (1995). Attachment security and indiscriminately friendly behavior in children adopted from Romanian orphanages. *Development and Psychopathology, 7*, 283-294.

Chodorow, N. J. (1978). *The reproduction of mothering.* Berkeley: University of California Press.

Clark, K. E., & Ladd, G. W. (2000). Connectedness and autonomy support in parent-child relationships: Links to children's socio-emotional orientation and peer relationships. *Developmental psychology, 36*(4), 485-498.

Clark, M. S., & Mills, J. (1979). Interpersonal attraction in exchange and communal relationships. *Journal of personality and social psychology, 37*, 12-24.

Clutton-Brock, T. H. (1991). *The evolution of parental care.* Princeton: Princeton University Press.

Coleman, J. S. (1990). *Foundations of social theory.* Cambridge, MA: Harvard.

Collins, N. L. (1996). Working models of attachment: Implications for explanation, emotion and behavior. *Journal of personality and social psychology, 71*, 810-832.

Constantine, L. L. (1986). *Family paradigms: The practice of theory in family therapy.* New York: Guilford.

Conway, L. G., III, & Schaller, M. (2002). On the verifiability of evolutionary psychological theories: An analysis of the psychology of scientific persuasion. *Personality and social psychology review, 6*(2), 152-166.

Cowan, C. P., & Cowan, P. A. (1992). *When partners become parents: The big life change for couples.* New York: Basic.

Crist, E. (1999). *Images of animals: Anthropomorphism and animal mind.* Philadelphia: Temple University Press.

Crittenden, P. M. (1995). Attachment and psychopathology. In S. Goldberg, R. Muir & J. Kerr (Eds.), *Attachment theory: Social, developmental, and clinical perspectives* (pp. 367-406). Hillsdale, NJ: Analytic Press.

Dager, E. Z. (1964). Socialization and personality development in the child. In H. T. Christensen (Ed.), *Handbook of marriage and the family* (pp. 740-781). Chicago: Rand McNally.

Daly, M., & Wilson, M. (1983). *Sex, evolution and behavior* (2nd ed.). Belmont, CA: Wadsworth Publishing.

Daly, M., & Wilson, M. (1999). *The truth about Cinderella: A Darwinian view of parental love.* London: Weidenfeld & Nicolson.

Damasio, A. R. (1994). *Descartes' error: Emotion, reason, and the human brain*. New York: Avon.

Darwall, S. (1998). Empathy, sympathy, care. *Philosophical studies, 89*, 261-282.

Davidson, R. J. (1992). Emotion and affective style: Hemispheric substrates. *Psychological science, 3*, 39-43.

Davis, J. H., & Leinhardt, S. (1972). The structure of positive interpersonal relations in small groups. In J. Berger (Ed.), *Sociological theories in progress, Vol. 2* (pp. 218-251). Boston: Houghton Mifflin.

Davis, K. E., Kirkpatrick, L. A., Levy, M. B., & O'Hearn, R. E. (1994). Stalking the elusive love style: Attachment styles, love styles, and relationship development. In R. Erber & R. Gilmour (Eds.), *Theoretical frameworks for personal relationships* (pp. 179-210). Hillsdale, NJ: Erlbaum.

Dawkins, R. (1976/1989). *The selfish gene* (2nd ed.). Oxford: Oxford University Press.

Dawkins, R. (1987). *The blind watchmaker*. New York: Norton.

De Vries, G. J., & Villalba, C. (1999). Brain sexual dimorphism and sex differences in parental and other social behaviors. In C. S. Carter, I. I. Lederhendler & B. Kirkpatrick (Eds.), *The integrative neurobiology of affiliation* (pp. 155-168). Cambridge, MA: MIT Press.

Deacon, T. W. (1990). Rethinking mammalian brain evolution. *American zoologist, 30*, 629-705.

Del Cerro, M. C. R. (1998). Role of the vomeronasal input in maternal behavior. *Psychoneuroendocrinology, 23*, 905-926.

DeLosier, P. P. (1982). Attachment theory and child abuse. In C. M. Parkes & J. Stevenson-Hinde (Eds.), *The place of attachment in human behavior* (pp. 95-117). New York: Basic.

deMause, L. (1974). The evolution of childhood. In L. deMause (Ed.), *The history of childhood: The untold story of child abuse* (pp. 1-73). New York: Peter Bedrick.

Diamond, D., & Blatt, S. J. (1994). Internal working models and the representational world in attachment and psychoanalytic theories. In M. B. Sperling & W. H. Berman (Eds.), *Attachment in adults: Clinical and developmental perspectives* (pp. 72-97). New York: Guilford.

Diamond, M. J. (1995). Someone to watch over me: The father as the original protector of the mother-infant dyad. *Psychoanalysis and psychotherapy, 12*, 89-102.

Dickinson, A., & Dearing, M. F. (1979). Appetitive-aversive interactions and inhibitory processes. In A. Dickinson & R. A. Boakes (Eds.),

Mechanisms of learning and motivation (pp. 203-231). Hillsdale, NJ: Erlbaum.

Dinnerstein, D. (1976). *The mermaid and the minotaur: Sexual arrangements and human malaise*. New York: Harper & Row.

Doherty, W. J. (1997). *The intentional family: How to build family ties in our modern world*. New York: Addison Wesley.

Doherty, W. J., Kouneski, E. P., & Erickson, M. F. (1998). Responsible fathering: An overview and conceptual framework. *Journal of marriage and the family, 60*, 277-292.

Doi, T. (1981). *The anatomy of dependence* (J. Bester, Trans.). Tokyo: Kodansha International.

Doi, T. (1986). *The anatomy of self* (M. A. Harbison, Trans.). Tokyo: Kodansha International.

Doi, T. (1989). The concept of amae and its psychoanalytic implications. *International review of psycho-analysis, 16*, 349-354.

Dollahite, D. C. (1998). Fathering, faith, and spirituality. *Journal of men's studies, 7*, 3-15.

Dollahite, D. C., & Hawkins, A. J. (1998). A conceptual ethic of generative fathering. *Journal of men's studies, 7*, 109-132.

Domhoff, G. W. (1970). *The higher circles: The governing class in America*. New York: Random House.

Duck, S. (1994). *Meaningful relationships: Talking, sense, and relating*. Thousand Oaks, CA: Sage.

Dunbar, R. (1996). *Grooming, gossip, and the evolution of language*. Cambridge, MA: Harvard University Press.

Durkheim, E. (1933). *The division of labor in society* (G. Simpson, Trans.). New York: Free Press.

Eckman, P. (1984). Expression and the nature of emotion. In R. Scherer & P. Ekman (Eds.), *Approaches to emotion* (pp. 319-343). Hillsdale, NJ: Erlbaum.

Egeland, B., & Farber, E. A. (1984). Infant-mother attachment: Factors related to its development and changes over time. *Child Development, 55*(3), 753-771.

Eibl-Eibesfeldt, I. (1996). *Love and hate: The natural history of behavior patterns* (Translator, Trans.). New York: Aldine de Gruyter.

Eisenberger, N. I., Gable, S. L., & Lieberman, M. D. (2007). Functional magnetic resonance imaging responses relate to differences in real-world social experience. *Emotion, 7*(4), 745-754.

Eisenberger, N. I., Lieberman, M. D., & Williams, K. D. (2003). Does rejection hurt? An fMRI study of social exclusion. *Science, 302*, 290-292.

Eisler, R. (1987). *The chalice and the blade: Our history, our future*. San Francisco: Harper & Row.

Ekeh, P. P. (1974). *Social exchange theory: The two traditions*. Cambridge, MA: Harvard University Press.

Ekman, P. (1984). Expression and the nature of emotion. In K. R. Scherer & P. Ekman (Eds.), *Approaches to emotion* (pp. 319-343). Hillsdale, NJ: Erlbaum.

Elster, J. (1989). *The cement of society: A study of social order*. Cambridge: Cambridge University Press.

Emde, R. M. (1992). Amae, intimacy, and the early moral self. *Infant mental health journal, 13*(1), 34-42.

Emerson, R. M. (1962). Power-dependence relations. *American sociological review, 27*, 31-41.

Epstein, C. F. (1988). *Deceptive distinctions: Sex, gender, and the social order*. New Haven: Yale.

Erikson, E. H. (1963). *Childhood and society*. New York: Norton.

Etzioni, A. (1988). *The moral dimension: Toward a new economics*. New York: Free Press.

Etzioni, A. (1993). *The spirit of community: The reinvention of American society*. New York: Touchstone.

Fairbairn, W. R. D. (1952). *An object-relations theory of the personality*. New York: Basic.

Feeney, J., & Noller, P. (1996). *Adult attachment*. Thousand Oaks, CA: Sage.

Ferguson, L. R. (1970). Dependency motivation in socialization. In R. A. Hoppe, G. A. Milton & E. C. Simmel (Eds.), *Early experiences and the process of socialization* (pp. 59-79). New York: Academic.

Ferree, M. M. (1990). Beyond separate spheres: Feminism and family research. *Journal of marriage and the family, 52*, 866-884.

Filsinger, E. E., & Fabes, R. A. (1985). Odor communication, pheromones, and human families. *Journal of marriage and family, 47*(2), 349-359.

Fleming, A. S., & Anderson, V. (1987). Affect and nurturance: mechanisms mediating maternal behavior in two female mammals. *Progress in neuro-psychopharmacology & biological psychiatry, 11*(2-3), 121-127.

Fogel, A., Gail F. Melson, & Mistry, J. (1986). Conceptualizing the determinants of nurturance: A reassessment of sex differences. In A.

Fogel & G. F. Melson (Eds.), *Origins of nurturance: Developmental, biological and cultural perspectives on caregiving* (pp. 53-67). Hillsdale, NJ: Erlbaum.

Fontana, A. M., Diegnan, T., Villenueve, A., & Lepore, S. J. (1999). Nonevaluative social support reduces cardiovascular reactivity in young women during acutely stressful performance situations. *Journal of behavioral medicine, 22*, 75-91.

Forgas, J. P. (2000). Feeling is believing? The role of processing strategies in mediating affective influences on beliefs. In N. H. Frijda, A. S. R. Manstead & S. Bem (Eds.), *Emotions and beliefs: How feelings influence thoughts* (pp. 108-143). Cambridge: Cambridge University Press.

Fortey, R. (1997). *Life: A natural history of the first four billion years of life on earth.* New York: Knopf.

Forward, S., & Torres, J. (1986). *Men who hate women & the women who love them.* Toronto: Bantam.

Fraiberg, S. (1974). Blind infants and their mothers: An examination of the sign system. In M. Lewis & L. A. Rosenblum (Eds.), *The effect of the infant on its caregiver* (pp. 215-232). New York: Wiley.

Freie, J. F. (1998). *Counterfeit community: The exploitation of our longings for connectedness.* Lanham, MD: Rowman & Littlefield.

French, J. R. P., Jr.,, & Raven, B. (1968). The bases of social power. In D. Cartwright & A. Zander (Eds.), *Group dynamics* (pp. 259-269). Evanston, IL: Row, Peterson.

Freud, S. (1961). *A general introduction to psychoanalysis.* New York: Washington Square.

Friedrich, C. J. (1963). *Man and his government: An empirical theory of politics.* New York: McGraw-Hill.

Fries, A. W., & Pollak, S. (2004). Emotion understanding in postinstitutionalized Eastern European children. *Developmental Psychopathology, 16*(2), 355-369.

Fries, A. W., Ziegler, T. E., Kurian, J. R., Jacoris, S., & Pollak, S. D. (2005). Early experience in humans is associated with changes in neuropeptides critical for regulating social behavior. *Proceedings of the National Academy of Sciences, 102*(47), 17237-17240.

Gaylin, W. (1979). *Feelings: Our vital signs.* New York: Harper & Row.

Geary, D. C. (2000). Attachment, caregiving and parental investment. *Psychological inquiry, 11*(2), 84-86.

Gecas, V. (1976). The socialization and child care roles. In F. I. Nye (Ed.), *Role structure and analysis of the family* (pp. 33-59). Beverly Hills, CA: Sage.

Gelles, R. J., & Straus, M. A. (1988). *Intimate violence*. New York: Simon & Schuster.

George, C., & Solomon, J. (1999). Attachment and caregiving: The caregiving behavioral system. In J. Cassidy & P. R. Shaver (Eds.), *Handbook of attachment: Theory, research, and clinical applications* (pp. 649-670). New York: Guilford.

Giddens, A. (1979). *Central problems in social theory: Action, structure and contradiction in social analysis*. Berkeley: University of California Press.

Giddings, F. H. (1896). *Principles of sociology*. New York: Macmillan.

Gilgun, J. F. (1995). We shared something special: The moral discourse of incest perpetrators. *Journal of marriage and the family, 57*, 265-281.

Gillath, O., Shaver, P. R., Mikulincer, M., Nitzberg, R. E., Erez, A., & van IJzendoorn, M. H. (2005). Attachment, caregiving, and volunteering: Placing volunteerism in an attachment-theoretical framework. *Personal relationshps, 12*, 425-446.

Gilligan, C. (1982). *In a different voice: Psychological theory and women's development*. Cambridge, MA: Harvard University Press.

Gilligan, C., Ward, J. V., & Taylor, J. M. (1988). *Mapping the moral domain: A contribution of women's thinking to psychological theory and education*. Cambridge, MA: Harvard University Press.

Glasser, W. (1984). *Control theory: A new explanation of how we control our lives*. New York: Harper & Row.

Glenn, N. D. (1991). The recent trend in marital success in the United States. *Journal of marriage and the family, 53*, 261-270.

Goldberg, S., Grusec, J. E., & Jenkiins, J. M. (1999). Narrow view of attachment or broad view of protection? Rejoinder to the commentaries. *Journal of family psychology, 13*(4), 504-507.

Gollwitzer, P. M., & Bargh, J. A. (Eds.). (1996). *The psychology of action: Linking cognition and motivation to behavior*. New York: Guilford.

Goode, W. J. (1971). Force and violence in the family. *Journal of marriage and the family, 33*, 445-458.

Goode, W. J. (1982). Why men resist. In B. Thorne & M. Yalom (Eds.), *Rethinking the family: Some feminist questions* (pp. 131-150). New York: Longman.

Gould, S. J. (1991). Exaptation: A crucial tool for evolutionary psychology. *Journal of social issues, 47j*, 43-65.

Gouldner, A. W. (1960). The norm of reciprocity: A preliminary statement. *American sociological review, 25*, 161-178.

Greenberg, L. S., & Safran, J. D. (1987). *Emotion in psychotherapy: Affect, cognition, and the process of change*. New York: Guilford.

Greenberg, M. S. (1980). A theory of indebtedness. In K. J. Gergen, M. S. Greenberg & R. H. Willis (Eds.), *Social exchange: Advances in theory and research* (pp. 3-26). New York: Plenum.

Grewen, K. M., Girdler, S. S., Amico, J. A., & Light, K. C. (2005). Effects of partner support on resting oxytocin, cortisol, norepinephrine, and blood pressure before and after warm partner contact. *Psychosomatic medicine, 67*, 531-538.

Griffin, D., & Bartholomew, K. (1994). Models of the self and other: Fundamental dimensions underlying measures of adult attachment. *Journal of personality and social psychology, 67*, 430-445.

Grossmann, K. E., Karin Grossmann, & Zimmermann, P. (1999). A wider view of attachment and exploration: Stability and change during the years of immaturity. In J. Cassidy & P. R. Shaver (Eds.), *Handbook of attachment: Theory, research, and clinical applications* (pp. 760-786). New York: Guilford.

Groves, J. E. (1978). Taking care of the hateful patient. *New England journal of medicine, 298*, 883-887.

Gubernick, D. J., Sengelaub, D. R. & Kurz, E. M. (1993). Neuroanatomical correlate of paternal and maternal behavior in the biparental California mouse (Peromyscus californicus). *Behavioral neuroscience, 107(1)*, 194-201.

Guillamon, A., & Segovia, S. (1997). Sex differences in the vomeronasal system. *Brain research bulletin, 44*(4), 377-382.

Gump, B. B., Polk, D. E., Kamarck, T. W., & Shiffman, S. M. (2001). Partner interactions are associated with reduced blood pressure in the natural environment: Ambultory monitoring evidence from a healthy, multiethnic adult sample. *Psychosomatic medicine, 63*, 423-433.

Gurnell, J. (1987). *The natural history of squirrels*. New York: Facts on File Publications.

Habermas, J. (1981). *The theory of communicative action. Vol. 1. Reason and the rationalization of society* (T. McCarthy, Trans.). Boston: Beacon.

Hage, J. (1972). *Techniques and problems of theory construction in sociology*. New York: Wiley.

Hanh, T. N. (1999). *The miracle of mindfulness*. Boston: Beacon Press.

Harding, S. (1991). *Whose Science? Whose knowledge? Thinking from women's lives*. Ithaca, NY: Cornell.

Harlow, H. F., & Harlow, M. K. (1965). The effect of rearing conditins on behavior. *International journal of psychiatry, 1*, 43-51.

Harris, J. R. (1998). *The nurture assumption: Why children turn out the way they do*. New York: Touchstone.

Harris, P. L., & Saarni, C. (1989). Children's understanding of emotion: An introduction. In C. Saarni & P. L. Harris (Eds.), *Children's understanding of emotion* (pp. 3-24). Cambridge: Cambridge University Press.

Hatfield, E., Cacioppo, J. T., & Rapson, R. L. (1994). *Emotional contagion*. New York: Cambridge University Press.

Hawkins, A. J., & Dollahite, D. C. (1997). *Generative fathering: Beyond the deficit perspectives*. Thousand Oaks, CA: Sage.

Hazan, C., Campa, M., & Gur-Yaish, N. (2006). What is adult attachment? In M. Mikulincer & G. S. Goodman (Eds.), *Dynamics of romantic love: Attachment, caregiving, and sex* (pp. 47-70). New York: Guilford Press.

Hazan, C., & Shaver, P. (1994). Attachment as an organizational framework for research on close relationships. *Psychological inquiry, 5*, 1-22.

Heard, D., & Lake, B. (1997). *The challenge of attachment for caregiving*. London: Routledge.

Hechter, M. (1987). *Principles of group solidarity*. Berkeley: University of California Press.

Heckhausen, J. (2000). Evolutionary perspectives on human motivation. *American behavioral scientist, 43*(6), 1015-1029??

Heiss, J. (1981). Social roles. In M. Rosenberg & R. H. Turner (Eds.), *Social psychology: Sociological perspectives* (pp. 94-129). New York: Basic.

Hennessy, M. B. (1999). Social influences on endocrine activity in guinea pigs, with comparisons to findings in nonhuman primates. *Neuroscience and biobehavioral reviews, 23*, 687-698.

Hennessy, M. B., Hornschuh, G., Kaiser, S., & Sachser, N. (2006). Cortisol responses and social buffering: A study throughout the lifespan. *Hormones & behavior, 49*(3), 383-390.

Hennessy, M. B., & Kaplan, J. N. (1982). Influence of the maternal surrogate on pituitary-adrenal activity and behavior of infant squirrel monkeys. *Developmental psychobiology, 15*, 423-431.

Hess, R. D., & Handel, G. (1959). *Family worlds: A psychosocial approach to family life*. Chicago: University of Chicago Press.

Hewitt, J. P. (1988). *Self and society: A symbolic interactionist social psychology (4th Ed.)*. Boston: Allyn & Bacon.

Hill, R. (1971). Modern systems theory and the family: A confrontation. *Social science information, 10(5)*, 7-26.

Hill, R., & Hansen, D. A. (1969). The identification of conceptual frameworks utilized in family study. In R. J. R. King (Ed.), *Family relations: Concepts and theories* (pp. 19-41). Berkeley: Glendessary Press.

Hillman, J. (1962). *Emotion: A comprehensive phenomenology of theories and their meanings for therapy*. Evanston, IL: Northwestern.

Hinde, R. A. (1976). On describing relationships. *Journal of child psychology and psychiatry, 17*, 1-19.

Hinde, R. A. (1982). Attachment: Some conceptual and biological issues. In C. M. Parkes & J. Stevenson-Hinde (Eds.), *The place of attachment in human behavior* (pp. 60-76). New York: Basic.

Hirschi, T. (1969). *Causes of delinquency*. Berkeley: University of California Press.

Hochschild, A. R. (1983). *The managed heart: Commercialization of human feeling*. Berkeley: University of California Press.

Hofer, M. A. (1994). Hidden regulators in attachment, separation, and loss. *Monographs for the Society for Research in Child Development, 59*(2/3), 192-207.

Hoffman, M. L. (1981). The development of empathy. In J. P. Rushton & R. M. Sorrentino (Eds.), *Alruism and helping behavior: Social, personality, and developmental perspectives* (pp. 41-63). Hillsdale, NJ: Erlbaum.

Homans, G. C. (1950). *The human group*. New York: Harcourt, Brace & World.

Homans, G. C. (1974). *Social behavior: Its elementary forms*. New York: Harcourt, Brace, Jovanovich.

Hrdy, S. B. (1999). *Mother nature: A history of mothers, infants, and natural selection*. New York: Pantheon.

Hrdy, S. B. (2005). Evolutionary context of human development: The cooperative breeding model. In C. S. Carter, L. Ahnert, K. E. Grossmann, S. B. Hrdy, M. E. Lamb, S. W. Porges & N. Sachser (Eds.),

Attachment and bonding: A new synthesis (pp. 9-32). Cambridge, MA: MIT Press.

Hyde, L. (1983). *The gift: Imagination and the erotic life of property.* New York: Vintage.

Ickes, W. (1993). Empathic accuracy. *Journal of personality, 61*, 587-610.

Insel, T. R. (1997). A neurobiological basis of social attachment. *American journal of psychiatry, 154(6)*, 726-735.

Insel, T. R., & Winslow, J. T. (1998). Serotonin and neuropeptides in affiliative behaviors. *Biological psychiatry, 44(3)*, 207-219.

Insel, T. R., Young, L., & Wang, Z. (1999). Molecular aspects of monogamy. In C. S. Carter, I. I. Lederhendler & B. Kirkpatrick (Eds.), *The integrative neurobiology of affiliation* (pp. 183-197). London: MIT Press.

Isabella, R. A. (1993). Origins of attachment: Maternal interactive behavior across the first year. *Child development, 64*, 605-621.

Izard, C. E. (1993). Four systems for emotion activation: Cognitive and noncognitive processes. *Psychological review, 100*, 68-90.

Izard, C. E., & Ackerman, B. P. (2000). Motivational, organizational, and regulatory functions of discrete emotions. In M. Lewis & J. M. Haviland-Jones (Eds.), *Handbook of emotions* (2nd ed., pp. 253-264). New York: Guilford.

Jacob, F. (1977). Evolution and tinkering. *Science, 196*, 1161-1166.

James, W. (1884). What is an emotion? *Mind, 9*, 188-205.

Jeannerod, M. (1997). *The cognitive neuroscience of action.* Oxford: Blackwell Publishers.

Joas, H. (1987). Symbolic interactionism. In A. Giddens & J. Turner (Eds.), *Social theory today* (pp. 82-115). Cambridge: Polity Press.

Jordan, J. V. (1991). Empathy and self boundaries. In J. V. Jordan, A. G. Kaplan, J. B. Miller, I. P. Stiver & J. L. Surrey (Eds.), *Women's growth in connection: Writings from the Stone Center* (pp. 67-80). New York: Guilford Press.

Jordan, J. V., Surrey, J. L., & Kaplan, A. G. (1991). Women and empathy: Implications for psychological development and psychotherapy. In J. V. Jordan, A. G. Kaplan, J. B. Miller, I. P. Stiver & J. L. Surrey (Eds.), *Women's growth in connection: Writings from the Stone Center* (pp. 27-50). New York: Guilford Press.

Justice, B., & Justice, R. (1990). *The abusing family* (Rev. ed.). New York: Plenum.

Kagan, J. (1977). The child in the family. *Daedalus, 106*, 33-56.

Kahn, R. L., & Antonucci, T. C. (1980). Convoys over the life course: Attachment, roles, and social support. In P. B. Baltes & O. G. Brim (Eds.), *Life-span development and behavior* (pp. 253-286). Boston: Lexington.

Kanter, R. M. (1972). *Commitment and community: Communes and utopianism in sociological perspective*. Cambridge, MA: Harvard University Press.

Kantor, D., & Lehr, W. (1975). *Inside the family: Toward a theory of family process*. New York: Harper & Row.

Karen, R. (1994). *Becoming attached: Unfolding the mystery of the infant-mother bond and its impact on later life*. New York: Warner.

Katz, P. A. (1979). The development of female identity. *Sex roles, 5*, 155-178.

Kelsey, M. T. (1981). *Caring: How can we love one another?* New York: Paulist.

Kemper, T. D. (1978). *A social interactional theory of emotions*. New York: Wiley.

Kemper, T. D. (1984). Power, status, and emotions: A sociological contribution to a psychophysiological domain. In K. R. Scherer & P. Ekman (Eds.), *Approaches to emotion* (pp. 369-383). Hillsdale, NJ: Erlbaum.

Kendrick, K. M. (2000). Oxytocin, motherhood and bonding. *Experimental physiology, 85*(Special No.), 111S-124S.

Kendrick, K. M., Da Costa, A. P. C., Broad, K. D., Ohkura, S., Guevara, R., Levy, F., et al. (1997). Neural control of maternal behaviour and olfactory recognition of offspring. *Brain research bulletin, 44*(4), 383-395.

Kerlinger, F. N. (1973). *Foundations of behavioral research* (2nd ed.). New York: Holt, Rinehart and Winston.

Kerr, M., & Bowen, M. (1988). *Family evaluation*. New York: Norton.

Keverne, E. B., Nevison, C. M., & Martel, F. L. (1999). Early learning and the social bond. In C. S. Carter, I. I. Lederhendler & B. Kirkpatrick (Eds.), *The integrative neurobiology of affiliation* (pp. 263-273). Cambridge, MA: MIT Press.

Klaus, M. H., Jerault, R., Kreger, N. C., McAlpine, W., Steffa, M., & Kennell, J. H. (1972). Maternal attachment: Importance of the first postpartum days. *New England journal of medicine, 286*, 460-463.

Klaus, M. H., Kennell, J. H., & Klaus, P. H. (1995). *Bonding: Building the foundations of secure attachment and independence*. Reading, MA: Addison-Wesley.

Klein, D. M., & White, J. M. (1996). *Family theories: An introduction.* Thousand Oaks, CA: Sage.

Knudson-Martin, C. (1993). Gender-making and marital interaction: A process model. *Paper presented at Theory Preconference, National Council on Family Relations*, Baltimore.

Knudson-Martin, C. (2000). Gender, family competence, and psychological symptoms. *Journal of marital and family therapy, 26*(3), 317-328.

Kobak, R. (1999). The emotional dynamics of disruptions in attachment relationships: Implications for theory, research, and clinical intervention. In J. Cassidy & P. R. Shaver (Eds.), *Handbook of attachment: Theory, research, and clinical applications* (pp. 21-43). New York: Guilford.

Kohlberg, L. (1966). A cognitive-developmental analysis of children's sex-role concepts and attitudes. In E. E. Maccoby (Ed.), *The development of sex differences* (pp. 82-173). Stanford, CA: Stanford University Press.

Kohut, H. (1984). *How does analysis cure?* Chicago: University of Chicago Press.

Konarski, J. (1967). *Integrative activity of the brain: An interdisciplinary approach.* Chicago: University of Chicago Press.

Kotelchuck, M. (1976). The infant's relationship to the father: Experimental evidence. In M. E. Lamb (Ed.), *The role of the father in child development.* New York: Wiley.

Kovács, G. L., Sarnyai, Z., & Szabó, G. (1998). Oxytocin and addiction: A review. *Psychoneuroendocrinology, 23*, 945-962.

Kunz, G. (1998). *The paradox of power and weakness: Levinas and an alternative paradigm for psychology.* Albany, NY: State University of New York Press.

Lakatos, I. (1978). *The methodology of scientific research programmes.* Cambridge: Cambridge University Press.

Lakoff, R. T. (1990). *Talking power: The politics of language in our lives.* [No city]: Basic.

Lamb, M. E. (1978). The father's role in the infant's social world. In J. H. Stevens, Jr. & M. Mathews (Eds.), *Mother/child, father/child relationships* (pp. 87-108). Washington, DC: National Association for the Education of Young Children.

Lang, P. J., Bradley, M. M., & Cuthbert, B. N. (1990). Emotion, attention, and the startle reflex. *Psychological review, 97*, 377-398.

LaRossa, R. (1986). *Becoming a parent.* Beverly Hills: Sage.

LaRossa, R., & LaRossa, M. M. (1981). *Transition to parenthood: How infants change families*. Beverly Hills: Sage.

LaRossa, R., & Reitzes, D. C. (1993). Continuity and change in middle class fatherhood, 1925-1935: The culture-conduct connection. *Journal of marriage and the family, 55*, 455-468.

Lasch, C. (1977). *Haven in a heartless world: The family besieged*. New York: Basic.

Lasswell, H., & Kaplan, A. (1950). *Power and society: A framework for political inquiry*. New Haven: Yale.

Lavorgna, G., Patthy, L., & Boncinelli, E. (2001). Were protein internal repeats formed by 'bricolage'? *Trends in genetics, 17*(3), 120-123.

Lazarus, R. S., Coyne, J. C., & Folkman, S. (1984). Cognition, emotion and motivation: The doctoring of Humpty-Dumpty. In K. R. Scherer & P. Ekman (Eds.), *Approaches to emotion* (pp. 221-237). Hillsdale, NJ: Erlbaum.

Lebra, T. S. (1976). *Japanese patterns of behavior*. Honolulu: University of Hawaii Press.

Lebra, T. S. (1984). *Japanese women: Constraint and fulfillment*. Honolulu: University of Hawaii Press.

Lederer, W. J., & Jackson, D. D. (1968). *The mirages of marriage*. New York: Norton.

LeDoux, J. (1996). *The emotional brain: The mysterious underpinnings of emotional life*. New York: Touchstone.

Lee, A., Li, M., Watchus, J., & Fleming, A. S. (1999). Neuroanatomical basis of maternal memory in postpartum rats: Selective role for the nucleus accumbens. *Behavioral neuroscience, 113*(3), 523-538.

Leeper, R. W. (1970). The motivational and perceptual properties of emotions as indicating their fundamental character and role. In M. B. Arnold (Ed.), *Feelings and emotions: The Loyola Symposium* (pp. 151-168). New York: Academic.

Lenski, G. E. (1966). *Power and privilege: A theory of social stratification*. New York: McGraw-Hill.

Lerner, M. (1957). *America as a civilization: Life and thought in the United States today*. New York: Simon and Schuster.

Leslie, G. R., & Korman (1985). *The family in social context* (6th ed.). New York: Oxford.

Lester, B. M., M. Kotelchuck, E. Spelke, M. J. Sellers, & Klein, R. E. (1974). Separation protest in Guatemalan Infants: Cross-cultural and cognitive findings. *Developmental psychology, 10*, 79-85.

Leventhal, H. (1984). A perceptual motor theory of emotion. In K. R. Scherer & P. Ekman (Eds.), *Approaches to emotion* (pp. 271-291). Hillsdale, NJ: Erlbaum.

Levinas, E. (1969). *Totality and infinity* (A. Lingis, Trans.). Pittsburgh: Duquesne University Press.

Levinas, E., & Kearney, R. (1986). Dialogue with Emmanuel Levinas. In R. A. Cohen (Ed.), *Face to face with Levinas* (pp. 13-33). Albany: State University of New York.

Levinger, G. (1982). A social exchange view on the dissolution of pair relationships. In F. I. Nye (Ed.), *Family relationships: Rewards and costs* (pp. 97-121). Beverly Hills: Sage.

Levinger, G. (1983). Development and change. In H. H. Kelley, E. Berscheid, A. Christensen, J. H. Harvey, T. L. Huston, G. Levinger, E. McClintock, L. A. Peplau & D. R. Peterson (Eds.), *Close relationships* (pp. 315-359). New York: W. H. Freeman.

Levinger, G., & Rausch, H. L. (1977). *Close relationships: Perspectives on the meaning of intimacy*. Amherst: University of Massachusetts.

Levitt, M. J., Coffman, S., Guacci-Franco, N., & Loveless, S. C. (1994). Attachment relationships and life transitions: An expectancy model. In M. B. Sperling & W. H. Berman (Eds.), *Attachment in adults: Clinical and developmental perspectives* (pp. 232-255).

Levy, R. I. (1984). The emotions in comparative perspective. In K. R. Scherer & P. Ekman (Eds.), *Approaches to emotion* (pp. 397-412). Hillsdale, NJ: Erlbaum.

Lévy-Strauss, C. (1969). *The elementary structure of kinship*. Boston: Beacon.

Lewis, M., & Haviland-Jones, J. M. (Eds.). (2000). *Handbook of emotions* (2nd ed.). New York: Guilford.

Light, K. C., Grewen, K. M., & Amico, J. A. (2005). More frequent partner hugs and higher oxytocin levels are linked to lower blood pressure and heart rate in premenopausal women. *Biological psychiatry, 69*, 5-21.

Lindsley, D. B. (1951). Emotions. In S. S. Stevens (Ed.), *Handbook of experimental psychology*. New York: Wiley.

Linton, R. (1945). *The cultural background of personality*. New York: Appleton-Century.

Lockley, R. M. (1965). *The private life of the rabbit: An account of the life history and social behaviour of the wild rabbit*. London: Andre Deutsch.

Lopez, B. H. (1978). *Of wolves and men*. New York: Scribner's.

Lowenthal, M. F., Majda Thurnher, & Chiriboga, D. (1975). *Four stages of life*. San Francisco: Jossey-Bass.

Lyons, N. P. (1990). Listening to voices we have not heard: Emma Willard Girls' ideas about self, relationships, and morality. In C. Gilligan, N. P. Lyons & T. J. Hanmer (Eds.), *Making connections: The relational worlds of adolescent girls at Emma Willard School* (pp. 30-72). Cambridge, MA: Harvard University Press.

MacLean, P. D. (1990). *The triune brain in evolution: Role in paleo-cerebral functions*. New York: Plenum.

Macy, M. W., & Skvoretz, J. (1998). The evolution of trust and cooperation between strangers: A computational model. *American sociological review, 63*, 638-660.

Maestripieri, D. (1999). The biology of human parenting: Insights from nonhuman primates. *Neuroscience and biobehavioral reviews, 23*, 411-422.

Mahler, M. S., Pine, F., & Bergman, A. (1975). *The psychological birth of the human infant*. New York: Basic.

Main, M. (1999). Attachment theory: Eighteen points with suggestions for future studies. In J. Cassidy & P. R. Shaver (Eds.), *Handbook of attachment: Theory, research, and clinical applications* (pp. 845-887). New York: Guilford.

Mann, J. (1992). Nurturance or negligence: Maternal psychology and behavioral preference among preterm twins. In J. H. Barkow, L. Cosmides & J. Tooby (Eds.), *The adapted mind: Evolutionary psychology and the generation of culture* (pp. 267-290). New York: Oxford University Press.

Marsiglio, W. (1991). Paternal engagement activities with minor children. *Journal of marriage and the family, 53*, 973-986.

Marx, K. (1968). The eighteenth Brumaire of Louis Bonaparte. In K. Marx & F. Engels (Eds.), *Selected Works*. New York: International Publishers.

Maslow, A. H. (1971). *The farther reaches of human nature*. New York: Penguin.

Maslow, A. H. (1987). *Motivation and personality. (3rd Ed.)*. New York: Harper & Row.

Mason, W. A., & Mendoza, S. P. (1998). Generic aspects of primate attachments: Parents, offspring and mates. *Psychoneuroendo-crinology, 23*, 765-778.

Mason, W. A., & Sponholz, R. R. (1963). Behavior of rhesus monkeys raised in isolation. *Journal of psychiatric research, 81*, 299-306.

Massey, D. S. (2002). A brief history of human society: The origin and role of emotion in social life. *American sociological review, 67*(February), 1-29.

Masson, J. M., & McCarthy, S. (1995). *When elephants weep: The emotional lives of animals*. New York: Delta.

Matthews, G., Zeidner, M., & Roberts, R. D. (2002). *Emotional intelligence: Science and myth*. Cambridge, MA: MIT Press.

Maurer, T. W., & Pleck, J. H. (2006). Fathers' caregiving and bread-winning: A gender congruence analysis. *Psychology of men and masculinity, 7*(2), 101-112.

Mauss, M. (1967). *The gift: Forms and functions of exchange in archaic societies* (I. Cunnison, Trans.). New York: Norton.

McCall, G. J., & Simmons, J. L. (1978). *Identities and interactions: An examination of human associations in everyday life (Rev. Ed.)*. New York: Free Press.

McDonald, G. W. (1977). Parental identification by the adolescent: A social power approach. *Journal of marriage and the family, 39*, 705-719.

McDonald, G. W. (1980). Family power: The assessment of a decade of theory and research. *Journal of marriage and the family, 42*, 841-854.

McDougall, W. (1923). *An introduction to social psychology (16th Ed.)*. Boston: Luce.

Mead, G. H. (1934). *Mind, self, and society*. Chicago: University of Chicago Press.

Mellen, S. L. W. (1981). *The evolution of love*. Oxford: W. H. Freeman.

Mendoza, S. P., & Mason, W. A. (1999). Attachment relationships in New World primates. In C. S. Carter, I. I. Lederhendler & B. Kirkpatrick (Eds.), *The integrative neurobiololgy of affiliation* (pp. 93-99). London: MIT Press.

Merton, R. K. (1967). *On theoretical sociology*. New York: Free Press.

Mikulincer, M. (2006). Attachment, caregiving, and sex within romantic relationships: A behavioral systems perspective. In M. Mikulincer & G. S. Goodman (Eds.), *Dynamics of romantic love: Attachment, caregiving, and sex* (pp. 23-44). New York: Guilford Press.

Mikulincer, M., & Shaver, P. R. (2007). *Attachment in adulthood: Structure, dynamics, and change*. New York: Guilford.

Miller, A. (1984). *For your own good: Hidden cruelty in child-rearing and the roots of violence*. (Hildegarde & Hunter Hannum, Trans.) New York: Farrar-Straus-Giroux.

Miller, J. B. (1986). *Toward a new psychology of women* (2nd ed.). Boston: Beacon.

Miller, J. B. (1991). The development of women's sense of self. In J. V. Jordan, A. G. Kaplan, J. B. Miller, I. P. Stiver & J. L. Surrey (Eds.), *Women's growth in connection: Writings from the Stone Center* (pp. 11-26). New York: Guilford Press.

Miller, L. C., & Fishkin, S. A. (1997). On the dynamics of human bonding and reproductive success: Seeking windows on the adapted-for human-environment interface. In J. A. Simpson & D. T. Kenrick (Eds.), *Evolutionary social psychology* (pp. 197-235). Mahwah, NJ: Erlbaum.

Millman, M., & Kanter, R. M. (1987). Introduction to another voice: Feminist perspective on social life and social science. In S. Harding (Ed.), *Feminism and methodology: Social science issues* (pp. 29-36). Bloomington, IN: Indiana University Press.

Mishler, E. G., & Waxler, N. E. (1968). *Interaction in families: An experimental study of family processes and schizophrenia.* New York: Wiley.

Mitani, J. C., & Watts, D. (1997). The evolution of non-maternal caretaking among anthropoid primates: Do helpers help? *Behavioral ecology and sociobiology, 40*, 213-220.

Mitchell, S. A. (1988). *Relational concepts on psychoanalysis: An integration*. Cambridge: Harvard.

Molinaro, J., Woolfolk, T., & Palkovitz, R. (1997). Developing the fatherhood identity: Processes, themes & influences. *Paper presented at Theory Construction and Research Methodology Workshop, National Conference on Family Relations*, Crystal City, VA.

Molm, L. D. (1990). Structure, action, and outcomes: The dynamics of power in social exchange. *American sociological review, 55*, 427-447.

Molm, L. D., Collett, J. L., & Schaefer, D. R. (2007). Building solidarity through generalized exchange: A theory of reciprocity. *American journal of sociology, 113*, 205-242.

Molm, L. D., Schaefer, D. R., & Collett, J. L. (2009). Fragile and resilient trust: Risk and uncertainty in negotiated and reciprocal exchange. *Sociological theory, 27*(1), 1-32.

Moncher, F. J. (1996). The relationship of maternal adult attachment style and risk of physical child abuse. *Journal of interpersonal violence, 11*, 335-350.

Montagu, A. (1986). *Touching: The human significance of the skin* (3rd ed.). New York: Harper & Row.

Moody, M. (2008). Serial reciprocity: A preliminary statement. *Sociological theory, 26*(2), 130-151.

Moschetti, G. J. (1979). The Christmas potlach: A refinement on the sociological interpretation of gift exchange. *Sociological focus, 12*, 1-7.

Murray, H. A. (1938). *Explorations in personality*. New York: Oxford University Press.

Murstein, B. I. (1970). Stimulus-value-role: A theory of marital choice. *Journal of marriage and the family, 32*(3), 465-481.

Murstein, B. I. (1976). *Who will marry whom? Theories and research in marital choice*. New York: Springer.

Murstein, B. I., Cerreto, M., & MacDonald, M. G. (1977). A theory and investigation of the effect of exchange-orientation on marriage and friendship. *Journal of marriage and the family, 39*, 543-548.

Nelson, E. E., & Panksepp, J. (1998). Brain substrates of infant-mother attachment: Contributions of opioids, oxytocin, and norepinephrine. *Neuroscience and biobehavioral reviews, 22*(3), 437-452.

Nisbet, R. (1990). *The quest for community: A study in the ethics of order & freedom*. San Francisco: Institute for Contemporary Studies.

Nisbett, R. E., & Wilson, T. D. (1977). Telling more than we can know: Verbal reports on mental processes. *Psychological review, 84*, 231-259.

Nissen, E., Uvnäs-Moberg, K., Svensson, K., Stock, S., Widström, A. M., & Winberg, J. (1996). Different patterns of oxytocin, prolactin but not cortisol release during breastfeeding in women delivered by caesarean section or by the vaginal route. *Early human development, 45*, 301-305.

Noddings, N. (1984). *Caring: A feminine approach to ethics & moral education*. Berkeley: University of California Press.

Noirot, E. (1972). Ultrasounds and maternal behavior in small rodents. *Developmental psychobiology, 5*, 371-387.

Numan, M., & Sheehan, T. P. (1999). Neuroanatomical circuitry for mammalian maternal behavior. In C. S. Carter, I. I. Lederhendler & B. Kirkpatrick (Eds.), *The integrative neurobiology of affiliation* (pp. 275-299). Cambridge, MA: MIT Press.

Nye, F. I. (1979). Choice, exchange and the family. In W. R. Burr, R. Hill, F. I. Nye & I. L. Reiss (Eds.), *Contemporary theories about the family, Vol. 2: General theories/theoretical orientations* (pp. 1-41). New York: Free Press.

Nye, F. I. (1980). Family mini theories as special instances of choice and exchange theory. *Journal of marriage and the family, 42*, 479-489.

Nye, F. I. (1982). The basic theory. In F. I. Nye (Ed.), *Family relationships: Rewards and costs* (pp. 13-31). Beverly Hills: Sage.

Nye, F. I., & McLaughlin, S. (1982). Role competence and marital satisfaction. In F. I. Nye (Ed.), *Family relationships: Rewards and costs* (pp. 67-79). Beverly Hills: Sage.

Nygren, A. (1953). *Agape and eros* (P. S. Watson, Trans.). New York: Harper & Row.

O'Connor, T. G. (2005). Attachment disturbances associated with early severe deprivation. In C. S. Carter, L. Ahnert, K. E. Grossmann, S. B. Hrdy, M. E. Lamb, S. W. Porges & N. Sachser (Eds.), *Attachment and bonding: A new synthesis* (pp. 258-267). Cambridge, MA: MIT Press.

Oatley, K. (2000). The sentiments and beliefs of distributed cognition. In N. H. Frijda, A. S. R. Manstead & S. Bem (Eds.), *Emotions and beliefs: How feelings influence thoughts* (pp. 78-107). Cambridge: Cambridge University Press.

Okonogi, K. (1992). *Amae* as seen in diverse interpersonal interactions. *Infant mental health journal, 13(1)*, 18-25.

Oliner, S. P., & Oliner, P. M. (1988). *The altruistic personality: Rescuers of Jews in Nazi Europe*. New York: Free Press.

Olson, D. H., & Cromwell, R. E. (1975). Power in families. In R. E. Cromwell & D. H. Olson (Eds.), *Power in families* (pp. 3-11). New York: Wiley.

Orbuch, T. L. (1997). People's accounts count: The sociology of accounts. *Annual review of sociology, 23*, 455-478.

Ortony, A., Clore, G. L., & Collins, A. (1988). *The cognitive structure of emotions*. Cambridge: Cambridge University Press.

Osmond, M. W. (1978). Reciprocity: A dynamic model and a method to study family power. *Journal of marriage and the family, 40*, 49-61.

Panksepp, J. (1998). *Affective neuroscience: The foundations of human and animal emotions*. New York: Oxford University Press.

Panksepp, J. (2003). Feeling the pain of social loss. *Science, 302*, 237-239.

Parens, H., & Saul, L. J. (1971). *Dependence in man: A psychoanalytic study*. New York: International Universities.

Parkes, C. M., & Stevenson-Hinde, J. (Eds.). (1982). *The place of attachment in human behavior*. New York: Basic Books.

Parsons, T. (1937). *The structure of social action*. Glencoe, IL: Free Press.

Parsons, T. (1951). *The social system*. Glencoe, IL: Free Press.

Parsons, T., & Bales, R. F. (1955). *Family, socialization and interaction process*. Glencoe: Free Press.

Parsons, T., & Shils, E. A. (1951). *Toward a general theory of action*. New York: Harper & Row.

Pavlov, I. P. (1960). *Conditioned reflexes*. [No city]: Dover.

Peck, M. S. (1978). *The road less travelled: A new psychology of love, traditional values and spiritual growth*. New York: Simon & Schuster.

Pierce, G. R., Sarason, B. R., Sarason, I. G., Joseph, H. J., & Henderson, C. A. (1996). Conceptualizing and assessing social support in the context of the family. In G. R. Pierce, B. R. Sarason & I. G. Sarason (Eds.), *Handbook of social support and the family* (pp. 3-23). New York: Plenum.

Pitts, J. R. (1964). The structural-functional approach. In H. T. Christensen (Ed.), *Handbook of marriage and the family* (pp. 51-124). Chicago: Rand McNally.

Plato (1952). *The dialogues of Plato* (B. Jowett, Trans.). Chicago: Great Books.

Pleck, J. H. (1985). *Working wives/working husbands*. Beverly Hills: Sage.

Plotkin, H. (1997). *Evolution in mind: An introduction to evolutionary psychology*. Cambridge, MA: Harvard University Press.

Plutchik, R. (1980). *Emotion: A psychoevolutionary synthesis*. New York: Harper & Row.

Plutchik, R. (1984). Emotions: A general psychoevolutionary theory. In K. R. Scherer & P. Ekman (Eds.), *Approaches to emotion* (pp. 197-219). Hillsdale, NJ: Erlbaum.

Popper, K. R. (1965). *Conjectures and refutations: The growth of scientific knowledge*. New York: Harper & Row.

Porges, S. W. (1998). Love: An emergent property of the mammalian autonomic nervous system. *Psychoneuroendocrinology, 23*, 837-861.

Porges, S. W. (1999). Emotion: An evolutionary byproduct of the neural regulation of the autonomic nervous system. In C. S. Carter, I. I. Lederhendler & B. Kirkpatrick (Eds.), *The integrative neurobiology of affiliation* (pp. 65-80). Cambridge, MA: MIT Press.

Porges, S. W. (2005). The role of social engagement in attachment and bonding: A phylogenetic perspective. In C. S. Carter, L. Ahnert, K. E. Grossmann, S. B. Hrdy, M. E. Lamb, S. W. Porges & N. Sachser (Eds.), *Attachment and bonding: A new synthesis* (pp. 33-54). Cambridge, MA: MIT Press.

Preston, S. D., & de Waal, F. B. M. (2002). Empathy: Its ultimate and proximate bases. *Behavioral and brain sciences, 25*, 1-72.

Pruett, K. D. (1987). *The nurturing father: Journey toward the complete man*. New York: Warner.

Rapoport, R., Rapoport, R. N., & Strelitz, Z. (1977). *Fathers, mothers and others: Towards new alliances*. London: Routledge & Kegan Paul.

Restak, R. M. (1995). *Brainscapes: An introduction to what neuroscience has learned about the structure, function, and abilities of the brain*. New York: Hyperion.

Rheingold, H. L. (1963). Maternal behavior in the dog. In H. L. Rheingold (Ed.), *Maternal behavior in mammals* (pp. 169-202). New York: Wiley.

Rheingold, H. L. (1969). The effect of a strange environment on the behavior of infants. In B. M. Foss (Ed.), *Determinants of infant behavior* (Vol. 4, pp. 137-166). London: Methuen.

Rholes, W. S., & Simpson, J. A. (2004a). Attachment theory: Basic concepts and contemporary questions. In W. S. Rholes & J. A. Simpson (Eds.), *Adult attachment: Theory, research, and clinical implications* (pp. 3-14). New York: Guilford Press.

Rholes, W. S., & Simpson, J. A. (Eds.). (2004b). *Adult attachment: Theory, research, and clinical implications*. New York: Guilford Press.

Robson, K. S., & Kumar, R. (1980). Delayed onset of maternal affection after childbirth. *British journal of psychiatry, 136*, 347-353.

Robson, K. S., & Moss, H. A. (1970). Patterns and determinants of maternal attachment. *Journal of pediatrics, 77*, 976-985.

Rochlin, G. (1980). *The masculine dilemma: A psychology of masculinity*. Boston: Little, Brown.

Rodgers, R. H. (1973). *Family interaction and transaction: The developmental approach*. Englewood Cliffs, NJ: Prentice-Hall.

Roemer, L., & Orsillo, S. M. (2008). *Mindfulness- and acceptance-based behavioral therapies in practice*. New York: Guilford.

Roland, A. (1988). *In search of self in India and Japan: Toward a cross-cultural psychology*. Princeton, NJ: Princeton University.

Rollins, B. C., & Thomas, D. L. (1979). Parental support, power, and control techniques in the socialization of children. In W. R. Burr, R. Hill, F. I. Nye & I. L. Reiss (Eds.), *Contemporary theories about the family. Vol. 1. Research-based theories* (pp. 317-364). New York: Free Press.

Rolls, E. T. (1999). *The brain and emotion*. New York: Oxford University Press.

Roney, J. R. (1999). Distinguishing adaptations from by-products. *American psychologist, 54*, 435-436.

Rosenblatt, J. S. (1990). Landmarks in the physiological study of maternal behavior with special reference to the rat. In N. A. Krasnegor & R. S. Bridges (Eds.), *Mammalian parenting* (pp. 40-60). New York: Oxford University Press.

Ross, G., Zelazo, J., & Kotelchuck, M. (1975). Separation protest in infants in home and laboratory. *Developmental psychology, 11*, 256-257.

Ross, S., Sawin, P. B., Zarrow, M. X., & Denenberg, V. H. (1963). Maternal behavior in the rabbit. In H. L. Rheingold (Ed.), *Maternal behavior in mammals* (pp. 94-121). New York: Wiley.

Rossi, A. S., & Rossi, P. H. (1990). *Of human bonding: Parent-child relations across the life course*. New York: Aldine de Gruyter.

Rothbard, J. C., & Shaver, P. R. (1994). Continuity of attachment across the life span. In M. B. Sperling & W. H. Berman (Eds.), *Attachment in adults: Clinical and developmental perspectives* (pp. 31-71). New York: Guilford.

Rothbaum, F., & Kakinuma, M. (2004). *Amae* and attachment: Security in cultural context. *Human development, 47*, 34-39.

Rubin, Z. (1973). *Liking and loving*. New York: Rinehart & Winston.

Ruddick, S. (1989). *Maternal thinking: Toward a politics of peace*. New York: Ballantine.

Russell, B. (1938). *Power: A new social analysis*. New York: Norton.

Russell, J. A., & Leng, G. (1998). Sex, parturition and motherhood without oxytocin? *Journal of endocrinology, 157*(3), 343-359.

Sachser, N. (2005). Adult social bonding: Insights from studies in nonhuman mammals. In C. S. Carter, L. Ahnert, K. E. Grossmann, S. B. Hrdy, M. E. Lamb, S. W. Porges & N. Sachser (Eds.), *Attachment and bonding: A new synthesis* (pp. 119-135). Cambridge, MA: MIT Press.

Sachser, N., Dürslag, M., & Hirzel, D. (1998). Social relationships and the management of stress. *Psychoneuroendocrinology, 23*, 891-904.

Safilios-Rothschild, C. (1976). A macro- and micro-examination of family power and love: An exchange model. *Journal of marriage and the family, 37*, 355-362.

Salamon, S. (1986). "Male chauvinism" as a manifestation of love in marriage. In T. S. Lebra & W. P. Lebra (Eds.), *Japanese culture and behavior: Selected readings (Rev. Ed.)* (pp. 130-141). Honolulu: University of Hawaii Press.

Salovey, P., Bedell, B. T., Detweiler, J. B., & Mayer, J. D. (2000). Current directions in emotional intelligence research. In M. Lewis & J. M. Haviland-Jones (Eds.), *Handbook of emotions* (2nd ed., pp. 504-520). New York: Guilford.

Sampson, R. V. (1965). *The psychology of power*. New York: Pantheon.

Scanzoni, J. (1982). *Sexual bargaining: Power politics in the American marriage* (2nd ed.). Chicago: University of Chicago Press.

Scanzoni, J., Polonko, K., Teachman, J., & Thompson, L. (1989). *The sexual bond: Rethinking families and close relationships*. Newbury Park: Sage.

Scanzoni, J., & Szinovacz, M. (1980). *Family decision-making: A developmental sex role model*. Beverly Hills: Sage.

Schachter, D. L. (1999). The seven sins of memory: Insights from psychology and cognitive neuroscience. *American psychologist, 54*, 182-203.

Schachter, S., & Singer, J. E. (1962). Cognitive, social, and physiological determinants of emotional state. *Psychological review, 69*, 379-399.

Scheff, T. J. (1990). *Microsociology: Discourse, emotion, and social structure*. Chicago: University of Chicago Press.

Scherer, K. R. (1984). On the nature and function of emotion: A component process approach. In K. R. Scherer & P. Ekman (Eds.), *Approaches to emotion* (pp. 293-317). Hillsdale, NJ: Erlbaum.

Schneider, B. H., & Younger, A. J. (1996). Adolescent-parent attachment and adolescents' relations with their peers: A closer look. *Youth and society, 28*, 95-108.

Schneirla, T. C. (1959). An evolutionary and developmental theory of biphasic processes underlying approach and withdrawal. In M. Jones (Ed.), *Nebraska symposium on motivation* (pp. 1-42). Lincoln: University of Nebraska Press.

Schneirla, T. C., Rosenblatt, J. S., & Tobach, E. (1963). Maternal behavior in the cat. In H. L. Rheingold (Ed.), *Maternal behavior in mammals* (pp. 122-168). New York: Wiley.

Schwartz, G., & Merten, D. (1980). *Love and commitment.* Beverly Hills: Sage.

Scott, J. P. (1963). The process of primary socialization in canie and human infants. *Monographs of the Society for Research on Child Development, 28*, 1-47.

Scott, M. B., & Lyman, S. M. (1968). Accounts. *American sociological review, 33*(1), 46-62.

Secord, P. F., & Backman, C. (1964). *Social psychology.* New York: McGraw-Hill.

Seeley, J. R., Sim, R. A., & Looseley, E. W. (1956). *Crestwood Heights.* New York: Wiley.

Segal, Z. V., Williams, J. M. G., & Teasdale, J. D. (2002). *Mindfulness-based cognitive therapy for depression: A new approach to preventing relapse.* New York: Guilford.

Segalen, M. (1983). *Love and power in the peasant family: Rural France in the nineteenth century* (S. Matthews, Trans.). Chicago: University of Chicago Press.

Shaffer, L. S. (1983). Toward Pepitone's vision of a normative social psychology: What is a social norm? *Journal of mind and behavior, 4*, 275-294.

Shaver, P. R., & Fraley, R. C. (2000). Attachment theory and caregiving. *Psychological inquiry, 11*(2), 109-114.

Shaver, P. R., & Hazan, C. (1988). A biased overview of the study of love. *Journal of social and personal relationships, 5*, 473-501.

Shaver, P. R., Hazen, C., & Bradshaw, D. (1988). Love as attachment: The integration of three behavioral systems. In R. J. Sternberg & M. L. Barnes (Eds.), *The psychology of love* (pp. 68-99). New Haven: Yale University Press.

Shaver, P. R., & Klinnert, M. (1982). Schachter's theories of affiliation and emotions: Implications of developmental research. In L. Wheeler (Ed.), *Review of personality and social psychology* (Vol. 3, pp. 37-71). Beverly Hills, CA: Sage.

Simons, R. L., Beaman, J., Conger, R. D., & Chao, W. (1993). Childhood experience, conceptions of parenting, and attitudes of spouse as determinants of parental behavior. *Journal of marriage and the family, 55*, 91-106.

Simons, R. L., Whitbeck, L. B., Conger, R. D., & Melby, J. N. (1990). Husband and wife differences in determinants of parenting: A social learning and exchange model of parental behavior. *Journal of marriage and the family, 52*, 375-392.

Simpson, J. A., & Rholes, W. S. (2000). Caregiving, attachment theory, and the connection theoretical orientation. *Psychological inquiry, 11*(2), 114-117.

Simpson, J. A., & Rholes, W. S. (Eds.). (1998). *Attachment theory and close relationships*. New York: Guilford.

Singer, I. (1966/1984). *The nature of love. Vol. 1, Plato to Luther* (2nd ed.). Chicago: University of Chicago Press.

Singer, I. (1984). *The nature of love. Vol. 2, Courtly and romantic*. Chicago: University of Chicago Press.

Singer, I. (1987). *The nature of love. Vol. 3, The modern world*. Chicago: University of Chicago Press.

Skinner, B. F. (1953). *Science and human behavior*. New York: Macmillan.

Smith, J. C., & Sales, G. D. (1980). Ultrasonic behavior and mother-infant interactions in rodents. In R. W. Bell & W. P. Smotherman (Eds.), *Maternal influences and early behavior*. New York: Spectrum Publications.

Smith, T. E. (1970). Foundations of parental influence upon adolescents: An application of social power theory. *American sociological review, 35*, 860-872.

Snarey, J. (1993). *How fathers care for the next generation: A four decade study*. Cambridge, MA: Harvard University Press.

Sober, E., & Wilson, D. S. (1998). *Unto others: The evolution and psychology of unselfish behavior*. Cambridge, MA: Harvard University Press.

Solomon, J., & George, C. (1996). Defining the caregiving system: Toward a theory of caregiving. *Infant mental health journal, 17(3)*, 183-197.

Solomon, J., & George, C. (1999). The measurement of attachment security in infancy and childhood. In J. Cassidy & P. R. Shaver (Eds.), *Handbook of attachment: Theory, research, and clinical applications* (pp. 287-316). New York: Guilford.

Solomon, M. F. (1989). *Narcissism and intimacy: Love and marriage in an age of confusion*. New York: Norton.

Solomon, R. C. (1990). *Love: Emotion, myth, & metaphor*. Buffalo, NY: Prometheus.

Sperling, M. B., & Berman, W. H. (Eds.). (1994). *Attachment in adults: Clinical and developmental perspectives*. New York: Guilford.

Sprey, J. (1971). On the management of conflict in families. *Journal of marriage and the family, 33*, 722-731.

Sroufe, L. A. (1988). The role of infant-caregiver attachment in development. In J. Belsky & T. Nezworski (Eds.), *Clinical implications of attachment* (pp. 18-38). Hillsdale, NJ: Erlbaum.

Sroufe, L. A., & Fleeson, J. (1986). Attachment and the construction of relationships. In W. W. Hartup & Z. Rubin (Eds.), *Relationships and development* (pp. 51-71). Hillsdale, NJ: Erlbaum.

Sroufe, L. A., & Waters, E. (1977). Attachment as an organizational construct. *Child development, 48*, 1184-1199.

Steinmetz, S. K. (1979). Disciplinary techniques and their relationship to aggressiveness, dependency, and conscience. In W. R. Burr, R. Hill, F. I. Nye & I. L. Reiss (Eds.), *Contemporary theories about the family, Vol. 2: General theories/theoretical orientations* (pp. 405-438). New York: Free Press.

Stern, D. N. (1985). *The interpersonal world of the infant: A view from psychoanalysis and developmental psychology*. New York: Basic.

Stets, J. E. (1992). Interactive processes in dating aggression: A national study. *Journal of marriage and the family, 54*, 165-177.

Stinchcombe, A. L. (1968). *Constructing social theories*. New York: Harcourt, Brace & World.

Stiver, I. P. (1991). The meanings of "dependency" in female-male relationships. In J. V. Jordan, A. G. Kaplan, J. B. Miller, I. P. Stiver & J. L. Surrey (Eds.), *Women's growth in connection: Writings from the Stone Center* (pp. 143-161). New York: Guilford Press.

Straus, M. A. (1964). Power and support structure of the family in relation to socialization. *Journal of marriage and the family, 26*, 318-326.

Strong, B., & Vault, C. D. (1989). *The marriage and family experience (4th ed.). St.* Paul: West.

Stryker, S. (1994). Identity theory: Its development, research base, and prospects. *Studies in symbolic interaction, 16*, 9-20.

Surrey, J. L. (1991). The "self-in-relation": A theory of women's development. In J. V. Jordan, A. G. Kaplan, J. B. Miller, I. P. Stiver & J. L. Surrey (Eds.), *Women's growth in connection: Writings from the Stone Center* (pp. 51-66). New York: Guilford Press.

Tannen, D. (1990). *You just don't understand: Women and men in conversation*. New York: Ballantine.

Tattersall, I. (1998). *Becoming human: Evolution and human uniqueness*. New York: Harcourt Brace.

Taylor, R. (1966). *Action and purpose*. Englewood Cliffs, NJ: Prentice-Hall.

Taylor, S. E. (2006). Tend and befriend: Biobehavioral bases of affiliation under stress. *Current directions in psychological science, 15*(6), 273-277.

Thevenin, T. (1987). *The family bed.* Wayne, NJ: Avery.

Thibaut, J. W., & Kelley, H. H. (1959). *The social psychology of groups.* New York: Wiley.

Thomas, L. (1989). *Living morally: A psychology of moral character.* Philadelphia: Temple.

Thorne, B., & Yalom, M. (1982). *Rethinking the family: Some feminist questions.* New York: Longman.

Toennies, F. (1961). Gemeinschaft and Gesellschaft (C. P. Loomis, Trans.). In T. Parsons, E. Shils, K. D. Naegele & J. R. Pitts (Eds.), *Theories of society: Foundations of modern sociological theory* (pp. 191-201). New York: Free Press.

Tomkins, S. S. (1984). Affect theory. In K. R. Scherer & P. Ekman (Eds.), *Approaches to emotion* (pp. 163-195). Hillsdale, NJ: Erlbaum.

Tooby, J., & Cosmides, L. (1992). The psychological foundations of culture. In J. H. Barkow, L. Cosmides & J. Tooby (Eds.), *The adapted mind: Evolutionary psychology and the generation of culture* (pp. 19-136). New York: Oxford University Press.

Trivers, R. (1972). Parental investment and sexual selection. In B. Campbell (Ed.), *Sexual selection and the descent of man 1871-1971.* Chicago: Aldine.

Trivers, R. (1985). *Social evolution.* Menlo Park, CA: Benjamin/Cummings.

Troll, L. E., & Smith, J. (1976). Attachment through the life-span: Some questions about dyadic bonds among adults. *Human development, 19*, 156-170.

Tudge, C. (2000). *The variety of life.* Oxford: Oxford University Press.

Turner, J. H. (1985). The concept of "action" in sociological analysis. In G. Seeba & R. Toumea (Eds.), *Analytical and sociological theories of action.* Dordrecht, Holland: Reidel.

Turner, J. H. (1991). *The structure of sociological theory* (5th ed.). Belmont, CA: Wadsworth.

Turner, J. H. (2000). *On the origins of human emotions: .* Stanford, CA: Stanford University Press.

Turner, R. H. (1962). Role-taking: Process vs conformity. In A. M. Rose (Ed.), *Human behavior and social processes: An interactionist approach* (pp. 20-40). Boston: Houghton Mifflin.

Turner, R. H. (1970). *Family interaction*. New York: Wiley.

Turner, S. (2002). *Brains/practices/relativism: Social theory after cognitive science*. Chicago: University of Chicago Press.

Uvnäs Moberg, K. (2003). *The oxytocin factor: Tapping the hormone of calm, love, and healing* (R. W. Francis, Trans.). Cambridge, MA: Da Capo Press.

Uvnäs-Moberg, K. (1997). Oxytocin linked antistress effects--the relaxation and growth response. *Acta psychologica scandinavica, 640 (Suppl.)*(38-42).

Uvnäs-Moberg, K. (1998). Oxytocin may mediate the benefits of positive social interaction and emotion. *Psychoneuroendocrinology, 23*, 819-835.

Uvnäs-Moberg, K. (1999). Physiological and endocrine effects of social contract. In C. S. Carter, I. I. Lederhendler & B. Kirkpatrick (Eds.), *The integrative neurobiology of affiliation* (pp. 245-262). Cambridge, MA: MIT Press.

Uvnäs-Moberg, K., Arn, I., & Magnusson, D. (2005). The psychobiology of emotion: The role of the oxytocinergic system. *International journal of behavioral medicine, 12*(2), 59-65.

Van IJzendoorn, M. H., & Tavecchio, L. W. C. (1987). The development of attachment theory as a Lakatosian research program: philosophical and methodological aspects. In L. W. C. Tavecchio & M. H. van IJzendoorn (Eds.), *Attachment in social networks: Contributions to the Bowlby-Ainsworth attachment theory* (pp. 3-31). Amsterdam: North-Holland.

Vannoy, D., & Philliber, W. W. (1992). Wife's employment and quality of marriage. *Journal of marriage and family, 54*, 387-398.

Vaughn, B., Egeland, B., Sroufe, L. A., & Waters, E. (1979). Individual differences in infant-mother attachment at twelve and eighteen months: Stability and change in families under stress. *Child development, 50*, 971-975.

Viorst, J. (1986). *Necessary losses*. New York: Simon & Schuster.

Vogel, E. F. (1963). *Japan's new middle class: The salary man and his family in a Tokyo suburb*. Berkeley: University of California Press.

Vom Saal, F. S., Franks, P., Boechler, M., Palanza, P., & Parmigiani, S. (1995). Nest defense and survival of offspring in highly aggressive wild Canadian female house mice. *Physiology & behavior, 58(4)*, 669-678.

Waller, W. (1937). The rating and dating complex. *American sociological review, 2*, 727-734.

Walster, E., Walster, G. W., & Berscheid, E. (1978). *Equity theory*. Boston: Allyn & Bacon.

Watson, J. B. (1930). *Behaviorism*. Chicago: University of Chicago Press.

Weber, M. (1946). *From Max Weber: Essays in sociology* (H. H. Gerth & C. W. Mills, Trans.). New York: Oxford.

Weber, M. (1947). *The theory of social and economic organization* (A. M. Henderson & T. Parsons, Trans.). New York: Free Press.

Weiss, R. S. (1974). The provisions of social relationships. In Z. Rubin (Ed.), *Doing unto others* (pp. 17-26). Englewood Cliffs: Prentice-Hall.

Weiss, R. S. (1982). Attachment in adult life. In C. M. Parkes & J. Stevenson-Hinde (Eds.), *The place of attachment in human behavior* (pp. 171-184). New York: Basic Books.

Wellman, J., Carr, D., Graham, A., Jones, H., Humm, J. L., Ruscio, M., et al. (1997). Preoptic area infusions of morphine disrupt - and naloxone restores - parental-like behavior in juvenile rats. *Brain research bulletin, 44(2)*, 183-191.

West, M. L., & Sheldon-Keller, A. E. (1994). *Patterns of relating: An adult attachment perspective*. New York: Guilford.

White, M. (1993). *The material child: Coming of age in Japan and America*. New York: Free Press.

Williams, G. C. (1966). *Adaptation and natural selection*. Princeton, NJ: Princeton University Press.

Wilson, E. O. (1975). *Sociobiology: The new synthesis*. Cambridge, MA: Belknap Press.

Wilson, J. Q. (1993). *The moral sense*. New York: Free Press.

Winnicott, D. W. (1965a). *The family and individual development*. London: Tavistock.

Winnicott, D. W. (1965b). *The maturational process and the facilitating environment*. New York: International Universities Press.

Wiseman, R. S. (1975). Crisis theory and the process of divorce. *Social casework, 56*(4), 205-212.

Wispé, L. (1986). The distinction between sympathy and empathy: To call forth a concept a word is needed. *Journal of personality and social psychology, 50*, 314-321.

Wright, R. (1994). *The moral animal: The new science of evolutionary psychology*. New York: Pantheon.

Wrong, D. H. (1961). The over-socialized conception of man in modern sociology. *American sociological review, 26*, 183-193.

Wrong, D. H. (1988). *Power: Its forms, bases, and uses*. Chicago: University of Chicago Press.

Wundt, W. (1897). *Outlines of psychology* (C. H. Judd, Trans.). Leipzig: Engelmann.

York, P., York, D., & Wachtel, T. (1982). *Toughlove*. New York: Bantam.

Young, L. J., & Wang, Z. (2004). The neurobiology of pair bonding. *Nature neuroscience, 7*(10), 1048-1054.

Zahn-Waxler, C., Robinson, J. L., & Emde, R. N. (1992). The development of empathy in twins. *Developmental psychology, 28*, 1038-1047.

Zajonc, R. (1980). Feeling and thinking: Preferences need no inferences. *American psychologist, 35*, 151-175.

Zeanah, C. H., Smyke, A. T., Koga, S. F., & Carlson, E. (2005). Attachment in institutionalized and community children in Romania. *Child development, 76*(5), 1015-1028.

Zeifman, D., & Hazan, C. (1997). Attachment: The bond in pair-bonds. In J. A. Simpson & D. T. Kenrick (Eds.), *Evolutionary social psychology* (pp. 237-263). Mahwah, NJ: Erlbaum.

Breinigsville, PA USA
18 March 2010

234358BV00004B/4/P

9 780739 143520